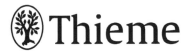

Measurements and Classifications in Musculoskeletal Radiology

Simone Waldt, MD
Associate Professor
Department of Radiology
Klinikum rechts der Isar der Technischen Universität
München
Munich, Germany

Klaus Woertler, MD
Professor
Department of Radiology
Klinikum rechts der Isar der Technischen Universität
München
Munich, Germany

With contributions by Matthias Eiber

423 illustrations

Thieme
Stuttgart · New York

Library of Congress Cataloging-in-Publication Data
Waldt, Simone, author.
[Messverfahren und Klassifikationen in der muskuloskel-
ettalen Radiologie. English]
  Measurements and classifications in musculoskeletal
radiology / Simone Waldt, Klaus Woertler ; translator,
Terry C. Telger ; illustrators, Christiane and Dr. Michael
Solodkoff.
      p. ; cm.
"This book is an authorized translation of the 1st German
edition, Messverfahren und Klassifikationen in der
muskuloskelettalen Radiologie."
Includes index.
  ISBN 978-3-13-169271-9 (alk. paper)—ISBN 978-3-13-
169281-8 (e-book)
  I. Woertler, Klaus, author. II. Telger, Terry C., translator.
III. Title.
  [DNLM: 1. Musculoskeletal Diseases—classification. 2.
Diagnostic Imaging—classification. WE 15]
RC925.7
616.7'075—dc23
                                                    2013039501

This book is an authorized translation of the 1st German
edition, published 2011 by Georg Thieme Verlag KG,
Stuttgart, Germany. Title of the German edition:
*Messverfahren und Klassifikationen in der muskuloskelet-
talen Radiologie.*

Translator: Terry C. Telger, Fort Worth, Texas, USA

Illustrators: Christiane and Dr. Michael Solodkoff,
Neckargemünd, Germany

Contributor: Matthias Eiber, MD, Department of
Radiology, Klinikum rechts der Isar der Technischen
Universität München, Munich, Germany

© 2014 Georg Thieme Verlag KG,
Rüdigerstrasse 14, 70469 Stuttgart, Germany
http://www.thieme.de
Thieme Medical Publishers, Inc., 333 Seventh Avenue,
New York, NY 10001, USA
http://www.thieme.com

Cover design: Thieme Publishing Group
Typesetting by Prepress Projects, Perth, UK
Printed in Germany by Beltz Grafische Betriebe

ISBN 978-3-13-169271-9

Also available as an e-book:
eISBN 978-3-13-169281-8

Important note: Medicine is an ever-changing science
undergoing continual development. Research and clinical
experience are continually expanding our knowledge, in
particular our knowledge of proper treatment and drug
therapy. Insofar as this book mentions any dosage or
application, readers may rest assured that the authors,
editors, and publishers have made every effort to ensure
that such references are in accordance with **the state of
knowledge at the time of production of the book.**
Nevertheless, this does not involve, imply, or express any
guarantee or responsibility on the part of the publishers
in respect to any dosage instructions and forms of ap-
plications stated in the book. **Every user is requested to
examine carefully** the manufacturers' leaflets accompa-
nying each drug and to check, if necessary in consultation
with a physician or specialist, whether the dosage sched-
ules mentioned therein or the contraindications stated by
the manufacturers differ from the statements made in the
present book. Such examination is particularly important
with drugs that are either rarely used or have been newly
released on the market. Every dosage schedule or every
form of application used is entirely at the user's own risk
and responsibility. The authors and publishers request
every user to report to the publishers any discrepancies or
inaccuracies noticed. If errors in this work are found after
publication, errata will be posted at www.thieme.com on
the product description page.

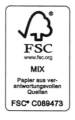

Preface

"The best books are those whose readers believe they themselves could have written."

Blaise Pascal, French mathematician, physicist and philosopher (1623–1662)

There is scarcely any subspecialty of clinical medicine in which we find such a bewildering array of measuring techniques and classification systems as in orthopedics. They are so numerous that every radiologist, orthopedist, or trauma surgeon cannot possibly keep all the methods and reference values "in their head." This problem, like the concept for this book, is not new.

When I began studying orthopedic radiology during my training at the University of Münster, an important tool in our reading room was a ring binder stuffed with separate pages that had been copied from various textbooks and journals. The pages, assembled in random order by my predecessors, covered important measurements and classifications that, while used with some frequency, were apparently difficult for the users to retain in their long-term memory. The ring binder and its contents, which had become tattered and unsightly over the years, was referred to by my colleagues and me simply as the "binder." We considered it an indispensible aid, guarded it jealously, and were constantly adding new pages and notes of our own.

Later, residents in orthopedic radiology training at the Technische Universität München compiled a very similar collection, though in digital form. While I never felt that it matched the charm of the old binder, the digital collection was surely more modern, better organized, more accessible, and definitely more sanitary than the original. Moreover, it was the direct precursor of this book.

While not exhaustive, this book presents a great variety of measuring techniques and classification systems drawn from all areas of musculoskeletal radiology (except for fractures, which would fill another book). The authors have tried to refer back to original publications whenever possible in order to eliminate any inaccuracies that may have been introduced over time. Besides explaining measurement techniques and classification criteria, we have tried to note the actual, practical value of specific methods. Outmoded practices and systems were either excluded from this collection or were included with appropriate comments.

This book cannot replace a textbook. It is intended as a handy reference for everyday use that will provide students and instructors with an "external memory" for things that are difficult to remember and, in many cases, need not be committed to memory. Of course, it is not enough simply to measure angles and juggle classifications. We suggest that you take the time saved by using this book, and spend it gaining a sound basic knowledge of orthopedic diagnosis or expanding the knowledge that you already have. There are many ways of doing this.

I hope that this book will serve its readers as effectively as the "binder" served me in its time. I plan to use it, anyway.

Klaus Woertler
Munich, Germany

Abbreviations

AASA	Anterior acetabular sector angle	IKDC	International Knee Documentation Committee
AHD	Acromiohumeral distance	in	Inch(es)
AHL	Anterior humeral line	IS, ISP	Infraspinatus
AJCC	American Joint Committee on Cancer	JC	Joint cartilage
aLDFA	Anatomic lateral distal femoral angle	LBC	Labral–bicipital complex
aMPFA	Anatomic medial proximal femoral angle	LDTA	Lateral distal tibial angle
		LI	Lumbar index
ALPSA	Anterior labral periosteal sleeve avulsion	LLC	Labral–ligamentous complex
		LPFA	Lateral proximal femoral angle
AP	Anteroposterior	LUCL	Lateral ulnar collateral ligament
ARCO	Association Research Circulation Osseous	MCS	Medial clear space
		MCP	Metacarpophalangeal
ASNR	American Society of Neuroradiology	MHz	Megahertz
ASSR	American Society of Spine Radiology	mLDFA	Mechanical lateral distal femoral angle
ASRS	American Scoliosis Research Society	mLPFA	Mechanical lateral proximal femoral angle
AT angle	Angle of femoral anteversion		
BHAGL	Bony humeral avulsion of glenohumeral ligaments	MPFA	Medial proximal femoral angle
		MPNST	Malignant peripheral nerve sheath tumor
CCD angle	Projected femoral neck–shaft angle (NSA)	MPTA	Medial proximal tibial angle
		MRI	Magnetic resonance imaging
CE angle	Center–edge angle (of Wiberg)	MT	Main thoracic
CIC	Carpal instability complex	MTP	Metatarsophalangeal
CID	Concealed interstitial delamination; carpal instability dissociative	MUCL	Medial ulnar collateral ligament
		NASS	North American Spine Society
CLIP	Capitolunate instability pattern	NOS	Not otherwise specified
CIND	Carpal instability, nondissociative	OARS	Osteoarthritis Research Society
CSV	Central sacral vertical line	OCD	Osteochondritis dissecans
CT	Computed tomography	OMERACT	Outcome Measures in Rheumatoid Arthritis Clinical Trials
DDH	Developmental dysplasia of the hip		
DISI	Dorsiflexed intercalated segment instability	PA	Posteroanterior
		PAINT	Partial articular-sided with intratendinous extension
DM	Double major		
DMAA	Distal metatarsal articular angle	PASA	Posterior acetabular sector angle
DT	Double thoracic	PASTA	Partial articular-sided supraspinatus tendon avulsion
DXA	Dual X-ray absorptiometry		
ED angle	Epiphyseal–diaphyseal angle	PIP	Proximal interphalangeal joint
ET angle	Epiphyseal torsion angle	PISI	Palmar-flexed intercalated segment instability
FAI	Femoroacetabular impingement		
FDP	Flexor digitorum profundus	PNET	Primitive neuroectodermal tumor
FDS	Flexor digitorum superficialis	PPL	Parallel pitch lines
GCTTS	Giant cell tumor of tendon sheaths	PTS	Posterior tibial slope
GLAD	Glenolabral articular disruption	PVNS	Pigmented villonodular synovitis
HAGL	Humeral avulsion of glenohumeral ligaments	QCT	Quantitative computed tomography
		ROI	Region of interest
HASA	Horizontal acetabular sector angle	RUS	Radius, ulna, and short bones
HTE angle	Horizontal toit externe (acetabular index of the weight-bearing zone)	SCFE	Slipped capital femoral epiphysis
		SCOI	Southern California Orthopedic Institute
HU	Hounsfield unit		
ICRS	International Cartilage Repair Society		
IGHL	Inferior glenohumeral ligament		

SD	Standard deviation	TFO	Tibiofibular overlap
SGHL	Superior glenohumeral ligament	TM	Teres minor, triple major
SLAC	Scapholunate advanced collapse	TMT	Tarsometatarsal
SLAP lesion	Superior labral anterior to posterior lesion	TT angle	Tibial torsion angle
		TTTG	Tibial tuberosity trochlear groove
SMS	Skeletal maturity score	UICC	Union Internationale Contre le Cancer
SSC	Subscapularis	UTL	Ulnar translation
SS, SSP	Supraspinatus	V	Volt(s)
STAS	Supraspinatus tendon articular-sided partial tear, not at the footprint	WHO	World Health Organization
		WOMAC score	Western Ontario and McMaster osteo-arthritis score
TCS	Total clear space		
TFCC	Triangular fibrocartilage complex		

Contents

Contents

15 Rheumatoid Arthritis 184

M. Eiber

16 Muscle Injuries 189

S. Waldt

17 Skeletal Age 192

M. Eiber, K. Woertler

Index 205

1 Lower Limb Alignment

Full-Length Anteroposterior Standing Radiograph

The full-length standing radiograph in the anteroposterior (AP) projection is the basic tool for the radiologic analysis of lower limb alignment.

To correctly evaluate the alignment of the lower limbs in the frontal plane, the femoral condyles must be oriented parallel to the X-ray film. This is accomplished by directing the patellae forward while keeping both knee joints in a neutral position. The most important quality criterion for a full-length AP standing radiograph is to have the patellae centered between the femoral condyles (**Fig. 1.1**).

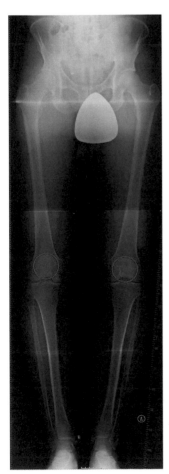

Fig. 1.1 Full-length anteroposterior standing radiograph. The patellae are correctly centered between the femoral condyles.

Usually this position requires 8–10° of external rotation of the feet. With torsional deformities of the tibia that cause lateralization or medialization of the patella, the joint position is adjusted by rotating the lower leg internally or externally until the patella is pointing forward (regardless of the foot position, **Fig. 1.2**).

The lower limb has both anatomic and mechanical axes, which are distinguished as follows:

- *Anatomic axes* (**Fig. 1.3**): The anatomic axes of the femur and tibia coincide with the mid-diaphyseal line of each bone. They are defined by the midpoints of two widely spaced lines drawn perpendicular to the shaft.

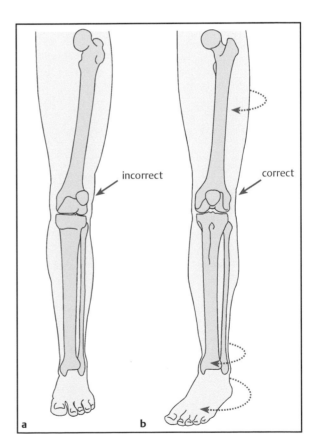

Fig. 1.2a,b Correction for rotational deformity of the tibia in the full-length standing radiograph. The patella must be oriented forward to position the femoral condyles parallel to the X-ray film. Rotational deformities of the tibia (**a**) are corrected by internal or external rotation of the lower leg (**b**).

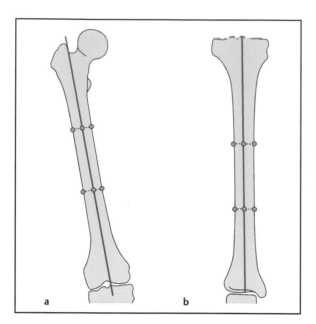

Fig. 1.3a,b Anatomic axes of the lower limb.
a Femur.
b Tibia.

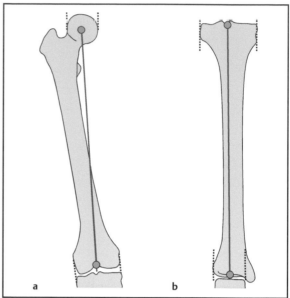

Fig. 1.4a,b Mechanical axes of the lower limb.
a Femur.
b Tibia.

- *Mechanical axes* (**Fig. 1.4**): The mechanical axes of the femur and tibia are defined by the center points of the adjacent joints. The mechanical axes of the femur and tibia form a physiologic varus angle of 1.2°.

Mechanical and Anatomic Axes of the Lower Limb

■ Mechanical Axis of the Lower Limb (Mikulicz Line)

The mechanical axis of the lower limb (**Fig. 1.5**) is determined on the full-length AP standing radiograph. The axis passes through the center point of the hip joint (center of the femoral head) and through the center point of the ankle joint (midpoint of the tibial plafond). The mechanical axis should pass just medial to the center point of the knee joint. The lateral or medial mechanical axis deviation (MAD) from the center of the joint is measured in millimeters (mm).

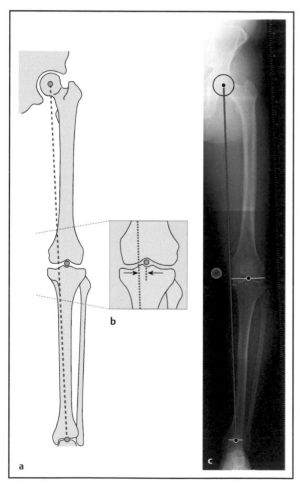

◀ **Fig. 1.5a–c** Mechanical axis of the lower limb (Mikulicz line). The mechanical axis runs through the center of the femoral head and through the midpoint of the tibial plafond.
a Diagram.
b Enlarged diagram of the axis passing through the knee joint.
c Determination of the axis on a radiograph.

Mechanical axis of the lower limb

- *Normal values (medial deviation of the mechanical axis):* 4 mm ± 4 mm (after Bhave et al) or 10 mm ± 7 mm (after Paley et al)
- *Genu valgum:* greater lateral deviation (> normal value – standard deviation)
- *Genu varum:* greater medial deviation (> normal value + standard deviation)

! Physiologically, the anatomic axes of the femur and tibia form a slight varus angle. A perfectly straight lower limb axis is therefore considered unphysiological. If the tibiofemoral angle is negative, genu varum is present.

Bhave A, et al. Unpublished results

Paley D, Herzenberg JE, Tetsworth K, McKie J, Bhave A. Deformity planning for frontal and sagittal plane corrective osteotomies. Orthop Clin North Am 1994;25(3):425–465

Paley D. Principles of deformity correction. Berlin: Springer; 2001

■ Anatomic Axis of the Lower Limb

The anatomic axis of the lower limb (**Fig. 1.6**) is evaluated on the full-length AP radiograph by measuring the anatomic tibiofemoral angle, i.e., the upper acute angle formed by the anatomic axes of the femur and tibia.

Anatomic axis of the lower limb

- *Normal values (anatomic tibiofemoral angle):*   6.85° ± 1.4°
- *Genu valgum:*   > 8.3°
- *Genu varum:*   < 0°

Basic Measuring Techniques for Planning Osteotomies

The deformity underlying an axial malalignment is analyzed by calculating the *joint orientation angles*. The basic reference lines for measuring these angles are the joint orientation lines shown in **Fig. 1.7**. The joint orientation angle is measured between the joint orientation line and either the mechanical or anatomic axis. Paley introduced nomenclature that is useful for identifying a particular measurement based on the abbreviation of the joint orientation angle. The prefix "m" or "a" states whether an

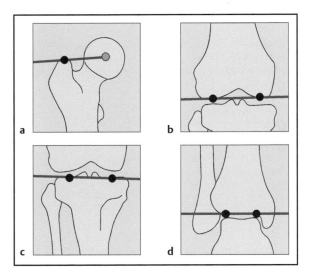

Fig. 1.7a–d Joint orientation lines of the lower limb (basic reference lines for determining joint orientation angles).
a Hip joint orientation line.
b Distal femoral knee joint orientation line.
c Proximal tibial knee joint orientation line.
d Ankle joint orientation line.

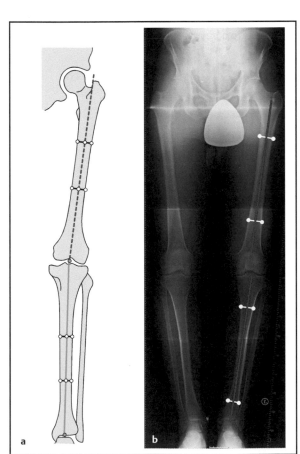

◀ **Fig. 1.6a,b** Anatomic axis of the lower limb. The anatomic axis is defined by the axis of the femoral and tibial shafts.
a Diagrammatic representation.
b Determination of the axis on a radiograph.

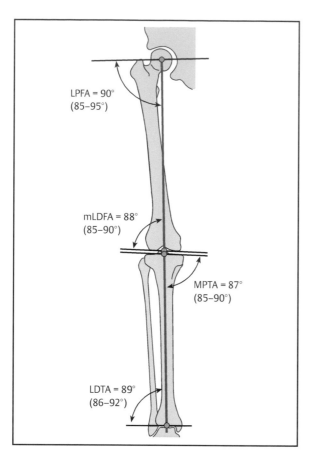

Fig. 1.8 Joint orientation angles described by Paley, measured relative to the mechanical axes of the femur and tibia. The numbers indicate normal values with range of variation shown in parentheses.

LDTA = Lateral distal tibial angle
LPFA = Lateral proximal femoral angle
mLDFA = Mechanical lateral distal femoral angle
MPTA = Medial proximal tibial angle

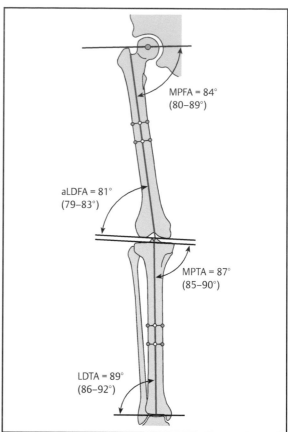

Fig. 1.9 Joint orientation angles described by Paley, measured relative to the anatomic axes of the femur and tibia. The numbers indicate normal values with range of variation shown in parentheses.

aLDFA = Anatomic lateral distal femoral angle
LDTA = Lateral distal tibial angle
MPFA = Medial proximal femoral angle
MPTA = Medial proximal tibial angle

angle is measured relative to a mechanical or anatomic axis. The second letter indicates whether the angle is measured medial (M) or lateral (L) to the axis line. The next letters indicate whether the proximal (P) or distal (D) joint orientation angle has been measured for the femur (F) or the tibia (T). Because the anatomic and mechanical axes of the tibia are generally parallel, the "m" or "a" prefix may be omitted in the lower leg.

Logically, the medial and lateral angles relative to an axis add up to 180°. The usual practice is to state the angle that normally measures less than 90°. By general consensus, the proximal femoral angles are measured relative to the anatomic axis on the medial side and relative to the mechanical axis on the lateral side.

Figs. 1.8 and **1.9** and **Table 1.1** show the angles relative to the joint orientation lines that are used in the planning of corrective osteotomies.

Paley D. Principles of deformity correction. Berlin: Springer; 2001

Limb Length

The length of the lower limb can be measured on a standard full-length AP standing radiograph using the following technique (**Fig. 1.10**): first a horizontal line is drawn tangent to the superior margin of the femoral head to define its highest point. Next the length of the femur is measured between that point and the most distal point of the medial femoral condyle, defined by a horizontal line tangent to the medial femoral condyle. Tibial length is measured from the most distal point of the medial femoral condyle to the center of the tibial plafond. Limb length is then determined by measuring the total length from

Table 1.1 Normal values and range of variation of joint orientation angles, after Paley

Angle		Normal value (°)	Range of variation (°)
aMPFA	Anatomic medial proximal femoral angle	84	80–89
mLPFA	Mechanical lateral proximal femoral angle	90	85–95
mLDFA	Mechanical lateral distal femoral angle	88	85–90
aLDFA	Anatomic lateral distal femoral angle	81	79–83
MPTA	Medial proximal tibial angle	87	85–90
LDTA	Lateral distal tibial angle	89	86–92

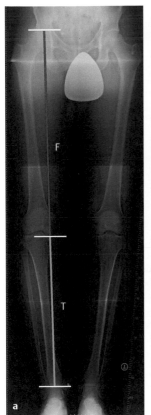
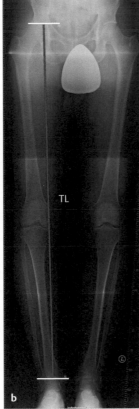

Fig. 1.10a,b Limb length measurement on the standing anteroposterior radiograph.
a The lengths of the femur (F) and tibia (T) are determined.
b Total limb length (TL) is determined.

the superior border of the femoral head to the center of the tibial plafond.

Sabharwal S, Zhao C, McKeon JJ, McClemens E, Edgar M, Behrens F. Computed radiographic measurement of limb-length discrepancy. Full-length standing anteroposterior radiograph compared with scanogram. J Bone Joint Surg Am 2006;88(10):2243–2251

Computed Tomographic Measurement of Torsion and Length

■ Femoral Anteversion

Femoral anteversion, also called the antetorsion (AT) angle, is measured on transverse computed tomography (CT) sections of the proximal and distal femur acquired at the level of the joints. The lower limb is in the neutral position during the examination. To determine the femoral neck axis with greatest accuracy and reproducibility, the scans should be acquired with a large section thickness (10 mm is recommended).

The AT angle is measured between the femoral neck axis and a line tangent to the posterior margin of the femoral condyles (**Fig. 1.11**). The tangent line is drawn on the CT section that displays the femoral condyles in their greatest diameter.

Various methods have been proposed for determining the femoral neck axis:

- The approximate femoral neck axis can be measured on a CT section that cuts portions of both the femoral head and the femoral neck (see **Fig. 1.11**).
- The femoral neck axis can be determined more precisely by using special software to superimpose CT sections on the monitor and calculate mean values.
- In the method of Murphy et al, the femoral neck axis is drawn as a straight line passing between the center of the femoral head and the center of the base of the femoral neck (**Fig. 1.12**). The base of the femoral neck appears as an ellipse on a CT section acquired at a relatively low level. These sections are superimposed, and the femoral neck axis is drawn by connecting the center of the ellipse to the center of the femoral head, which is located with a circle template.

The analysis can be simplified by measuring the proximal and distal femoral angles separately relative to a horizontal reference line and then adding the angles together or subtracting them. If the angles have the same sign relative to the horizontal (frontal) plane, they are subtracted; if they have different signs as in **Fig. 1.11**, they are added.

Lower Limb Alignment

1

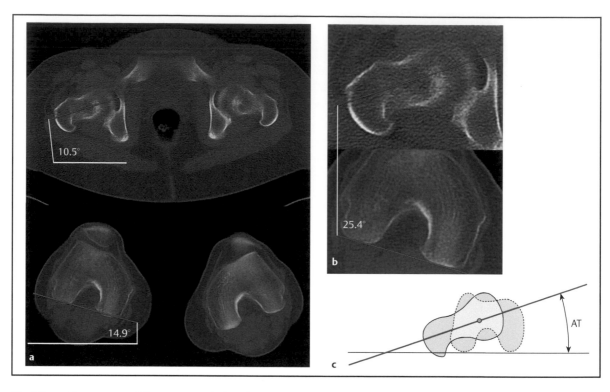

Fig. 1.11a–c Measurement of the antetorsion (AT) angle on transverse computed tomography sections.

a Determine the angles between the femoral neck axis and the horizontal reference line and between a line tangent to the posterior border of the femoral condyles and the horizontal reference line.

b The angles are added together to yield the AT angle.
c Diagram showing how the AT angle is determined.

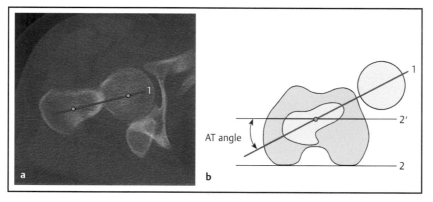

Fig. 1.12a,b Determining the antetorsion (AT) angle by the Murphy method. The femoral neck axis is defined on superimposed computed tomography (CT) images by the center of the femoral head and the center of the base of the femoral neck.
a Determining the femoral neck axis on the CT image.
b Schematic drawing.
   1 = Femoral neck axis
   2 = Line tangent to the posterior border of the femoral condyles
   2' = Line parallel to 2

The following normal value for the AT angle has been reported by Dihlmann and published in textbooks of anatomy:

Femoral neck axis	
• *Normal value:*	α = 10–15° of anteversion

Table 2.3 (see p. 14) shows age-adjusted normal values and analytic criteria proposed by the Commission for the Study of Hip Dysplasia of the German Society for Orthopedics and Traumatology. **Table 1.2** lists various studies in which normal values were established and tabulated based on reference populations. The divergent results are due mainly to the large range of variation that exists in AT angles. In addition, the AT angle is strongly age-dependent and decreases from infancy (> 30°) to the normal values for the adult population stated above.

> ! Even large discrepancies in the AT angles of adolescents will often normalize spontaneously with aging. No specific criteria are available for accurately predicting the progression of AT angles over time.

Table 1.2 Study results on normal values of the antetorsion angle in adults

Study	Method	Number	Mean value of AT angle (± standard deviation) (°)	Range (°)
Dunlap et al 1953	Conventional radiographs	200	10	5–26
Budin and Chandler 1957	Review of available literature	–		8–15
Tomczak et al 1997	MRI	25	22.2	0–37
	CT	25	15.7	3–48
Schneider et al 1997	MRI	98	10.4 ± 6.2	
Strecker et al 1997	CT	505	24.1 ± 17.4	
Jend 1986	CT	32	15.3 ± 11.9	

AT = Antetorsion
CT = Computed tomography
MRI = Magnetic resonance imaging

Budin E, Chandler E. Measurement of femoral neck anteversion by a direct method. Radiology 1957;69(2):209–213

Dunlap K, Shands AR Jr, Hollister LC Jr, Gaul JS Jr, Streit HA. A new method for determination of torsion of the femur. J Bone Joint Surg Am 1953;35-A(2):289–311

Jend HH. Computed tomographic determination of the anteversion angle. Premises and possibilities. [Article in German] Rofo 1986;144(4):447–452

Keats TE. Atlas of Radiologic Measurement. St. Louis: Mosby; 2001

Murphy SB, Simon SR, Kijewski PK, Wilkinson RH, Griscom NT. Femoral anteversion. J Bone Joint Surg Am 1987;69(8):1169–1176

Schneider B, Laubenberger J, Jemlich S, Groene K, Weber HM, Langer M. Measurement of femoral antetorsion and tibial torsion by magnetic resonance imaging. Br J Radiol 1997;70(834):575–579

Strecker W, Keppler P, Gebhard F, Kinzl L. Length and torsion of the lower limb. J Bone Joint Surg Br 1997;79(6):1019–1023

Tomczak RJ, Guenther KP, Rieber A, Mergo P, Ros PR, Brambs HJ. MR imaging measurement of the femoral antetorsional angle as a new technique: comparison with CT in children and adults. AJR Am J Roentgenol 1997;168(3):791–794

■ Tibial Torsion

Like femoral anteversion, tibial torsion, also called tibial torsion (TT) angle, is measured with the lower limb in the neutral position. To avoid errors, the longitudinal axis of the tibia should be parallel to the z-axis of the CT scanner during the examination.

Transverse images are acquired through the proximal and distal tibia at the levels of the knee and ankle joints. The TT angle is measured between one reference line at the level of the tibial plateau and another line at the level of the tibial pilon. The proximal section should be just above the fibular head, and the distal section should display the tibial pilon in its largest dimension.

Several methods for defining the reference lines on these images have been described and evaluated in the literature (**Fig. 1.13**):

● The *proximal* reference line is drawn tangent to the posterior border of the tibial condyles. A less precise method is to draw a longitudinal axis through the cross-section of the tibial plateau.

● The *distal* reference line is drawn through the centers of the tibial pilon and the fibula. Another option is to

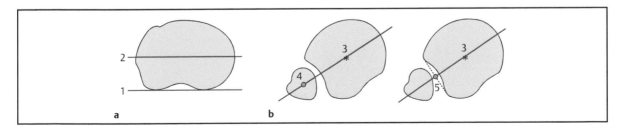

Fig. 1.13a,b Reference lines for the computed tomographic measurement of tibial torsion.

a Proximal reference lines (above the fibular head).
1 = Tangent to posterior border of tibial plateau
2 = Longitudinal axis through cross-section of tibial plateau

b Distal reference lines at the level of the tibial pilon.
3 = Center of tibial pilon
4 = Center of fibula
5 = Center of fibular notch

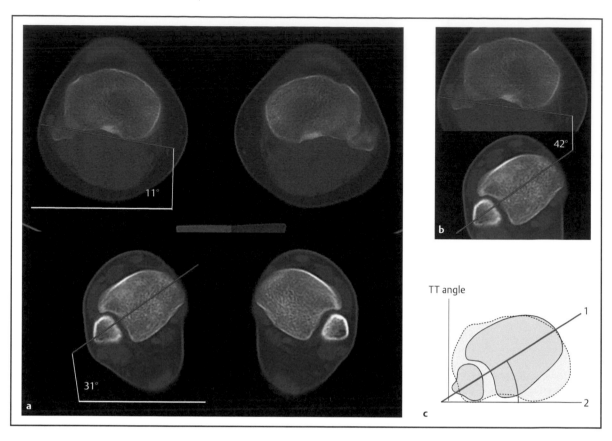

Fig. 1.14a–c Measurement of the tibial torsion (TT) angle on transverse computed tomography sections.

a Determine the angles between the posterior border of the tibial plateau and the horizontal reference line and between a line through the tibial and fibular centers and the horizontal reference line.

b These angles are added to yield the TT angle.

c Schematic representation of the TT angle.
1 = Line through the center of the tibial pilon and fibula (distal reference line)
2 = Line tangent to the tibial condyles (proximal reference line)

draw a line through the center of the fibular notch of the tibia and the center of the tibial pilon.

!
Measuring between the posterior border of the tibial plateau and a line through the centers of the tibia and fibula is the most widely used method and was found to be the most accurate in a comparative study (**Fig. 1.14**; see also **Fig. 1.13**).

!
The variation of normal values reported in the literature results from significant differences in study populations and methods of measurement (**Table 1.3**). The following standard is recommended for routine clinical assessments: the normal range of tibial torsion is from 0 to 40°. Larger angles and negative angles are definitely abnormal. Another method is to evaluate tibial torsion in a side-to-side comparison: as noted by Jend et al, a difference > 8° should be considered abnormal.

TT angle

• *Mean value:*	~20–30°
• *Physiologic range of variation:*	0–40°
• *Increased torsion:*	> 40°
• *Medial torsion:*	Negative angles

Tibial torsion describes the lateral rotation of the distal tibia relative to the proximal portion of the bone. If the distal portion is rotated medially, the TT angle has a negative value.

Clementz BG. Tibial torsion measured in normal adults. Acta Orthop Scand 1988;59(4):441–442

Hutter CG Jr, Scott W. Tibial torsion. J Bone Joint Surg Am 1949;31A(3):511–518

Jakob RP, Haertel M, Stüssi E. Tibial torsion calculated by computerised tomography and compared to other methods of measurement. J Bone Joint Surg Br 1980;62-B(2):238–242

Jend HH, Heller M, Dallek M, Schoettle H. Measurement of tibial torsion by computer tomography. Acta Radiol Diagn (Stockh) 1981;22(3A):271–276

Table 1.3 Study results on normal values of the tibial torsion angle in children and adults

Study	Method	Age group	Number	Tibial torsion (°)
Staheli and Engel 1972	Clinical examination	Children:	160	
		• Birth to 1 year		4–7
		• 2–8 years		9–11
		• 9–13 years		12–14
		Adults	20	14 ± 5
Hutter and Scott 1949	Cadaver study	Adults	40	20 (0–40)
Jakob et al 1980	CT	Adults	45	30
Schneider et al 1997	MRI	Adults	98	41.7 ± 8.8
Strecker et al 1997	CT	Adults	504	34.9 ± 15.9
Clementz 1988	Fluoroscopy	Adults	200	
		• Right	100	30.7 ± 7.8
		• Left	100	28.6 ± 7.6

CT = Computed tomography

MRI = Magnetic resonance imaging

Keats TE. Atlas of Radiologic Measurement. St. Louis: Mosby; 2001

Schneider B, Laubenberger J, Jemlich S, Groene K, Weber HM, Langer M. Measurement of femoral antetorsion and tibial torsion by magnetic resonance imaging. Br J Radiol 1997;70(834):575–579

Staheli LT, Engel GM. Tibial torsion: a method of assessment and a survey of normal children. Clin Orthop Relat Res 1972;86:183–186

Strecker W, Keppler P, Gebhard F, Kinzl L. Length and torsion of the lower limb. J Bone Joint Surg Br 1997;79(6):1019–1023

■ Measurement of Femoral and Tibial Length

The lengths of the femur and tibia can be measured on a CT scout view just as on a full-length AP radiograph, with the legs placed in the neutral position (**Fig. 1.15**).

- *Femoral length:* Femoral length is measured between the superior border of the femoral head and the most distal point on the medial femoral condyle. Both points are located most accurately by drawing horizontal tangents.
- *Tibial length:* The reference points for measuring tibial length are the medial femoral condyle and the center of the tibial plafond.
- *Total length:* Total limb length is measured as the distance from the superior border of the femoral head to the center of the tibial plafond.

Sabharwal S, Zhao C, McKeon JJ, McClemens E, Edgar M, Behrens F. Computed radiographic measurement of limb-length discrepancy. Full-length standing anteroposterior radiograph compared with scanogram. J Bone Joint Surg Am 2006;88(10):2243–2251

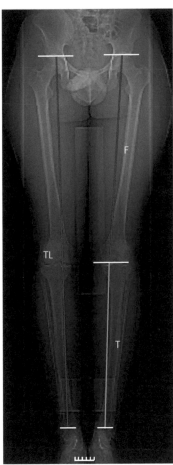

Fig. 1.15 Computed tomographic measurement of limb length.

F = Length of the femur

T = Length of the tibia

TL = Total limb length

2 Hip

Radiographic Landmarks of the Hip

The following radiographic landmarks and their inter-relationships are helpful in diagnosing congenital and acquired abnormalities of the acetabulum (**Fig. 2.1**):

- *Iliopectineal line* (arcuate line, linea terminalis): The iliopectineal line is the radiographic reference line for the anterior column.
- *Ilioischial line:* The upper portion of this line is formed by the posterior part of the quadrilateral plate, its lower portion by the ischium (medial boundary). The ilioischial line is the landmark for the posterior column.
- *Acetabular roof line.*
- *Acetabular teardrop:* This is a teardrop-shaped figure formed laterally by the medial portion of the acetabulum and medially by the antero-inferior portion of the quadrilateral plate. The quadrilateral plate is the posterior wall of the acetabulum, which faces inward on

the pelvic inlet and presents an approximately square, flat surface.

- *Anterior rim of the acetabulum.*
- *Posterior rim of the acetabulum.*

Armbuster TG, Guerra J Jr, Resnick D, et al. The adult hip: an anatomic study. Part I: the bony landmarks. Radiology 1978;128(1):1–10

Femoral Neck–Shaft Angle and Anteversion Angle

Projected Neck–Shaft Angle

The projected femoral neck–shaft angle (NSA, called also the caput–collum–diaphyseal (CCD) angle; **Fig. 2.2**) is determined on the anteroposterior (AP) pelvic radiograph or the AP radiograph of the hip and femur. It is the angle formed by the longitudinal axes of the neck and shaft of the femur.

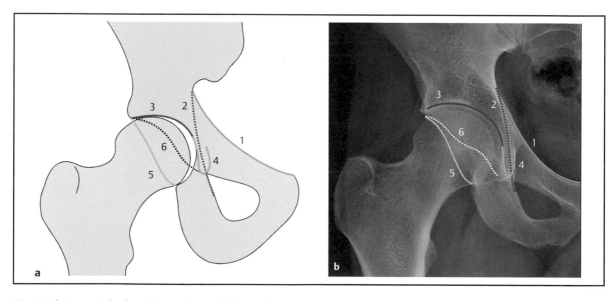

Fig. 2.1a,b Anatomic landmarks for evaluating the hip in the anteroposterior pelvic radiograph.

1 = Iliopectineal line
2 = Ilioischial line
3 = Acetabular roof line
4 = Acetabular teardrop
5 = Posterior rim of acetabulum
6 = Anterior rim of acetabulum
a Schematic drawing.
b Anteroposterior pelvic radiograph.

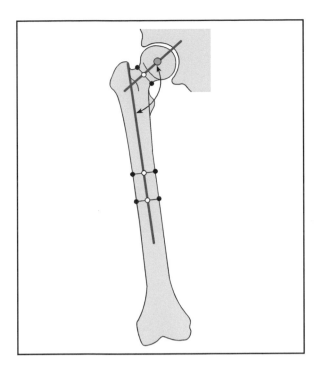

Fig. 2.2 Neck–shaft angle. Schematic drawing.

The femoral neck axis can be determined as follows (**Fig. 2.3**): first the center of the femoral head is located with a circle template or computer-assisted technique at a workstation. Next a line is drawn connecting the points where the circle intersects the medial and lateral borders of the femoral neck. A line drawn perpendicular to that

line through the center of the femoral head represents the femoral neck axis.

M.E. Müller uses the following method for an accurate reconstruction of the NSA:

1. The center of the femoral head is located with a circle template or a computer-assisted technique. Reference points for the circular arc are the lateral portion (outermost point) of the epiphysis and the medial corner of the femoral neck.
2. The point of deepest concavity on the lateral border of the femoral neck is marked.
3. Another arc through that point using the center of the femoral head as the center is drawn.
4. The points where the circle intersects the femoral neck are connected.
5. A line is drawn perpendicular to that line through the center of the femoral head. That line represents the femoral neck axis.
6. The femoral shaft axis is drawn midway between the lateral and medial borders of the femoral shaft.

Projected NSA	
• *Normal values in adults:*	~ 120–130°
• *Coxa valga:*	> 130°
• *Coxa vara:*	< 120°

!
The anteversion of the proximal femur causes the NSA to appear larger on radiographs than it really is.

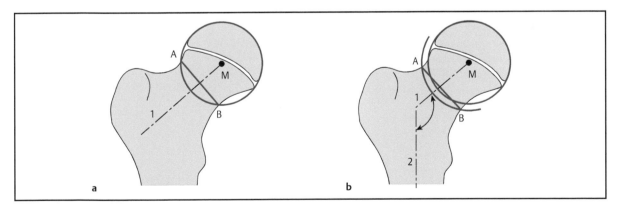

Fig. 2.3a,b Determining the femoral neck axis on an anteroposterior radiograph of the hip or pelvis.

a Approximate determination of the femoral neck axis.
  M = Center of the femoral head
  A = Point where the circle intersects the lateral cortex of the femoral neck
  B = Point where the circle intersects the medial cortex of the femoral neck
  1 = Femoral neck axis (line perpendicular to AB through M)

b M. E. Müller method for accurate reconstruction of the femoral neck axis.
  M = Center of the femoral head
  A = Deepest point in lateral concavity of the femoral neck
  B = Point on medial border of the femoral neck defined by the second arc
  1 = Femoral neck axis (line perpendicular to AB through M)
  2 = Femoral shaft axis

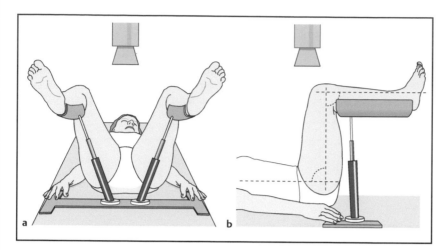

Fig. 2.4a,b Dunn–Rippstein–Müller method of determining the anteversion angle on conventional radiographs. Schematic illustration.
a View from the foot of the table.
b Side view.

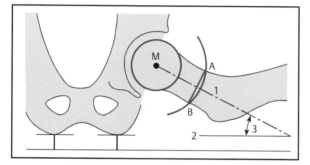

Fig. 2.5 Dunn-Rippstein-Müller method of reconstructing the anteversion angle.
M = Center of the femoral head
A = Deepest point in lateral concavity of the femoral neck
B = Point where the second arc intersects the medial femoral neck
1 = Femoral neck axis (line perpendicular to AB through M)
2 = Horizontal plane (defined by the positioning frame)
3 = Projected anteversion angle

Müller ME. Die hüftnahen Femurosteotomien. 1st ed. Stuttgart: Thieme; 1957

Projected Anteversion Angle (Dunn–Rippstein–Müller Method)

Today the Dunn–Rippstein–Müller method is widely used to assess rotational deformity by calculating the true NSA and femoral anteversion (AV) angle. The projected AV angle is measured on a radiograph in the Rippstein projection (called also the Rippstein II view). This projection is standardized by using a positioning frame that holds the hip in 90° of flexion and 20° of abduction (**Fig. 2.4**).

The AV angle is measured between the horizontal plane (defined by the positioning frame) and the femoral neck axis (**Fig. 2.5**). The Müller method (see p. 11) is best for determining the femoral neck axis. When calculated in this way, the AV angle is determined relative to the transverse axis of the femoral condyles.

True Neck–Shaft Angle and Anteversion Angle

Geometric formulae are available for converting the projected NSA and AV angle to the true angles.

Calculation of the true AV angle:

$$\tan\alpha = \frac{\alpha_2 \cdot \cos\left(\beta_2 - 90° - \gamma\right)}{\cos\beta_2 - 90°}$$

Calculation of the true NSA:

$$\cot\beta = \cot\beta_2 \cdot \cot\alpha$$

where:
α = true AV angle
α_2 = projected AV angle
β_2 = projected NSA
γ = abduction angle of the femur = 20°

The use of conversion charts will facilitate the rapid calculation of values in everyday practice. The chart published by Müller in 1957 is a well-established clinical tool (**Table 2.1**). Another current option is the use of computer software.

Both the NSA and AV angle change with aging and show a large range of variation. **Tables 2.2** and **2.3** list age-adjusted normal values and analytic criteria proposed by the Commission for the Study of Developmental Dysplasia of the Hip of the German Society for Orthopedics and Traumatology. These tables can be helpful in routine clinical decision-making. Prognostic assessments are difficult, however, because spontaneous normalization often occurs during growth and cannot be predicted with certainty.

Table 2.1 Chart for finding the true values of the anteversion (AV) angle (horizontal numbers) and neck–shaft angle (NSA) (vertical numbers) based on the projected angles (source: Müller 1957)

Projected NSA (°)	Projected AV angle (°)															
	5	10	15	20	25	30	35	40	45	50	55	60	65	70	75	80
100	4	9	15	20	25	30	35	40	45	50	55	60	65	70	75	80
	101	100	100	100	100	99	99	98	97	96	95	94	94	93	92	91
105	5	9	15	20	25	31	35	41	46	51	56	60	65	70	75	80
	105	105	104	104	103	103	102	100	100	99	98	97	96	95	94	92
110	5	10	16	21	27	32	36	42	47	52	56	61	66	71	76	80
	110	110	109	108	108	106	106	105	104	103	101	99	98	97	95	93
115	5	10	16	21	27	32	37	43	48	52	57	62	67	71	76	81
	115	115	114	112	112	111	110	109	107	105	104	102	101	99	96	94
120	6	11	16	22	28	33	38	44	49	53	58	63	68	72	77	81
	120	119	118	117	116	115	114	112	110	108	106	104	103	101	98	95
125	6	11	17	23	28	34	39	44	50	54	58	63	68	72	77	81
	125	124	123	121	120	119	118	116	114	112	109	107	105	103	100	95
130	6	12	18	24	29	35	40	46	51	55	60	64	69	73	78	82
	130	129	127	126	125	124	122	120	117	116	112	109	107	104	101	96
135	7	13	19	25	31	36	42	47	52	56	61	65	70	74	78	82
	135	133	132	131	130	129	126	124	120	118	114	112	109	105	102	96
140	7	13	20	27	32	38	44	49	53	58	63	67	71	75	79	83
	139	138	137	135	134	132	130	127	124	120	117	114	111	107	103	97
145	8	14	21	28	34	40	45	50	55	59	64	68	72	75	79	83
	144	142	141	139	138	136	134	131	128	124	120	117	114	110	104	98
150	8	15	22	29	35	42	47	52	56	61	65	69	73	76	80	84
	149	147	146	144	143	141	138	136	134	129	124	120	116	112	105	100
155	9	17	24	32	38	44	50	54	58	63	67	71	74	77	81	84
	154	152	151	149	148	145	142	139	137	132	128	124	119	115	108	103
160	10	18	27	34	44	46	52	57	61	65	69	73	76	79	82	82
	159	158	157	155	153	151	147	144	141	134	132	128	122	116	111	105
165	13	23	33	40	47	53	57	62	67	69	73	76	78	81	83	86
	164	162	160	159	158	156	153	148	144	140	135	130	122	119	113	106
170	15	27	37	46	53	58	63	67	70	73	76	78	80	83	84	87
	169	167	166	164	163	159	157	154	150	145	142	134	130	122	118	113

Hip

2

Dunn DM. Anteversion of the neck of the femur; a method of measurement. J Bone Joint Surg Br 1952;34-B(2):181–186

Müller ME. Die hüftnahen Femurosteotomien. 1st ed. Stuttgart: Thieme; 1957

Rippstein J. Determination of the antetorsion of the femur neck by means of two x-ray pictures. [Article in German] Z Orthop Ihre Grenzgeb 1955;86(3):345–360

Tönnis D. Die angeborene Hüftdysplasie und Hüftluxation im Kindes- und Erwachsenenalter. Chapter 9: Allgemeine Röntgendiagnostik des Hüftgelenks. Berlin: Springer; 1984; 129–134

Hip

2

Table 2.2 Classification of true neck–shaft angles (NSAs) (Commission for the Study of DDH, German Society for Orthopedics and Traumatology; MV = mean value; source: Tönnis 1984)

Age (years)	Grade –4 (extremely abnormal)	Grade –3 (severely abnormal)	Grade –2 (slightly abnormal)	Grade 1 (normal to borderline)	Grade +2 (slightly abnormal)	Grade +3 (severely abnormal)	Grade +4 (extremely abnormal)
> 1 to < 3	< 105	≥ 105 to < 115	≥ 115 to < 125	≥ 125 to < 150 (MV 140)	≥ 150 to < 155	≥ 155 to < 160	≥ 160
> 3 to < 5	< 105	≥ 105 to < 115	≥ 115 to < 125	≥ 125 to < 145 (MV 135)	≥ 145 to < 150	≥ 150 to < 155	≥ 155
> 5 to < 10	< 100	≥ 100 to < 110	≥ 110 to < 120	≥ 120 to < 145 (MV 132)	≥ 145 to < 150	≥ 150 to < 155	≥ 155
> 10 to < 14	< 100	≥ 100 to < 110	≥ 110 to < 120	≥ 120 to < 140 (MV 130)	≥ 140 to < 145	≥ 145 to < 155	≥ 155
14 or more	< 100	≥ 100 to < 110	≥ 110 to < 120	≥ 120 to < 135 (MV 128)	≥ 135 to < 140	≥ 140 to < 150	≥ 150

Table 2.3 Classification of true anteversion (AV) angles (Commission for the Study of DDH, German Society for Orthopedics and Traumatology; MV = mean value; source: Tönnis 1984)

Age (years)	Grade –4 (extremely abnormal)	Grade –3 (severely abnormal)	Grade –2 (slightly abnormal, borderline)	Grade 1 (normal)	Grade +2 (slightly abnormal, borderline)	Grade +3 (severely abnormal)	Grade +4 (extremely abnormal)
> 1 to < 3	< 20	≥ 20 to < 25	≥ 25 to < 35	≥ 35 to < 55 (MV 45)	≥ 55 to < 60	≥ 60 to < 75	≥ 75
≥ 3 to < 7	< 15	≥ 15 to < 20	≥ 20 to < 30	≥ 30 to < 50 (MV 40)	≥ 50 to < 55	≥ 55 to < 70	≥ 70
≥ 7 to < 9	< 10	≥ 10 to < 15	≥ 15 to < 25	≥ 25 to < 45 (MV 35)	≥ 45 to < 50	≥ 50 to < 65	≥ 65
≥ 9 to < 11	< 5	≥ 5 to < 10	≥ 10 to < 20	≥ 20 to < 40 (MV 30)	≥ 40 to < 45	≥ 45 to < 60	≥ 60
≥ 11 to < 13	< 5	≥ 5 to < 10	≥ 10 to < 15	≥ 15 to < 35 (MV 25)	≥ 35 to < 40	≥ 40 to < 55	≥ 55
≥ 13 to <15	< 0	≥ 0 to < 5	≥ 5 to < 10	≥ 10 to < 30 (MV 20)	≥ 30 to < 35	≥ 35 to < 50	≥ 50
≥ 15	< 0	≥ 0 to < 5	≥ 5 to < 10	≥ 10 to < 25 (MV 15)	≥ 25 to < 30	≥ 30 to < 45	≥ 45

Acetabular Anteversion

Conventional Radiograph

The AP pelvic view itself can suggest whether the acetabulum has a normal or abnormal degree of anteversion. The pelvis should not be rotated laterally or tilted when the radiograph is taken (symmetrical obturator foramina, middle of sacrococcygeal joint and pubic symphysis are defined). Some degree of acetabular anteversion is present in a normal hip.

Distance between Anterior and Posterior Acetabular Rims

A perpendicular line is drawn from the center of the femoral head to the acetabular rims, and the distance between the anterior and posterior rims is measured (**Fig. 2.6**). Because the rims of the acetabulum are not parallel, this value is only an approximation.

Distance between anterior and posterior rims of the acetabulum	
• *Normal value:*	~ 1.5 cm
• *Decreased anteversion:*	< 1.5 cm
• *No anteversion:*	≈ 0
• *Increased anteversion:*	>> 1.5 cm

Cross-over Sign

This sign is an indicator of acetabular retroversion, which can predispose to femoroacetabular impingement. Normally the anterior acetabular rim projects superior and medial to the posterior acetabular rim on the AP pelvic radiograph, and both projected lines converge at the level of the superior rim. With acetabular retroversion, the two lines cross before that point, creating a propeller-shaped figure called the "cross-over sign" or figure-of-eight configuration (**Fig. 2.7**).

Posterior Wall Sign

In a normal hip the posterior rim of the acetabulum descends approximately through the center of the femoral head on the AP pelvic radiograph. When the posterior acetabular rim is very prominent, it will typically project lateral to the center of the femoral head, creating a "posterior wall sign" (**Fig. 2.8**). A prominent posterior rim may cause posterior femoroacetabular impingement to occur during extension and external rotation of the hip. If the posterior acetabular rim is deficient, it will project medial to the center of the femoral head (e.g., in a patient with acetabular retroversion or hip dysplasia).

Tannast M, Siebenrock KA, Anderson SE. Femoroacetabular impingement: radiographic diagnosis—what the radiologist should know. AJR Am J Roentgenol 2007;188(6):1540–1552

Hip

2

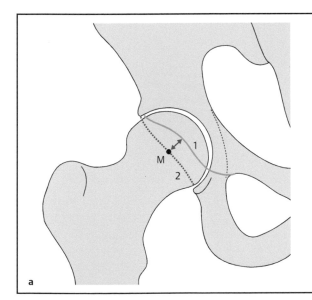
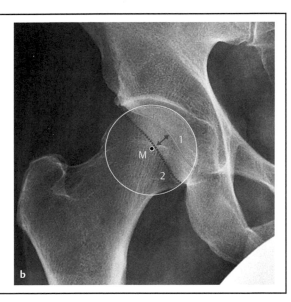

Fig. 2.6a,b Measuring the distance between the anterior and posterior acetabular rims.

M = Center of the femoral head
1 = Anterior acetabular rim
2 = Posterior acetabular rim

a Schematic drawing.
b Measurement on a radiograph.

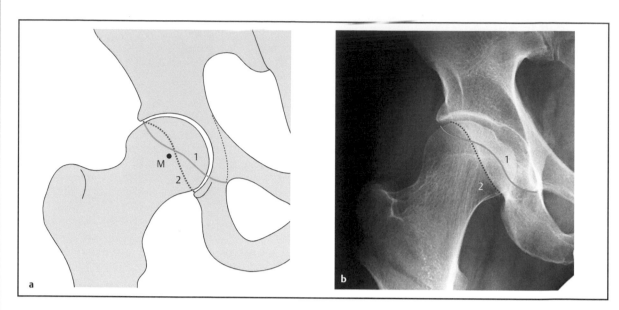

Fig. 2.7a,b Cross-over sign.

M = Center of the femoral head
1 = Anterior acetabular rim
2 = Posterior acetabular rim

a Schematic drawing.
b Radiographic appearance.

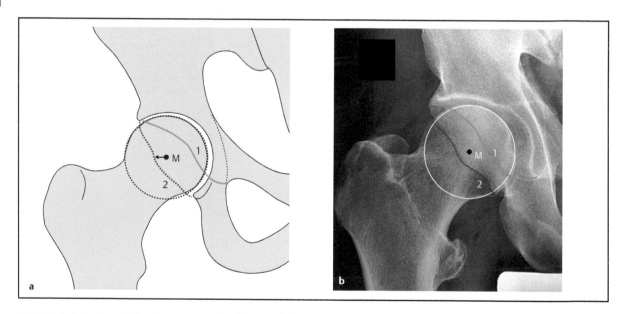

Fig. 2.8a,b Posterior wall sign. The posterior rim of the acetabulum projects lateral to the center of the femoral head.

M = Center of the femoral head
1 = Anterior acetabular rim
2 = Posterior acetabular rim

a Schematic drawing.
b Radiographic appearance.

Computed Tomographic Measurement of Acetabular Anteversion

Anda Method

Acetabular anteversion can be measured on transverse computed tomography (CT) scans using a method introduced by Anda et al (**Fig. 2.9**). Transverse CT sections are obtained at the level of the hip joint, and the acetabula are measured on a transverse section passing through the centers of the femoral heads. The center (M) of each femoral head is located with a template, and a straight connecting line (g) is drawn between the femoral head centers. A line (s) perpendicular to g is drawn through the posterior rim of the acetabulum (P). The angle between the perpendicular line (s) and a straight line tangent to the anterior (A) and posterior (P) acetabular rims equals the degree of acetabular anteversion. While the AP pelvic radiograph can provide only signs that are suggestive of abnormal acetabular version, the deformity can be accurately quantified by CT.

Anda S, Terjesen T, Kvistad KA. Computed tomography measurements of the acetabulum in adult dysplastic hips: which level is appropriate? Skeletal Radiol 1991;20(4):267–271

Anda S, Terjesen T, Kvistad KA, Svenningsen S. Acetabular angles and femoral anteversion in dysplastic hips in adults: CT investigation. J Comput Assist Tomogr 1991;15(1):115–120

Method of Tönnis and Heinecke

Because the anterior rim of the acetabulum undergoes considerable regression in its lower portion, some authors prefer to measure acetabular anteversion in the upper part of the hip joint (**Fig. 2.10**). As in the Anda method, measurements are performed on transverse CT sections. The hip should be scanned in the prone position to obtain a neutral, reproducible pelvic tilt. The measurement of acetabular anteversion, which closely follows the Anda method, is then performed on the section that displays a sharply tapered bony rim anterior to the femoral head. That section is located slightly above the center of the femoral head.

Acetabular anteversion	
• *Normal mean value in men:*	*18.5° ± 4.5°*
• *Normal mean value in women:*	*21.5° ± 5°*

Acetabular anteversion	
Normal range:	*~ 15–20°*

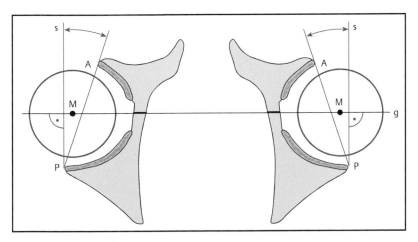

Fig. 2.9 CT measurement of acetabular anteversion by the Anda method.
M = Center of the femoral head
A = Anterior acetabular rim
P = Posterior acetabular rim
g = Straight line through the centers of both femoral heads
s = Line perpendicular to g through the posterior acetabular rim P

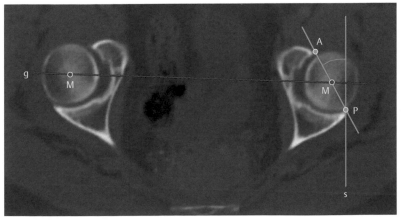

Fig. 2.10 Measurement of acetabular anteversion by the method of Tönnis and Heinecke.
M = Center of the femoral head
A = Anterior acetabular rim
P = Posterior acetabular rim
g = Straight line through the centers of both femoral heads
s = Line perpendicular to g through the posterior acetabular rim P

Tönnis D, Heinecke A. Antetorsion und Anteversion als pathogene Faktoren. In: Tschauner C. Hüfte und Becken. Stuttgart: Thieme; 2003

Coxa profunda

Relationship of the Acetabular Line to the Ilioischial Line

Coxa profunda is a condition in which the acetabular fossa is too deep. The depth of the acetabulum can be evaluated on the AP pelvic radiograph by measuring the distance between the medial acetabular roof line and the ilioischial line (**Fig. 2.11**).

> ! The interrelationship of the pelvic reference lines should be evaluated on the AP pelvic radiograph (**Fig. 2.12**). Do not use an AP radiograph of the hip with the beam centered on the joint, because this projection can give a false impression of coxa profunda or protrusio acetabuli.

A horizontal line is drawn between the centers of both femoral heads on the pelvic radiograph. The distance from the ilioischial line to the medial acetabular line, which is continuous inferiorly with the acetabular teardrop, is measured at the level where they intersect the horizontal line between the femoral head centers.

If the ilioischial line is medial to the acetabular line, the measured distance has a positive value. If the acetabular line is medial, the measurement has a negative value.

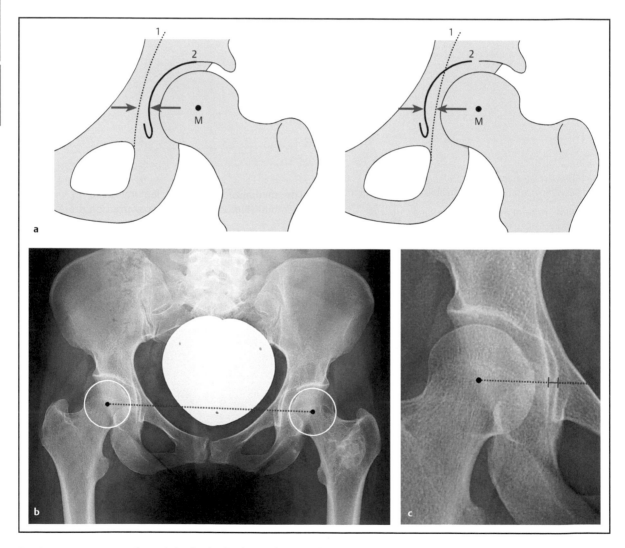

Fig. 2.11a–c Assessment of acetabular depth. The distance between the ilioischial line and acetabular line is measured.

a Schematic drawing. The measurement has a positive value on the left side, a negative value on the right.
  1 = Ilioischial line

2 = Acetabular roof line
b AP pelvic radiograph.
c AP pelvic radiograph, magnified view.

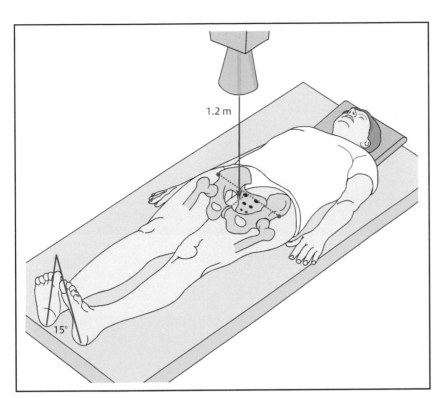

Fig. 2.12 Positioning technique and central ray orientation for the anteroposterior pelvic radiograph.

Coxa profunda

- *Critical value in men, coxa profunda:* distance between acetabular line and ilioischial line < −3 mm
- *Critical value in women, coxa profunda:* distance between acetabular line and ilioischial line < −6 mm

Armbuster TG, Guerra J Jr, Resnick D, et al. The adult hip: an anatomic study. Part I: the bony landmarks. Radiology 1978;128(1):1–10

CE Angle of Wiberg

The center-edge (CE) angle of Wiberg (see also p. 29 and **Fig. 2.27**) describes the position of the femoral head in relation to the acetabulum. The deeper the acetabulum, the greater the CE angle. As the acetabulum becomes flatter and steeper (dysplastic), the CE angle decreases.

Typically the CE angle is increased in coxa profunda and protrusio acetabuli. A CE angle > 39° is considered an indicator of coxa profunda or protrusio acetabuli in adults.

Indicator of coxa profunda in adults

CE angle: > 39°

Protrusio acetabuli

The medialization of the femoral head in protrusio acetabuli (**Fig. 2.13**) can be recognized on the AP pelvic radiograph by noting the relationship of the medial border of the femoral head to the ilioischial line. Protrusio acetabuli is present if the medial border of the femoral head is medial to the ilioischial line.

> ! Both coxa profunda and protrusio acetabuli are characterized by increased depth of the acetabulum. Many authors use both terms synonymously. The relationship of the changes is unclear, however, and coxa profunda may be a precursor of protrusio acetabuli. Strictly speaking, coxa profunda refers to a deep acetabular fossa while protrusio acetabuli refers to medialization of the femoral head as described above.

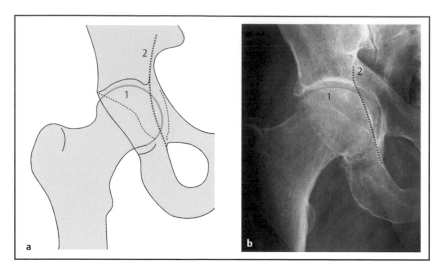

Fig. 2.13a,b Protrusio acetabuli. The femoral head line is projected medial to the ilioischial line.
1 = Femoral head line
2 = Ilioischial line
a Schematic drawing.
b Radiographic appearance.

Developmental Dysplasia of the Hip

Imaging of Developmental Dysplasia of the Hip

The following methods are used in the imaging evaluation of developmental dysplasia of the hip (DDH) at various ages:

- *Birth to 12 months:* ultrasound.
  - Many countries have implemented ultrasound screening (for example in Germany ultrasound is routinely performed in the 4th to 6th week of life).
  - Used in newborns with risk factors:
    - positive family history
    - breech presentation
    - clinical abnormalities
  - Ultrasound is rewarding until ~ 1 year of age.
- *After 12 months:* radiographs. Generally it is sufficient to obtain one AP pelvic radiograph.
- *Small children (up to 4 years of age):*
  - The most important parameter for evaluating DDH in small children is the acetabular index.
  - The following parameters can also be calculated or assessed:
    - Shenton–Ménard line
    - Calvé line
    - Grade of dislocation according to Tönnis
    - Smith migration index
    - Reimer migration index
    - Acetabular teardrop
    - Acetabular angle of Sharp
- *Useful parameters after 4 years of age:*
  - Center-edge angle (CE angle), ACM angle of Idelberger and Frank, summarized hip factor (SHF)
  - False profile view →VCA angle (anterior center-edge angle) of Lequesne and De Sèze

- *After closure of the triradiate cartilage:* The following angles can be used to evaluate for residual dysplasia in the skeletally mature patient:
  - CE angle, horizontal toit externe angle (HTE angle, acetabular index of the weight-bearing zone), SHF, ACM angle, acetabular angle of Sharp
  - False profile view → VCA angle
  - If necessary, femoral head coverage by the acetabulum can be quantified on transverse CT sections using the Anda method.

Ultrasound Evaluation in the First Year of Life

While the Graf method is widely used in Europe for evaluating the infant hip and has become a routine screening study in several European countries, the Harcke method has become widely established in the United States. The Graf method is a static morphologic evaluation whereas the Harcke method is a dynamic technique that evaluates the stability of the joint.

■ Graf Method

The Graf method for sonographic evaluation of the infant hip follows a standard technique based on the use of a high-resolution transducer (at least 7 MHz). The infant is scanned in a lateral decubitus position with the examiner on the right side. The acetabulum appears on the right side of the image, the greater trochanter on the left side. The hip joint is evaluated in a standard coronal plane (**Fig. 2.14**). Three key landmarks should be visualized in this plane:

1. The inferior border of the ilium in the acetabular fossa
2. The central weight-bearing zone of the acetabular roof
3. The acetabular labrum

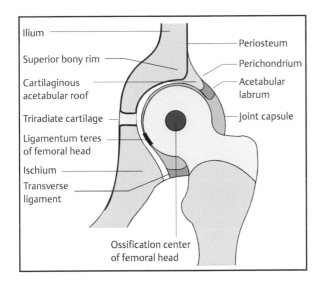

Ilium
Periosteum
Superior bony rim
Perichondrium
Cartilaginous acetabular roof
Acetabular labrum
Triradiate cartilage
Joint capsule
Ligamentum teres of femoral head
Ischium
Transverse ligament
Ossification center of femoral head

Fig. 2.14 Schematic drawing of the infant hip in the standard ultrasound plane.

To evaluate the sonogram in the standard Graf plane, all angles are measured in relation to the "baseline," which is tangent to the lateral border of the ilium (**Fig. 2.15**). Two more reference lines are drawn along the bony roof of the acetabulum (acetabular roof line) and along the acetabular labrum (labral line). The acetabular roof line is drawn from the superior bony rim of the acetabulum to the lower edge of the ilium in the acetabular fossa. The labral line runs from the labrum to the superior bony rim of the acetabulum or to the transition point from the convexity of the superior bony rim to the concave acetabular roof.

The intersections of these lines form the alpha (α) and beta (β) angles of the hip. The α angle is formed by the baseline and acetabular roof line and reflects the bony coverage of the femoral head. The β angle, formed by the baseline and labral line, is a criterion for evaluating the cartilaginous acetabular roof (**Table 2.4**).

> ! The routine interpretation of standard hip sonograms is usually aided by a "sonometer." This special gauge is used to perform the angle measurements and also provides a direct readout of hip type based on the Graf classification.

Graf R. Sonographie der Säuglingshüfte. 5th ed. Stuttgart: Thieme; 2000
Graf R. Hip Sonography. Diagnosis and Management of Infant Hip Dysplasia. 2nd ed. Berlin Heidelberg: Springer; 2006

■ Harcke Method

The Harcke method is a dynamic ultrasound examination that includes stress maneuvers based on accepted clinical examination techniques (Barlow and Ortolani maneuvers). The infant is scanned in the supine position with the feet directed toward the examiner. The study employs a four-step scanning technique with two standard orthogonal planes (coronal and transverse views), each of which is evaluated with the hip in a neutral and flexed position at rest and during stress.

The coronal neutral view corresponds to the standard Graf plane. The examiner assesses femoral head coverage and acetabular and labral morphology in this view without taking any quantitative measurements.

In the coronal flexion view, the hip and knee joints are flexed 90° and the transducer is placed at a slightly more posterior site over the center of the triradiate cartilage. Hip stability is then assessed by "pistoning" the hip anteroposteriorly. In a normal flexion view the femoral head should not be visible above the triradiate cartilage. If the femoral head subluxates during stress (pulling the knee), it will be visible above the triradiate cartilage.

In the transverse neutral view, which corresponds to a transverse CT section at that level, the femoral head in a normal hip will be centered over the triradiate cartilage

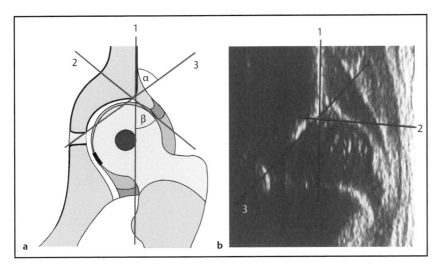

Fig. 2.15a,b Graf technique for ultrasound evaluation of the hip.
1 = Baseline
2 = Labral line
3 = Acetabular roof line
α = Alpha angle
β = Beta angle
a Schematic drawing.
b Sonographic appearance.

21

Table 2.4 Graf sonographic classification of infant hips

Classification	Bony roof / Bony roof angle α	Superior bony rim (bony promontory)	Cartilaginous roof / Cartilage roof angle β
Type I (mature hip, any age)	Good α angle ≥ 60°	Angular/slightly rounded ("blunt")	Covers the femoral head Type Ia → β angle < 55° Type Ib → β angle > 55°
Type IIa (+) (physiologically immature → appropriate for age, age < 12 weeks)	Adequate (satisfactory) α angle 50–59° appropriate for age	Rounded	Covers the femoral head
Type IIa (–) (physiologically immature → maturation deficit, age 6–12 weeks)	Deficient α angle 50–59° not appropriate for age	Rounded	Covers the femoral head
Type IIb (delayed ossification, age > 12 weeks)	Deficient α angle 50–59°	Rounded	Covers the femoral head
Type IIc (critical zone, any age)	Severely deficient α angle 43–49°	Rounded to flattened	Still covers the femoral head β angle < 77°
Type IId (decentering hip, any age)	Severely deficient α angle 43–49°	Rounded to flattened	Displaced β angle < 77°
Type IIIa (eccentric hip, any age)	Poor α angle < 43°	Flattened	Pressed upward, without structural alteration
Type IIIb (eccentric hip, any age)	Poor α angle < 43°	Flattened	Pressed upward, with structural alteration
Type IV (eccentric hip, any age)	Poor α angle < 43°	Flattened	Pressed downward
Exception: Type II coming to maturity	Deficient	Angular (!)	Covers the femoral head

with the bony margin of the pubis anteriorly and the ischium posteriorly.

In the transverse flexion view (**Fig. 2.16**), in which the hip and knee are again held in 90° of flexion, the femoral head appears between the echogenic (ossified) limbs of the femoral metaphysis anteriorly and the ischium at the posterior rim of the acetabulum. These form a v-shape with the hip in adduction and a u-shape with the hip in abduction. Instability can be assessed by adducting the hip and applying stress (gentle posterior traction, Barlow maneuver), and the reduction of a dislocated hip can be assessed by abduction (Ortolani maneuver).

The Graf and Harcke methods have shown comparable dependable results in many studies. The Harcke method has a somewhat longer learning curve, however. It requires more training and greater clinical experience.

Harcke HT, Grissom LE. Performing dynamic sonography of the infant hip. AJR Am J Roentgenol 1990;155(4):837–844

Martinoli C, Valle M. Pediatric musculoskeletal ultrasound. In: Ultrasound of the Musculoskeletal System. 1st ed. Berlin Heidelberg: Springer; 2007: 921–959

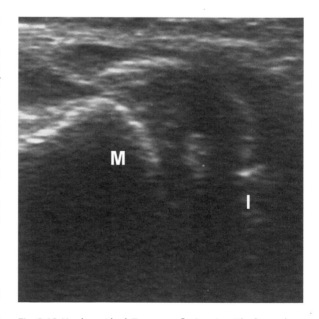

Fig. 2.16 Harcke method: Transverse flexion view. The femoral head is located between the femoral metaphysis (M) and the ischium (I). These form a v-shape with adduction and a u-shape with abduction.

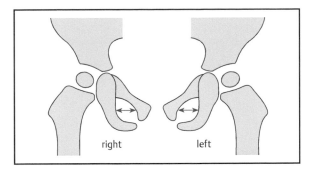

Fig. 2.17 Pelvic rotation ratio (Q) of Tönnis and Brunken. The ratio is defined as Q = diameter of the right obturator foramen/diameter of the left foramen. The normal range is between 0.56 and 1.8.

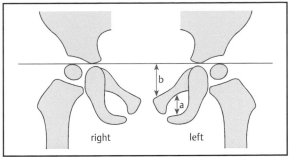

Fig. 2.18 Pelvic tilt index (I) of Ball and Kommenda. The index is defined as I = a/b (a = vertical diameter of obturator foramen, b = distance between superior border of pubis and the Hilgenreiner line). The normal range is between 0.75 and 1.2.

Radiographic Evaluation in Small Children (up to Age 4)

The X-ray evaluation of hip dysplasia in small children from 1 to ~ 4 years of age is usually based on the AP pelvic radiograph, which is used for various measurements and calculations. The most important parameter, and by far the most widely used, is the acetabular index (AC angle of Hilgenreiner). A selection of other parameters, some of which yield complementary information, is presented below.

■ Anteroposterior Pelvic Radiograph— Correct Positioning

For the AP pelvic radiograph in infants, the legs are held in a neutral position with the knees pointing forward; up to 10–15° of knee flexion is allowed. The following indices can be used to confirm correct positioning.

Pelvic Rotation Ratio (of Tönnis and Brunken)

This is the ratio of the apparent diameters of both obturator foramina (**Fig. 2.17**). The ratio should be between 0.56 and 1.8.

> **!**
> A rotated projection will distort the acetabular index (acetabular roof inclination). If the ratio is between 0.56 and 1.87, the acetabular index will be distorted by no more than 2°. If the view is rotated to the right, the acetabular index measured on the right side will be too low while the acetabular index on the left will be too high.

Tönnis D. On changes in the acetabular vault angle of the hip joint in rotated and tilted positions of the pelvis in children. [Article in German] Z Orthop Ihre Grenzgeb 1962;96:462–478

Pelvic Tilt Index (of Ball and Kommenda)

This index is the ratio of the vertical diameter of the obturator foramen to the distance between the superior border of the pubic bone and the Hilgenreiner line (**Fig. 2.18**). The index should be between 0.75 and 1.2.

Ball F, Kommenda K. Sources of error in the roentgen evaluation of the hip in infancy. [Article in Multiple languages] Ann Radiol (Paris) 1968;11(5):298–303

■ Auxiliary Lines and Measurements for the Evaluation of Hip Dysplasia and Hip Dislocation

All the parameters listed below are determined on the AP pelvic radiograph with the legs in the neutral position and the knees pointing forward. Up to 10–15° of knee flexion is allowed.

Hilgenreiner Line (Y-Line)

The Hilgenreiner line (**Fig. 2.19**) is a horizontal line drawn across the lowest points of both iliac wings, tangent to the inferolateral edge of the ilium above the triradiate cartilage. It serves as a reference line for various measurements used in the detection and classification of hip dysplasia.

Perkins–Ombrédanne Line

The Perkins–Ombrédanne line (see **Fig. 2.19**) is drawn perpendicular to the Hilgenreiner line and passes through the most lateral point of the acetabular roof. It is used to determine various parameters for evaluating hip dysplasia.

Hip

2

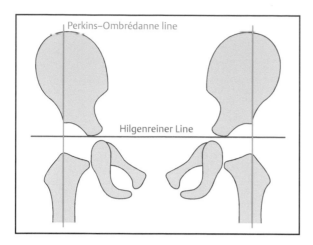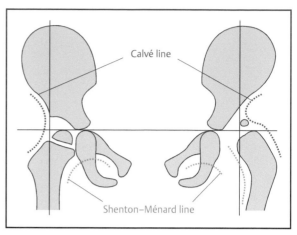

Fig. 2.19 Hilgenreiner line and Perkins–Ombrédanne line. The Hilgenreiner line and Perkins–Ombrédanne line serve as reference lines for various measurements used in the evaluation of developmental dysplasia of the hip.

Fig. 2.20 Shenton–Ménard line and Calvé line. These lines are illustrated for a healthy hip (left) and for a dysplastic hip (right).

Shenton–Ménard Line

A line traced along the medial aspect of the femoral neck and the superior border of the obturator foramen normally forms a smooth, unbroken arc called the Shenton–Ménard line (**Fig. 2.20**). When the hip is dislocated, the arc is broken because the femoral neck occupies an abnormally high position (as it also does in Perthes disease). An externally rotated position of the lower limb will also cause a break in the Shenton–Ménard line.

> The Shenton–Ménard line dates from the older literature and is no longer widely used today.

Calvé Line

The Calvé line (see **Fig. 2.20**) is a curved line drawn along the lateral border of the iliac wing, the superior acetabular rim to the femoral neck. It should form a smooth, uniform arc. If the proximal femur creates a break or bulge in the line, this is considered evidence that the hip is dislocated.

> The Calvé line, like the Shenton–Ménard line, is largely of historic interest today.

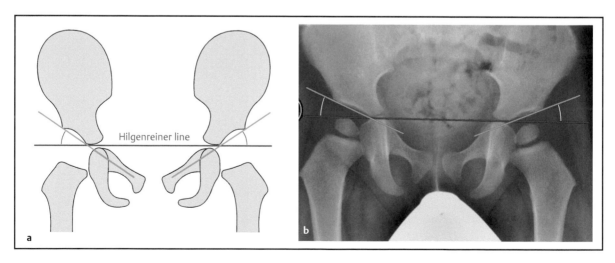

Fig. 2.21a,b Acetabular index (AC angle of Hilgenreiner). This angle is formed by the Hilgenreiner line and a line tangent to the acetabular roof.

a Schematic drawing.

b Radiographic appearance.

Table 2.5 Mean values of the acetabular index in normal and borderline hips at various ages, with single standard deviations (source: Tönnis and Brunken 1968)

Age	Number of girls examined (n)	Girls		Number of boys examined (n)	Boys	
		Right hip	Left hip		Right hip	Left hip
1–2 months	25	30.0 ± 5.8	30.6 ± 5.5	13	23.6 ± 4.1	27.2 ± 4.0
3–4 months	90	26.5 ± 4.9	27.7 ± 5.5	54	23.4 ± 4.5	24.5 ± 4.6
5–6 months	96	22.8 ± 4.5	24.5 ± 4.8	62	19.4 ± 4.8	22.0 ± 4.8
7–9 months	143	21.2 ± 4.1	22.7 ± 4.2	65	20.3 ± 4.3	21.3 ± 4.1
10–12 months	84	20.8 ± 3.9	22.8 ± 4.3	42	19.4 ± 3.8	21.3 ± 3.9
13–15 months	62	20.2 ± 4.4	22.1 ± 4.8	26	18.7 ± 4.4	20.3 ± 3.7
16–18 months	44	20.7 ± 4.3	21.8 ± 4.3	28	19.5 ± 4.3	21.6 ± 4.2
19–24 months	59	19.8 ± 4.3	22.0 ± 4.4	33	16.8 ± 3.8	19.1 ± 4.1
2–3 years	59	18.0 ± 3.8	19.5 ± 3.8	46	16.7 ± 4.3	18.5 ± 4.2
3–5 years	33	14.5 ± 3.4	16.6 ± 4.6	36	14.9 ± 4.3	15.8 ± 4.0
5–7 years	24	15.2 ± 4.1	15.8 ± 4.0	23	12.7 ± 4.1	15.4 ± 3.9

Table 2.6 Evaluation of the acetabular index: normal limits of acetabular angles based on standard deviation data (SD = one standard deviation from normal population of equal age and gender; source: Tönnis and Brunken 1968)

Age	Girls				Boys			
	Mildly dysplastic (SD)		Severely dysplastic (2 SD)		Mildly dysplastic (SD)		Severely dysplastic (2 SD)	
	Right	Left	Right	Left	Right	Left	Right	Left
1–2 months	36.0	36.0	41.5	41.5	29.0	31.0	33.0	35.0
3–4 months	31.5	33.0	36.5	38.5	28.0	29.0	32.5	33.5
5–6 months	27.5	29.5	32.0	34.0	24.5	27.0	29.0	31.5
7–9 months	25.5	27.0	29.5	31.5	24.5	25.5	29.0	29.5
10–12 months	24.5	27.0	29.0	31.5	23.5	25.0	27.0	29.0
13–15 months	24.5	27.0	29.0	31.5	23.0	24.0	27.5	27.5
16–18 months	24.5	26.0	29.0	30.5	23.0	24.0	26.5	27.5
19–24 months	24.0	25.5	28.0	30.5	21.5	23.0	26.5	27.0
2–3 years	22.0	23.5	25.5	27.0	21.0	22.5	25.0	27.0
3–5 years	18.0	21.0	22.5	25.5	19.0	20.0	23.5	24.0
5–7 years	18.0	20.0	23.0	23.5	17.0	19.0	21.0	23.0

Acetabular Index (AC Angle of Hilgenreiner)

The acetabular index is the angle formed by the Hilgenreiner line (see above) and a line tangent to the acetabular roof (**Fig. 2.21**). The tangent appears as a straight line passing through the inferior edge of the ilium and the lateral rim of the acetabulum. The acetabular index is age-dependent. Normal values can be derived from percentile curves or tables (**Tables 2.5** and **2.6**).

Acetabular index

The values are classified as follows:

- *Normal finding:* Angle < (mean value + SD)
- *Mild dysplasia:* (Mean value + SD) ≤ angle < (mean value + 2 SD)
- *Severe dysplasia:* Angle ≥ (mean value + 2 SD)

(SD = one standard deviation from the normal population of equal age and gender)

Table 2.7 Classification of acetabular index values (Commission for the Study of DDH, German Society for Orthopedics and Traumatology; source: Tönnis 1984)

Age	Normal mean value	Grade 1 (normal)	Grade 2 (slightly abnormal)	Grade 3 (severely abnormal)	Grade 4 (extremely abnormal)
3–4 months	25	< 30	≥ 30 to < 35	≥ 35 to < 40	≥ 40
5–24 months	20	< 25	≥ 25 to < 30	≥ 30 to < 35	≥ 35
2–3 years	18	< 23	≥ 23 to < 28	≥ 28 to < 33	≥ 33
3–7 years	15	< 20	≥ 20 to < 25	≥ 25 to < 30	≥ 30
7–14 years	10	< 15	≥ 15 to < 20	≥ 20 to < 25	≥ 25

Values within one standard deviation are classified as definitely normal. Angles between one and two standard deviations are classified as mildly dysplastic and require follow-up. Values in this range may improve spontaneously (in ~ 40% of cases) or may worsen over time (in ~ 20% of cases). Values outside two standard deviations are definitely abnormal.

The Commission for the Study of DDH of the German Society for Orthopedics and Traumatology published grades of deviation for the acetabular index shown in **Table 2.7**.

Tönnis D, Brunken D. Differentiation of normal and pathological acetabular roof angle in the diagnosis of hip dysplasia. Evaluation of 2294 acetabular roof angles of hip joints in children. [Article in German] Arch Orthop Trauma Surg 1968;64(3):197–228

Tönnis D. Die angeborene Hüftdysplasie und Hüftluxation im Kindes- und Erwachsenenalter. Chapter 9: Allgemeine Röntgendiagnostik des Hüftgelenks. Berlin: Springer; 1984; 129–134

Grade of dislocation	Findings	
1	Normal findings. The capital femoral ossification center is medial to the Perkins–Ombrédanne line	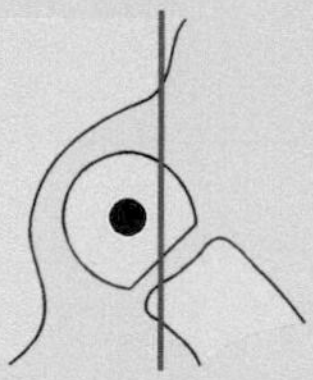
2	Dislocation. The capital femoral ossification center is lateral to the Perkins–Ombrédanne line and below the superior acetabular rim (lower outer quadrant)	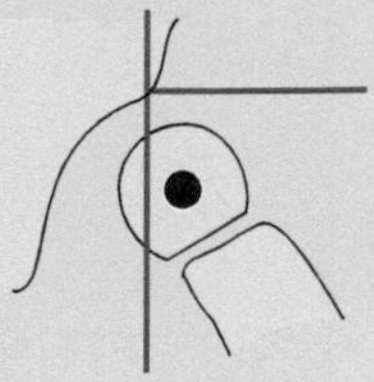
3	Dislocation. The capital femoral ossification center is lateral to the Perkins–Ombrédanne line and is at the level of the superior acetabular rim	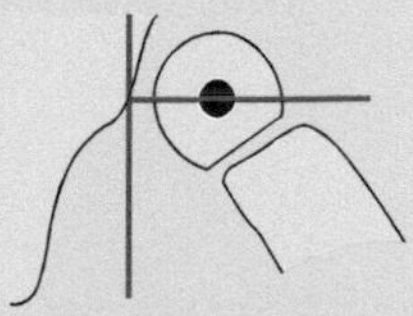
4	Complete high dislocation. The capital femoral ossification center is lateral to the Perkins–Ombrédanne line and above the superior acetabular rim	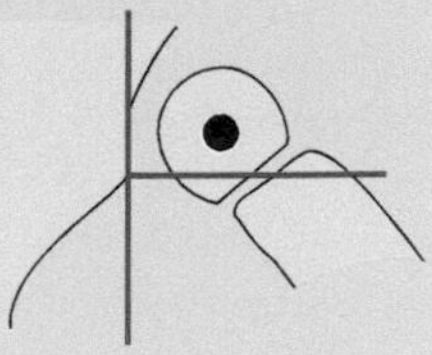

Fig. 2.22 Grades of hip dislocation according to Tönnis.

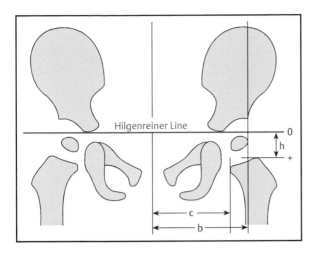

Fig. 2.23 Smith migration index. Reference lines for this index are the Hilgenreiner line, the Perkins–Ombrédanne line, and the vertical midline through the sacrum and pubic symphysis.
Lateral displacement   = c/b
Superior displacement   = h/b

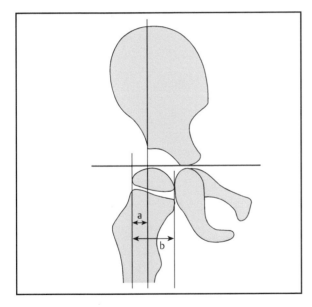

Fig. 2.24 Reimers migration index. A ruler placed across the lines bordering the femoral head can give a direct readout of the percentage of the head not covered by the acetabulum. The index is defined as I = a/b × 100% (a = distance from lateral border of femoral head to Perkins–Ombrédanne line, b = width of femoral head parallel to Hilgenreiner line).

Grades of Hip Dislocation According to Tönnis

The Hilgenreiner line and Perkins–Ombrédanne line divide the hip joint into four quadrants. The four grades of hip dislocation are based on the position of the femoral head ossification center in relation to the four quadrants (**Fig. 2.22**).

Tönnis D, et al. Hüftluxation und Hüftkopfnekrose. Eine Sammelstatistik des Arbeitskreises für Hüftdysplasie. Bücherei des Orthopäden, Vol. 21. Stuttgart: Enke, 1978

Smith Migration Index

The Smith index (**Fig. 2.23**) quantifies the lateral and superior displacement of the proximal femur. Reference lines are the pelvic midline passing through the center of the sacrum and pubic symphysis, the Perkins–Ombrédanne line, and a horizontal line through the center of both triradiate cartilages. The distance from the midline to the medial femoral spike is designated as c, the distance to the Perkins line as b. The distance from the Hilgenreiner line to the superolateral femoral border is designated as h.

Smith migration index	
• *Normal values:*	
• Lateral displacement:	b/c = 0.6–0.9
• Superior displacement:	h/b = 0.1–0.2
• *Abnormal values suggesting hip dislocation:*	
• Lateral displacement:	b/c > 0.9
• Superior displacement:	h/b = 0 to –0.7

Smith WS, Badgley CE, Orwig JB, Harper JM. Correlation of post-reduction roentgenograms and thirty-one-year follow-up in congenital dislocation of the hip. J Bone Joint Surg Am 1968;50(6):1081–1098

Reimer Migration Index

This index expresses how deeply the femoral head is seated in the acetabulum (**Fig. 2.24**). It is found by calculating the ratio of the distance of the lateral femoral head margin from the Perkins–Ombrédanne line (a) to the width of the femoral head parallel to the Hilgenreiner line (b):

Percentage of femoral head uncovered by the acetabular roof is

a/b • 100%

Reimer migration index	
• *Normal values:*	
• Age 0–14 years:	0%
• Age 4–16 years:	< 10%
• *In subluxation:*	33–99%
• *In dislocation:*	100%

Hip

2

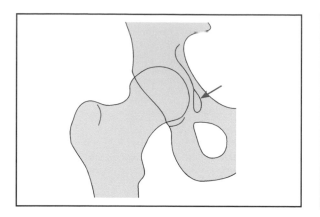

Fig. 2.25 Acetabular teardrop. Schematic drawing (arrow).

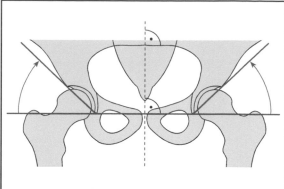

Fig. 2.26 Acetabular angle of Sharp. This angle describes the inclination of the acetabular roof relative to the horizontal plane.

The advantage of the Reimer migration index is that it is relatively insensitive to rotational deformities of the pelvis and leg.

> ! The Reimer index indicates the percentage of femoral head left uncovered by the acetabular roof. By placing a ruler obliquely across the lines bordering the femoral head so that one line is at 0 cm and the other is at 10 cm, you can read the percentage coverage deficit at the point where the ruler intersects the Perkins–Ombrédanne line.

Reimers J. The stability of the hip in children. A radiological study of the results of muscle surgery in cerebral palsy. Acta Orthop Scand Suppl 1980;184(Suppl.):1–100

Acetabular Teardrop

Distortion or nondelineation of the acetabular teardrop figure (**Fig. 2.25**) may signify hip instability or an abnormal position of the femoral head.

The medial portion of the teardrop is formed by the cortex of the medial pelvic wall at the level of the posterior acetabular rim. Its lateral portion is formed by the acetabular fossa. It develops in response to functional stimuli during the 4th to 6th months of life. The teardrop figure will not develop unless the femoral head is fully contained within the acetabulum. With subluxation of the femoral head, the teardrop assumes a widened, v-shaped appearance at its tip instead of a narrow, rounded shape.

Acetabular Angle of Sharp

This angle is formed by a horizontal line through the lowest point of both acetabular teardrops and a straight line through the superior acetabular rim and the lowest point of the teardrop (**Fig. 2.26**).

> **Acetabular angle of Sharp**
> - *Normal values:*
>   - Age 1–10 years: ≤ 45°
>   - Age > 10 years and adults: ≤ 40°
> - *Dysplasia:*
>   - Age 1–10 years: > 45°
>   - Age > 10 years and adults: > 40°

The classification system shown in **Table 2.8** was developed by the Commission for the Study of DDH of the German Society for Orthopedics and Traumatology. The acetabular angle of Sharp can still be measured after the cessation of skeletal growth (ossification of the triradiate cartilage).

Table 2.8 Normal values and grades of deviation of the Sharp acetabular angles (Commission for the Study of DDH, German Society for Orthopedics and Traumatology; source: Tönnis 1984)

Age (years)	Normal mean value	Grade 1 (normal)	Grade 2 (slightly abnormal)	Grade 3 (severely abnormal)	Grade 4 (extremely abnormal)
1–11	46	≤ 49	50–52	53–55	≥ 56
11–13	44	≤ 47	48–51	52–54	≥ 55
13–14	42	≤ 45	46–49	50–52	≥ 53
14 or over	40	≤ 43	44–46	47–49	≥ 50

Hip

2

Table 2.9 Classification of center-edge angles (Commission for the Study of DDH, German Society for Orthopedics and Traumatology; source: Tönnis 1984)

Age (years)	Normal mean value	Grade 1 (normal)	Grade 2 (slightly abnormal)	Grade 3 (severely abnormal)	Grade 4 (extremely abnormal)
≥ 0 to ≤ 8	25	≥ 20	≥ 15 to < 20	≥ 0 to < 15	< 0
≥ 8 to ≤ 18	32	≥ 25	≥ 20 to < 25	≥ 5 to < 20	< 5
≥ 18 to 50	35	≥ 30	≥ 20 to < 30	≥ 5 to < 20	< 5

Sharp IK. Acetabular dysplasia. The acetabular angle. J Bone Joint Surg Br 1961;43:268–272

Tönnis D. Die angeborene Hüftdysplasie und Hüftluxation im Kindes- und Erwachsenenalter. Chapter 9: Allgemeine Röntgendiagnostik des Hüftgelenks. Berlin: Springer; 1984; 129–134

Radiographic Evaluation after 4 Years of Age

Center-edge (CE) Angle of Wiberg (Lateral Coverage)

The CE angle is calculated on the AP pelvic radiograph (**Fig. 2.27**). It is measured between a line parallel to the longitudinal body-axis and a line connecting the center (C) of the femoral head to the outer edge (E) of the superior acetabular rim.

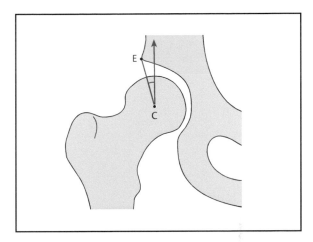

Fig. 2.27 CE angle of Wiberg.
C = Center of the femoral head
E = Edge of the superior acetabular rim

CE angle of Wiberg	
• *Mean values:*	
• Age 5–8 years:	~ 25°
• Age 9–12 years:	~ 30°
• Age > 12 years:	~ 35°
• *Normal values:*	
• Age 5–8 years:	> 20°
• Age ≥ 9 years:	> 25°

Normal value studies have been performed in various populations. The Commission for the Study of DDH of the German Society for Orthopedics and Traumatology compiled the normal values and grades of deviation shown in **Table 2.9**. The CE angle describes the position of the femoral head in relation to the acetabulum. The deeper the acetabulum, the greater the CE angle. As the acetabulum becomes flatter and steeper (dysplastic), the CE angle decreases.

> **!** The CE angle is of key importance in evaluating hip dysplasia and is considered the principal angle for evaluating residual hip dysplasia in children and adults.

Tönnis D. Die angeborene Hüftdysplasie und Hüftluxation im Kindes- und Erwachsenenalter. Chapter 9: Allgemeine Röntgendiagnostik des Hüftgelenks. Berlin: Springer; 1984; 129–134

Wiberg G. Studies on dysplastic acetabula and congenital subluxation of the hip joint: with special reference to the complication of osteoarthritis. Acta Chir Scand 1939;58(Suppl.):7–38

VCA Angle of Lequesne and De Sèze

The VCA angle, which reflects the anterior coverage of the femoral head, is measured in the false profile view (**Fig. 2.28**). This radiograph is taken in the standing position with the pelvis rotated 65° relative to the cassette. The foot is parallel to the film cassette, and weight is borne on the affected leg. The central beam is directed to the femoral head (**Fig. 2.29**). The VCA angle is formed by a vertical line (V, parallel to the longitudinal body-axis) drawn through the center of the femoral head and an oblique line drawn from the femoral head center to the anterior rim of the acetabulum (A; see **Fig. 2.28**).

Hip

2

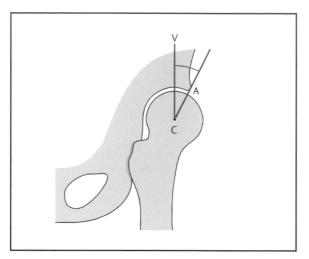

Fig. 2.28 VCA angle of Lequesne and De Sèze.
V = Vertical line through femoral head center (parallel to longitudinal body axis)
C = Center of the femoral head
A = Anterior border of the acetabulum

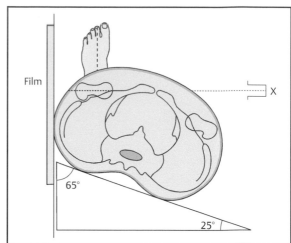

Fig. 2.29 Positioning technique for the false profile view.

VCA angle in adults	
• *Normal values:*	*> 25°*
• *Slightly abnormal:*	*20° ≤ VCA angle ≤ 25°*
• *Severely abnormal:*	*< 20°*

The VCA angle is used to evaluate the anterior coverage of the femoral head by the acetabulum. It can detect deficient anterior coverage, which is usually less pronounced than the lateral component of hip dysplasia, as well as very rare instances of isolated anterior dysplasia. In measuring the angle, it may be difficult to identify point A owing to the difficulty of locating the most anterior point of the acetabular roof.

Lequesne M; de Sèze S. False profile of the pelvis. A new radiographic incidence for the study of the hip. Its use in dysplasias and different coxopathies. [Article in French] Rev Rhum Mal Osteoartic 1961;28:643–652

ACM Angle of Idelberger and Frank

The ACM angle is calculated on the AP pelvic radiograph. Several points are identified in constructing this angle (**Fig. 2.30**).

ACM angle	
• *Mean value in adults (according to Busse):*	*45° ± 3°*
• *Abnormal by approximately age 4:*	*> 50°*

The Commission for the Study of DDH of the German Society for Orthopedics and Traumatology published the normal values and grades of deviation for the ACM angle shown in **Table 2.10**.

The ACM angle reflects the depth of the acetabulum. Large angles denote a very shallow acetabulum (dysplasia), while small angles mean that the acetabulum has a spherical or hemispherical shape. One advantage of the ACM angle is that it is relatively independent of pelvic tilt and rotation. One disadvantage is that it gives no information on the inclination of the acetabulum relative to the horizontal plane.

Idelberger K, Frank A. A new method for determination of the angle of the pelvic acetabulum in child and in adult. [Article in German] Z Orthop Ihre Grenzgeb 1952;82(4):571–577

Tönnis D. Die angeborene Hüftdysplasie und Hüftluxation im Kindes- und Erwachsenenalter. Chapter 9: Allgemeine Röntgendiagnostik des Hüftgelenks. Berlin: Springer; 1984; 129–134

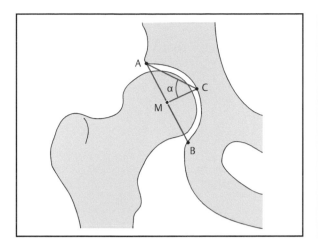

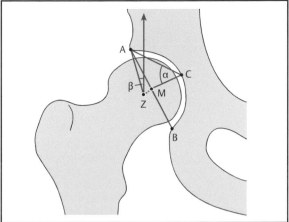

Fig. 2.30 ACM Angle of Idelberger and Frank.
A = Superior rim of the acetabulum
B = Inferior rim of the acetabulum
M = Midpoint of connecting line AB
C = Point on the acetabulum intersected by a line perpendicular to AB and through M
α = ACM angle (formed by AC and CM)

Fig. 2.31 Measurements for calculating the summarized hip factor.
A = Superior rim of the acetabulum
B = Inferior rim of the acetabulum
M = Midpoint of connecting line AB
C = Point on the acetabulum intersected by a line perpendicular to AB
Z = Center of the femoral head
MZ = Off-center distance (in mm)
α = ACM angle (formed by AC and CM)
β = CE angle

Table 2.10 Classification of ACM angles (Commission for the Study of DDH, German Society for Orthopedics and Traumatology; source: Tönnis 1984)

Age (years)	Normal mean value	Grade 1 (normal)	Grade 2 (slightly abnormal)	Grade 3 (severely abnormal)	Grade 4 (extremely abnormal)
> 2	45	< 50	≥ 50 to < 55	≥ 55 to < 60	≥ 60

Summarized Hip Factor

The summarized hip factor (SHF, **Fig. 2.31**) is a combination of several values used to make a more accurate prognosis of hip dysplasia. The SHF is calculated on the AP pelvic radiograph. Points A, B, C, M and Z are defined as in the measurement of the ACM angle (see **Fig. 2.30**).

The following formula is used to calculate the SHF:

SHF = A + B + C + 10

where

$$A = \frac{\sqrt{3} \cdot \left(ACM - \text{mean value of ACM} \right)}{\text{standard deviation of ACM}}$$

$$B = \frac{\sqrt{3} \cdot \left(\left[\text{mean value of CE} \right] - CE \right)}{\text{standard deviation of CE}}$$

$$C = \frac{\sqrt{3} \cdot \left(MZ - \text{mean value of MZ} \right)}{\text{standard deviation of MZ}}$$

and ACM = ACM angle, CE = CE angle, MZ = off-center distance (mm).

The mean values and standard deviations in **Table 2.11** can be used to calculate the SHF from the above formula (using computer software or a pocket calculator).

For routine clinical work, the SHF can be quickly determined from age-adjusted nomograms (see Appendix to this Chapter, pp. 48 and 49). First calculate the ACM and CE angles and mark them on the two scales on the left side of the nomogram. Draw a connecting line between those points and extend it across the center scale. Next draw a second line connecting that point on the center scale to the off-center distance MZ marked on the fourth scale. The point where that line crosses the right-hand scale will indicate the summarized hip factor.

Table 2.11 Mean values and standard deviations for calculating the summarized hip factor (source: Tönnis 1984)

Age (years)	Measurements	Number	Mean value ± standard deviation	Normal range
5 through 8	ACM angle	326	45.9° ± 2.7°	<49°
	CE angle	326	24.7° ± 6.3°	>20°
	MZ distance	326	3.2 mm ± 1.7 mm	<5 mm
9 through 12	ACM angle	326	45.0° ± 2.4°	<46°
	CE angle	326	31.3° ± 5.0°	>26°
	MZ distance	326	2.9 mm ± 1.5 mm	<4 mm
13 through 16	ACM angle	254	45.6° ± 2.8°	<47°
	CE angle	254	34.3° ± 5.7°	>30°
	MZ distance	254	3.1 mm ± 1.5 mm	<5 mm
17 through 20	ACM angle	204	44.6° ± 3.0°	<47°
	CE angle	204	35.1° ± 5.4°	>30°
	MZ distance	204	3.6 mm ± 1.5 mm	<6 mm
21 through 50	ACM angle	358	45.0° ± 3.2°	<49°
	CE angle	358	35.7° ± 6.5°	>30°
	MZ distance	358	3.9 mm ± 1.7 mm	<6 mm

ACM = Angle of Idelberger and Frank
CE = Center-edge
MZ = Off-center distance

Table 2.12 Classification of the summarized hip factor (Commission for the Study of DDH, German Society for Orthopedics and Traumatology; source: Tönnis 1984)

Age (years)	Normal mean value	Grade 1 (normal)	Grade 2 (slightly abnormal)	Grade 3 (severely abnormal)	Grade 4 (extremely abnormal)
≥ 5 to ≤ 18	10	≥ 6 to < 15	≥ 15 to < 20	≥ 20 to < 30	≥ 30
Adults	10	≥ 6 to < 16	≥ 16 to < 21	≥ 21 to < 31	≥ 31

Summarized hip factor

- *Mean values:*
  - Children ≥ 5 to ≤ 18 years: 10
  - Adults: 10
- *Normal values:*
  - Children ≥ 5 to ≤ 18 years: 6 ≤ SHF < 15
  - Adults: 6 ≤ SHF < 16

! Calculation of the SHF is relatively complex, so it is not routinely included in the follow-up of known DDH. The advantage of the SHF is that "false-positives" for preosteoarthritic deformity are much less common than when the CE angle, for example, is calculated alone.

Table 2.12 lists the ranges of values for grading the SHF based on data from the Commission for the Study of DDH.

The SHF takes into account several aspects that are important for age-appropriate development of the joint. The ACM angle reflects the depth of the acetabulum, while the CE angle indicates coverage. The off-center distance MZ measures how far the center point of the femoral head has decentered from the acetabulum.

Tönnis D. Die angeborene Hüftdysplasie und Hüftluxation im Kindes- und Erwachsenenalter. Chapter 9: Allgemeine Röntgendiagnostik des Hüftgelenks. Berlin: Springer; 1984; 129–134

Tönnis D. Normal values of the hip joint for the evaluation of X-rays in children and adults. Clin Orthop Relat Res 1976;119(119):39–47

Radiographic Measurements after Skeletal Maturity (Residual Hip Dysplasia)

The CE angle of Wiberg (lateral coverage; see **Fig. 2.27**) and the VCA angle of Lequesne and De Sèze (see **Fig. 2.28**) are useful parameters in patients who have reached skeletal maturity. The acetabular angle of Sharp (**Fig. 2.26**) also plays a key role. Other important values are described below.

Horizontal Toit Externe (HTE) Angle (Acetabular Index of the Weight-Bearing Zone)

The HTE angle (**Fig. 2.32**) is measured on the AP pelvic radiograph. It reflects the slope of the sclerotic zone of the acetabular roof (weight-bearing surface) relative to the horizontal plane. A line is drawn tangent to the acetabular roof, passing through the most lateral and inferior points of the sclerotic zone. Then a horizontal line is drawn through the lowest point of both sclerotic zones. The angle formed by the two lines is the HTE angle.

HTE angle
• *Normal value in adolescents and adults: – 10° to + 10°*
• *Tschauner classification of the HTE angle:*

• Grade 1 (normal):	< 9°
• Grade 2 (slightly abnormal):	10–15°
• Grade 3 (severely abnormal):	16–25°
• Grade 4 (extremely abnormal):	> 25°

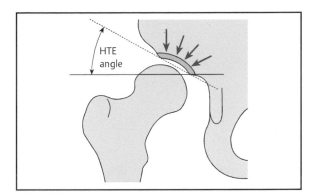

Fig. 2.32 Horizontal toit externe angle of the acetabular weight-bearing zone.

> **!** The acetabular index can no longer be determined after the triradiate cartilage has closed, but the sclerotic weight-bearing zone of the acetabular roof can still be seen on conventional radiographs. Its slope is of great functional importance because only a near-horizontal orientation of the weight-bearing surface will allow uniform pressure transfer across the joint.

CT Measurement of Acetabular Coverage

The degree of femoral head coverage by the acetabulum can be evaluated on transverse CT images using a technique established by Anda et al (**Fig. 2.33**). The measurement is performed on a transverse CT section acquired through the centers of both femoral heads. The center points (Z) are located with a circle template or a computer-assisted technique and interconnected by a straight line (g).

From the center of each femoral head, a line is drawn tangent to the anterior and posterior rims of the acetabulum. The angle formed by the tangent to the anterior acetabular rim and the line connecting the femoral head

Fig. 2.33 Quantification of femoral head coverage on transverse computed tomography sections.
Z = Center of the femoral head
A = Anterior rim of the acetabulum
P = Posterior rim of the acetabulum
g = Straight line through the femoral head centers
AASA = Anterior acetabular sector angle
PASA = Posterior acetabular sector angle
HASA = Horizontal acetabular sector angle

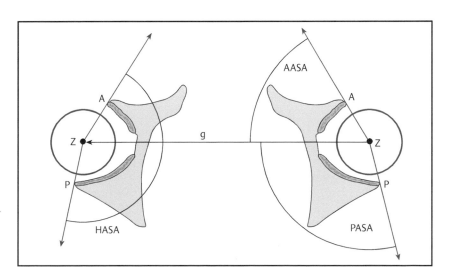

Hip

2

Table 2.13 Normal values for the anterior, posterior and horizontal acetabular sector angles

	Men	Women
AASA	64° ± 6°	63° ± 6°
PASA	102° ± 8°	105° ± 8°
HASA	167° ± 11°	169° ± 10°

AASA = Anterior acetabular sector angle
PASA = Posterior acetabular sector angle
HASA = Horizontal acetabular sector angle

centers (g) is called the anterior acetabular sector angle (AASA). Similarly, the tangent to the posterior acetabular rim forms the posterior acetabular sector angle (PASA). The AASA quantifies the anterior coverage of the femoral head, while the PASA quantifies its posterior coverage. The sum of both angles, called the horizontal acetabular sector angle (HASA), provides a parameter for assessing global acetabular coverage. Normal values for the AASA, PASA and HASA are shown in **Table 2.13**.

Anda S, Svenningsen S, Dale LG, Benum P. The acetabular sector angle of the adult hip determined by computed tomography. Acta Radiol Diagn (Stockh) 1986;27(4):443–447
Anda S, Terjesen T, Kvistad KA. Computed tomography measurements of the acetabulum in adult dysplastic hips: which level is appropriate? Skeletal Radiol 1991;20(4):267–271
Anda S, Terjesen T, Kvistad KA, Svenningsen S. Acetabular angles and femoral anteversion in dysplastic hips in adults: CT investigation. J Comput Assist Tomogr 1991;15(1):115–120

Perthes Disease

Perthes disease refers to aseptic (idiopathic) osteonecrosis of the femoral head in children. Its course differs markedly from osteonecrosis of the femoral head in adults owing to the high healing potential in the pediatric age group.

Stages of the Disease (Waldenström Stages)

Perthes disease passes through five consecutive stages, first described by H. Waldenström:

1. *Initial stage:* cessation of growth of the capital femoral epiphysis
2. *Condensation:* sclerosis of the epiphysis with initial subchondral fracture
3. *Fragmentation (resorption)*
4. *Reossification (repair)*
5. *Healing*

Catterall Classification

The extent of epiphyseal necrosis and metaphyseal involvement significantly affect the prognosis of Perthes disease. In 1971 Catterall introduced a radiographic classification that quantifies the extent of epiphyseal necrosis and assigns patients to prognostic groups (**Fig. 2.34**). The Catterall classification is based on conventional radiographs: the AP view and the frog lateral view (Lauenstein view). Patients in groups 1 and 2 have a good prognosis without treatment (> 90% of cases), but the prognosis for untreated patients in groups 3 and 4 is poor (> 90% of cases).

> **!** Besides the Catterall classification, the Herring and Salter–Thompson classification systems also quantify the extent of epiphyseal involvement and supply a corresponding prognosis. The Catterall classification is the most widely used, however. It is generally agreed that hips in Catterall groups 3 and 4, Salter–Thompson group B, or Herring group C have an unfavorable prognosis and therefore require treatment.

Catterall A. The natural history of Perthes' disease. J Bone Joint Surg Br 1971;53(1):37–53

"Head at Risk" Signs

Catterall described several radiographic signs of a "head at risk" for epiphyseal collapse that are separate from the Catterall classification. These criteria are particularly useful for identifying cases that, though assigned to group 2, would still have an unfavorable prognosis:

- *Lateral subluxation of the femoral head:* Decentering of the head leads to deficient anterolateral coverage and early deformity of the femoral head.
- *Gage sign:* The detection of a small, V-shaped osteolytic segment on the lateral side of the epiphysis.
- *Calcification lateral to the epiphysis:* Calcifications in the laterally displaced, cartilaginous portions of the epiphysis. Displacement of the epiphysis leads to eccentric growth of the femoral head.
- *Horizontal orientation of the growth plate:* Catterall interpreted a transversely oriented growth plate as an early sign of subluxation. More recent studies ascribe less importance to this finding, and some authors interpret it merely as a transient reorientation of the growth plate.
- *Metaphyseal involvement:* Pronounced metaphyseal changes may lead to premature closure of the growth plate, resulting in deformity of the proximal femur.

Group	Radiographic appearance
1	• Only a circumscribed anterior portion of the epiphysis is involved (frog lateral view) • No fracture or collapse • No sequestrum • Metaphyseal changes are unusual • (Regeneration from the periphery)
2	• Larger portions of the anterior epiphysis are involved • Fracture with formation of a sequestrum (sclerotic fragment) • Intact bone medial and lateral to the sequestrum (maintaining epiphyseal height) in the AP view
3	• Large portions of the epiphysis are necrotic, with only small peripheral areas of residual uninvolved bone • Only a small, posterior portion of the head is uninvolved in the lateral view • Pronounced metaphyseal changes are usually seen
4	• The whole epiphysis is involved • Early collapse of the epiphysis • Collapsed epiphysis appears as a dense line in the AP view • Extensive metaphyseal changes

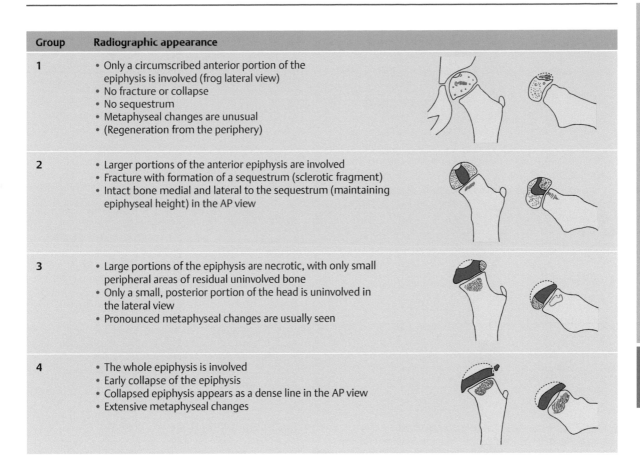

Fig. 2.34 Catterall classification of Perthes disease.

> ! Of the risk factors listed above, the following have the greatest prognostic significance: lateral subluxation of the femoral head, calcification lateral to the epiphysis, and metaphyseal involvement. Lateral subluxation is as important a prognostic factor as the extent of osteonecrosis. Gage sign and a transversely oriented growth plate are considered less relevant.

Catterall A. The natural history of Perthes' disease. J Bone Joint Surg Br 1971;53(1):37–53

Salter–Thompson Classification

The Salter–Thompson classification, like the Catterall classification, evaluates the degree of epiphyseal involvement. It assesses the extent of the subchondral fracture, which occurs relatively early in the course of the disease (during the condensation stage) and precedes the reossification stage. The subchondral fracture appears on conventional radiographs as a radiolucent line in the femoral head ("crescent sign").

The classification is based on conventional radiographs (**Table 2.14**) using the AP and frog lateral views. Group B is considered to have an unfavorable prognosis.

> ! The Salter–Thompson classification is limited by the fact that the subchondral fracture is not radiographically visible in a significant percentage of patients.

Salter RB, Thompson GH. Legg-Calvé-Perthes disease. The prognostic significance of the subchondral fracture and a two-group classification of the femoral head involvement. J Bone Joint Surg Am 1984;66(4):479–489

Table 2.14 Salter–Thompson classification of Perthes disease

Group	Radiographic criteria
A	Fracture involves less than half of the femoral head
B	Fracture involves more than half of the femoral head

Hip

2

Lateral Pillar Classification of Herring

Like Catterall and Salter–Thompson, Herring proposed a classification that would provide a long-term prognosis for Perthes disease (**Table 2.15**). The Herring classification evaluates only the involvement of the "lateral pillar" of the femoral head in semiquantitative terms. The underlying concept is that significant deformity and decentering of the femoral head will not occur as long as the lateral pillar remains intact.

The classification is based on conventional AP radiographs of the hip, on which the femoral head is divided into a lateral, central and medial pillar (**Fig. 2.35**). The prognosis is considered favorable for group A, indeterminate for group B, and unfavorable for group C.

Herring JA, Neustadt JB, Williams JJ, Early JS, Browne RH. The lateral pillar classification of Legg-Calvé-Perthes disease. J Pediatr Orthop 1992;12(2):143–150

Slipped Capital Femoral Epiphysis

Early Signs on the Anteroposterior Radiograph

The following are considered early signs of slipped capital femoral epiphysis (SCFE) on the AP radiograph of the hip (**Fig. 2.36**):

- *Loss of Capener sign:* In an AP projection of the hip in normal adolescents, a triangular area of decreased radiolucency can be seen on the medial side of the femoral neck. Caused by superimposed shadows from the posterior acetabular wall and medial side of the femoral neck, this sign usually disappears at an early stage in patients with SCFE.
- *Growth plate widened and ill-defined.*

Table 2.15 Lateral pillar classification (Herring classification) of Perthes disease

Group	Radiographic criteria
A	No involvement of the lateral pillar
B	> 50% of lateral pillar height maintained
C	< 50% of lateral pillar height maintained

- *Klein line:* A line tangent to the lateral cortex of the femoral neck no longer intersects the epiphysis.
- *Relative loss of epiphyseal height.*

Greenspan A. Orthopedic Imaging: A Practical Approach. 4th ed. Philadelphia: Lippincott Williams and Wilkins 2004

Klein A, Joplin RJ, Reidy JA, Hanelin J. Roentgenographic features of slipped capital femoral epiphysis. Am J Roentgenol Radium Ther 1951;66(3):361–374

Gekeler J. Radiology of adolescent slipped capital femoral epiphysis: measurement of epiphyseal angles and diagnosis. Oper Orthop Traumatol 2007;19(4):329–344

Epiphyseal Slip Angles

■ Southwick Method

The Southwick method is widely used in English-speaking countries for calculating epiphyseal slip angles, while the Gekeler method is used in German-speaking countries.

Measurements for determining the Southwick angles are performed on radiographs of the hip in two planes. The first radiograph is an AP pelvic view with the beam centered midway between both hip joints. The second is a frog lateral view obtained by positioning the hips in maximum external rotation and abduction and flexing the knees so that the soles of the feet are touching and the lateral sides of the feet are on the table surface.

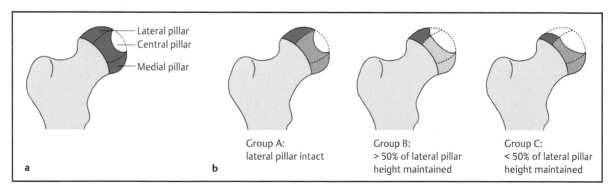

Fig. 2.35a,b Lateral pillar classification of Herring.

a The femoral head is divided into a lateral, central, and medial pillar.

b Groups A–C in the lateral pillar classification.

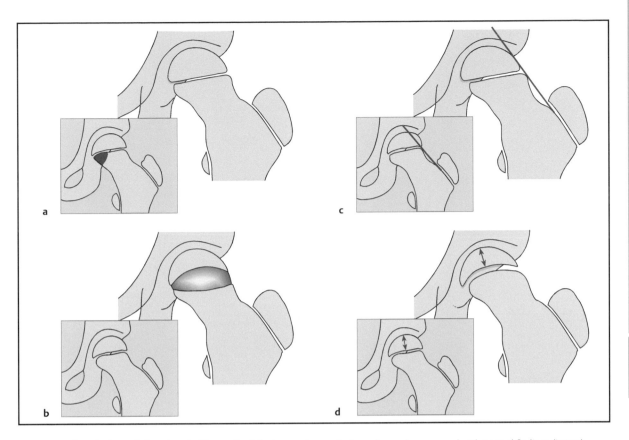

Fig. 2.36a–d Early signs of slipped capital femoral epiphysis on anteroposterior radiograph, compared with normal findings (insets).

a Loss of Capener sign.
b Growth plate is widened and ill-defined.

c Klein tangent no longer intersects the epiphysis.
d Relative loss of epiphyseal height.

The radiographs are interpreted exactly as in the Gekeler method (see below). The angles between the femoral shaft axis and a line perpendicular to the base of the epiphysis are measured in both views (**Fig. 2.38**).

> ! The advantage of the Gekeler method (below) is that the standard positioning technique and conversion table permit a more accurate conversion of the projected slip angles into true slip angles. In everyday practice, the conversion to true slip angles is relevant only in cases with a relatively large degree of slippage.

Southwick WO. Osteotomy through the lesser trochanter for slipped capital femoral epiphysis. J Bone Joint Surg Am 1967;49(5):807–835

Tins BJ, Cassar-Pullicino VN. Slipped upper femoral epiphysis. In: Imaging of the Hip and Bony Pelvis. 1st ed. Berlin Heidelberg: Springer; 2006: 173–194

■ Gekeler Method

The Gekeler method employs two standard, mutually perpendicular radiographic views to accurately evaluate the position of the slipped epiphysis. As projection errors cannot be avoided, even with a standard positioning technique, a conversion table is used to convert the measured projected slip angles into the true slip angles.

The standard views for determining the slip angles are an AP radiograph of the proximal femur and the Imhäuser flexion–abduction view (**Fig. 2.37**). The leg should be positioned in neutral rotation for the AP view. This is most easily confirmed by noting the position of the patella, which should point forward. The pelvis should be elevated to correct for any external rotation contracture at the hip joint. The second radiograph is taken in 90° of hip flexion and 45° of abduction (Imhäuser view). The lower leg should be in neutral rotation and parallel to the longitudinal axis of the table.

- *ED angle* (**Fig. 2.38**): The projected epiphyseal–diaphyseal (ED) angle is measured on the AP view. First the epiphysis baseline is defined by drawing a connecting line between the corners of the epiphysis. By definition, the line perpendicular to the epiphyseal baseline represents the epiphyseal axis. The ED angle is measured between the femoral shaft axis and epiphyseal axis.

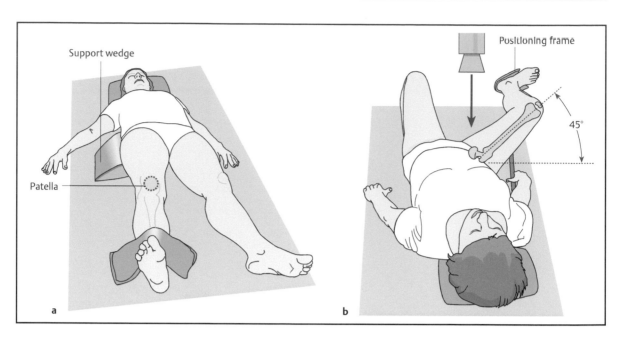

Fig. 2.37 Standard projections for measuring the angle of a slipped capital femoral epiphysis by the Gekeler method.
a Anteroposterior view of the proximal femur.
b Imhäuser view (hip is flexed 90° and abducted 45°).

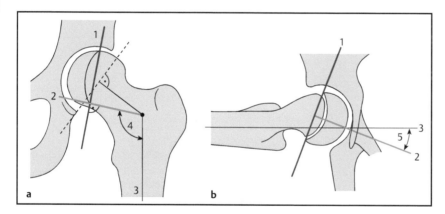

Fig. 2.38a,b Gekeler method for determining the epiphyseal slip angle.
1 = Epiphyseal baseline
2 = Epiphyseal axis (perpendicular to the baseline)
3 = Femoral shaft axis
4 = ED angle
5 = ET angle
a ED angle.
b ET angle.

● *ET angle* (**Fig. 2.38**): The projected epiphyseal torsion (ET) angle is measured on the flexion–abduction view. First the epiphyseal baseline is drawn through the corners of the epiphysis. The ET angle is formed by a line perpendicular to the epiphyseal baseline (= epiphyseal axis) and the femoral shaft axis.

Table 2.16 shows an excerpt from a conversion table published by Gekeler in 1977. The table, based on trigonometric calculations, can be used for the direct determination of true dislocation angles.

The discrepancies between the projected and true slip angles may be particularly great in patients with higher degrees of slippage in the usual posteroinferior direction. In patients with mild to moderate slips, the projection error is relatively small and generally is not clinically significant.

> **!**
> Until a few years ago, an ET angle of 30° was considered the critical cutoff point for the development of preosteoarthritic deformity of the proximal femur, and corrective surgery was generally withheld until that critical point was reached. Today, however, recent discoveries on femoroacetabular impingement have prompted many authors to recommend more rigorous tolerance limits and expand the indications for surgical intervention.

Table 2.16 Table for converting projected ED and ET angles into true ED and ET angles for the most common posteroinferior slip (after Gekeler)

Projected angles		True angles	
ED' (°) (antero-posterior view)	ET' (°) (flexion–abduction view, 90°/45°)	ED (°) (antero-posterior view)	ET (°) (flexion-abduction view, 90°/45°)
150	– 90	90	– 90
150	– 70	108	– 79
150	– 50	125	– 67
150	– 30	139	– 48
150	– 10	149	– 19
140	– 90	90	– 90
140	– 70	105	– 77
140	– 50	120	– 62
140	– 30	132	– 42
140	– 10	139	– 15
130	– 90	90	– 90
130	– 70	103	– 74
130	– 50	114	– 57
130	– 30	124	– 37
130	– 10	129	– 13
120	– 90	90	– 90
120	– 70	100	– 72
120	– 50	109	– 53
120	– 30	116	– 33
120	– 10	120	– 11
110	– 90	90	– 90
110	– 70	97	– 69
110	– 50	103	– 49
110	– 30	108	– 29
110	– 10	110	– 10
100	– 90	90	– 90
100	– 70	94	– 66
100	– 50	97	– 45
100	– 30	99	– 26
100	– 10	100	– 8
90	– 90	90	– 90
90	– 70	90	– 63
90	– 50	90	– 40
90	– 30	90	– 22
90	– 10	90	– 7

ED = Epiphyseal–diaphyseal

ET = Epiphyseal torsion

Gekeler J. Die Hüftkopfepiphysenlösung. Radiometrie und Korrekturplanung. Bücherei des Orthopäden, Vol. 19. Stuttgart: Enke; 1977

Gekeler J. Radiology and measurement in adolescent slipped capital femoral epiphysis. [Article in German] Orthopade 2002;31(9):841–850

Gekeler J. Radiology of adolescent slipped capital femoral epiphysis: measurement of epiphyseal angles and diagnosis. Oper Orthop Traumatol 2007;19(4):329–344

Southwick WO. Osteotomy through the lesser trochanter for slipped capital femoral epiphysis. J Bone Joint Surg Am 1967;49(5):807–835

Tins BJ, Cassar-Pullicino VN. Slipped upper femoral epiphysis. In: Imaging of the Hip and Bony Pelvis. 1st ed. Berlin Heidelberg: Springer; 2006: 173–194

Osteonecrosis of the Femoral Head

Ficat and Arlet Classification

The Ficat and Arlet classification is one of the oldest classifications of femoral head osteonecrosis, and today it is still the most widely used. The original Ficat and Arlet classification, which recognized only two stages, has been revised twice, and the current classification published by Ficat in 1985 defines a total of five stages (**Table 2.17**). The system takes into account clinical presentation in addition to conventional radiographic findings.

> **!** It is recommended that a frog lateral view be obtained in addition to the AP radiograph.

In the original 1985 publication, the detection of a subchondral fracture line ("crescent sign") and incipient segmental flattening of the femoral head were believed to mark the transition from stage 2 to stage 3 disease. But as the occurrence of a fracture (regardless of type or severity) is the most important prognostic factor, it is recommended that cases with a detectable fracture be classified as stage 3. The classification also appears in this form in many textbooks.

Ficat RP. Idiopathic bone necrosis of the femoral head. Early diagnosis and treatment. J Bone Joint Surg Br 1985;67(1):3–9

ARCO Classification of Osteonecrosis

The ARCO (Association Research Circulation Osseous) classification has become increasingly popular in Europe in recent years. Besides staging bony changes, the ARCO classification also takes into account the extent and location of necrosis based on various imaging modalities

Table 2.17 Ficat and Arlet classification of osteonecrosis of the femoral head

Stage	Radiographic findings	Clinical presentation
0	Normal	Asymptomatic
1	Normal	Symptomatic
2	• Sclerotic areas (linear, diffuse or localized) in the femoral head • Osteolytic or "cystoid" changes (usually more difficult to define) • Femoral head has normal shape and margins (!); no joint-space narrowing	Symptomatic
3	• Collapse and flattening of the femoral head with complete loss of bone structure • Large cyst-like lucencies, diffuse sclerotic changes	Symptomatic
4	Secondary osteoarthritic changes	Symptomatic

Imaging modalities, subclassifications	Stage 0	Stage 1	Stage 2	Stage 3	Stage 4
Imaging					
X-rays	Normal	Normal	Sclerosis and osteolysis in necrotic segment; sclerotic margin	(Subchondral) fracture; flattening of femoral dome	Osteoarthritis
MRI	Normal	Demarcated necrotic segment	Necrosis with reactive margin; "double-line" sign	(Subchondral) fracture	Osteoarthritis
CT	Normal	Normal	Sclerosis and osteolysis in necrotic segment; sclerotic margin; "asterisk" sign	(Subchondral) fracture; deterioration of spherical head shape	Osteoarthritis
Scintigraphy	Normal	Diffuse or cold spot	"Cold in hot" pattern	"Hot in hot" pattern	Hot spot
Subclassifications					
Location of necrosis	None	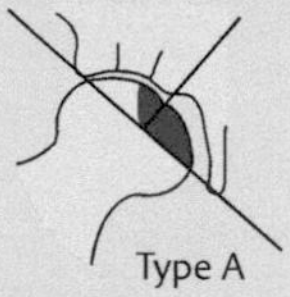 Type A	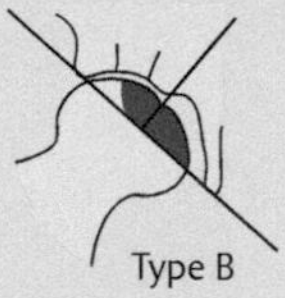 Type B	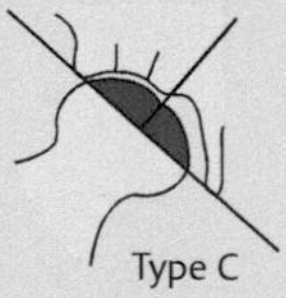 Type C	None
Quantitation of necrosis	None	Percentage area of femoral head involvement: • A < 15% • B 15–30% • C > 30%		Length of subchondral fracture: • A < 15% • B 15–30% • C > 30% Dome depression • A < 2 mm • B 2–4 mm • C > 4 mm	None

Fig. 2.39 Association Research Circulation Osseous stages of osteonecrosis.

Hip

2

(radiography, CT, magnetic resonance imaging [MRI], and scintigraphy; **Fig. 2.39**):

- *ARCO stage 0 (initial stage):* All imaging studies at this stage are negative. In theory, histology would show evidence of necrosis.
- *ARCO stage 1 (reversible early stage):* MRI and scintigraphy are already positive at this stage, whereas conventional radiographs and CT scans are still normal. Stage 1 is divided into three subcategories according to the location and extent of necrosis. The location is classified as medial (A), central (B), or lateral (C) and is designated by the corresponding letter. The extent of necrosis is quantified by estimating the percentage involvement of the femoral head, and this is indicated by a second letter: < 15% (A), 15–30% (B), and > 30% (C).
- *ARCO stage 2 (irreversible early stage):* This stage is characterized by an increasing demarcation of the necrotic area. A specific change is the "double line" sign on MRI which circumscribes the necrotic area (granulation tissue plus sclerotic bone bordering on healthy bone). The necrotic segment shows structural bone changes (sclerosis and osteolysis) on plain radiographs and CT. In time the healthy bone forms a sclerotic margin. This stage is subclassified using the same criteria as in stage 1.
- *ARCO stage 3 (transitional stage):* The hallmark of ARCO stage 3 is a radiographically visible fracture.

Most cases initially show a subchondral fracture, which forms a crescent-shaped lucency ("crescent sign") on radiographs and CT scans. This stage is marked by progressive flattening or distortion of the femoral dome, which will eventually collapse. There is still no evidence of joint-space narrowing or acetabular involvement. ARCO stage 3 is subclassified by the relative extent of the subchondral fracture line—< 15% (A), 15–30% (B), and > 30% (C)—or by the amount of flattening of the femoral dome: < 2 mm (A), 2–4 mm (B), and > 4 mm (C). As in stages 1 and 2, the location of the necrosis is classified as medial (A), central (B), or lateral (C).

- *ARCO stage 4 (late stage):* This stage is characterized by the development of secondary osteoarthritis. Joint-space narrowing is visible on radiographs, CT, and MRI. The classic signs of osteoarthritis are also visible on the acetabular side of the joint. Subclassification is no longer necessary in stage 4.

The main advantage of the ARCO classification is that it addresses and summarizes the factors that are relevant to therapeutic decision making.

> ! While all imaging modalities are listed in the ARCO classification, conventional radiographs will generally allow accurate staging and can be supplemented if needed by MRI. The main prognostic criterion is the detection of a fracture. Flattening of the femoral dome is a key preosteoarthritic change, and long-term preservation of the femoral head is rarely possible once flattening has occurred. Therefore, if a subchondral fracture cannot be excluded in stage 2, the femur should be investigated further by CT.

Subgroup C is unfavorable in any ARCO stage and will generally warrant advancing the treatment level to the next stage (**Table 2.18**).

Gardeniers JWM. Report of the committee of staging and nomenclature. ARCO News Letter 1993;5:79–82

Table 2.18 Treatment of osteonecrosis by stages

ARCO stage	Treatment
1	• Conservative • Decompression (group C)
2	• Decompression • Repositioning osteotomy • Bone grafting (group C)
3	• Bone grafting • Endoprosthesis • Endoprosthesis (group C)
4	• Endoprosthesis

Table 2.19 Marcus classification of osteonecrosis of the femoral head

Stage	Radiographic findings	Shape of femoral head	Grade of osteoarthritis
1	Mottled areas of increased density	Round	0
2	Sclerotic rim	Round	0
3	Subchondral radiolucency	Slightly flattened	0
4	Depression of lateral edge of infarct	Markedly flattened	0–1
5	Lateral and medial depression	Flattened and compressed	0–2
6	Secondary degenerative changes (signs of osteoarthritis)	Flattened and compressed	2–3

Marcus Classification of Osteonecrosis

The Marcus classification of avascular necrosis is less widely used than the first two classifications above but is included here for completeness. It is based on conventional radiographs in two planes (AP and frog lateral views; **Table 2.19**).

Marcus ND, Enneking WF, Massam RA. The silent hip in idiopathic aseptic necrosis. Treatment by bone-grafting. J Bone Joint Surg Am 1973;55(7):1351–1366

Femoroacetabular Impingement

Femoroacetabular impingement (FAI) denotes a condition of abnormal contact between the anterior or anterosuperior femoral head–neck junction and the acetabular rim. Even slight morphologic abnormalities may cause FAI to occur during flexion and internal rotation of the hip joint.

The classification of impingement is based on the underlying mechanism of the joint damage. A nonspherical femoral head leads to cam impingement, while overcoverage of the femoral head by the acetabulum leads to pincer impingement. Most patients with FAI are thought to have a mixed type of impingement with a combination of femoral and acetabular changes (**Fig. 2.40**). Characteristic features of cam and pincer impingement are listed and compared in **Table 2.20**.

Tannast M, Siebenrock KA, Anderson SE. Femoroacetabular impingement: radiographic diagnosis—what the radiologist should know. AJR Am J Roentgenol 2007;188(6):1540–1552

Cam Impingement

Cam impingement is caused by an aspherical shape of the femoral head. A bony hump at the femoral head–neck junction, usually directed anteriorly or anterosuperiorly, is jammed into the intact acetabulum during flexion and internal rotation. This creates shear forces in the corresponding portion of the acetabulum leading to circumscribed, often delaminating, cartilage lesions.

Alpha Angle

The α angle (**Fig. 2.41**) is a quantitative measure for describing the pathologic shape of the anterior femoral head–neck junction (aspherical femoral head shape with a decreased femoral head–neck offset).

MRI

The α angle is most accurately determined on transverse oblique MR images oriented parallel to the femoral neck. The angle is calculated on the slice that passes through the center of the femoral neck (**Fig. 2.42**). The α angle is formed by the femoral neck axis and a second line drawn from the center of the femoral head through the point where the head contour starts to become aspherical.

The femoral head outline and center are identified and drawn with a circle template. The femoral neck axis is

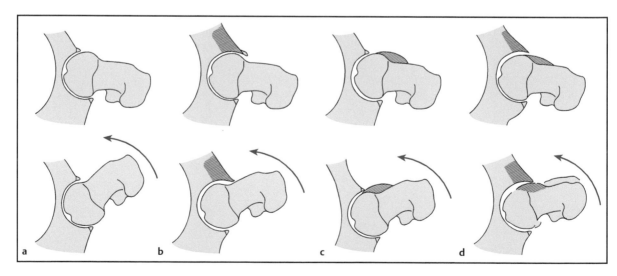

Fig. 2.40a–d Classification of femoroacetabular impingement.
a Normal configuration.
b Pincer impingement.
c Cam impingement.
d Mixed type.

Table 2.20 Characteristic features of femoroacetabular impingement

Criteria	Cam impingement	Pincer impingement
Mechanism	• Aspherical femoral head with decreased offset of head–neck junction • Spherical head portion is jammed into acetabulum during flexion and internal rotation	• Focal or general overcoverage • Linear contact between overcovering rim and head–neck junction
Lesions	• Circumscribed acetabular cartilage lesions at the 11 o'clock to 3 o'clock position (anterosuperior) • "Interface" lesions	• Early labral lesions involving long portions of the labrum • Linear cartilage lesions in a narrow strip parallel to acetabular rim • Contrecoup-like cartilage lesions on postero-inferior aspect of acetabulum and femoral head

Anteroposterior pelvic radiograph	• Pistol-grip deformity
	• Neck–shaft angle < 125°
		• Coxa profunda:
		  • Medial acetabular rim/ilioischial line < –3 or –6 mm
		  • Center-edge angle > 39°
		  • Horizontal toit externe angle negative
		• Protrusio acetabuli: femoral head medial to ilioischial line
		• Acetabular retroversion: "cross-over sign"

Lateral radiograph	• α angle > 55° • Femoral head–neck offset <10 mm • Femoral retrotorsion • Offset ratio < 0.18	• "Linear indentation sign"

Magnetic resonance arthrography	• Early: acetabular cartilage lesions
	• Labral lesions
	• Transverse oblique images:
	  • α angle > 55°
	  • Head–neck offset < 10 mm
	  • Femoral retrotorsion
	• Offset ratio < 0.18
	• Radial reformatting may be helpful
	• Assessment of superior and anterosuperior changes
		• Early: long labral lesions
		• Parallel strip of chondral lesions
		• Later: femoral neck abnormalities (see cam impingement)

Secondary changes	• Subchondral changes on anterolateral femoral neck, including herniation pits • Ossification of labrum	

Hip

2

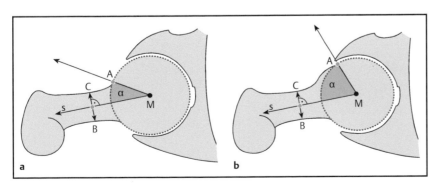

Fig. 2.41a,b Alpha angle. Schematic representation.
A = Point where the femoral head contour first becomes aspherical
M = Center of the femoral head
s = Femoral neck axis (perpendicular line through the midpoint of BC and the center of the femoral head)
a Normal hip joint.
b Cam impingement.

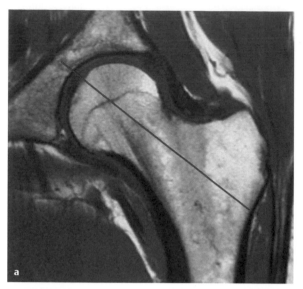

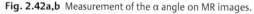

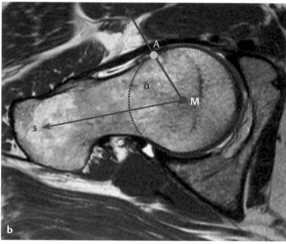

Fig. 2.42a,b Measurement of the α angle on MR images.
a Transverse oblique MR image through the center of the femoral neck.
b Measurement of the α angle.
A = Point where the femoral head contour first becomes aspherical
M = Center of the femoral head
s = Femoral neck axis

drawn through the femoral head center and the midpoint of a straight line drawn across the smallest diameter of the femoral neck. The Müller method (see p. 11) allows the most reproducible determination of the femoral neck axis.

Alpha angle	
• *Normal range:*	α < 55°
• *Cutoff value for FAI:*	α ≥ 55°

Some studies suggest a lower cutoff value of 50° for diagnosing FAI.

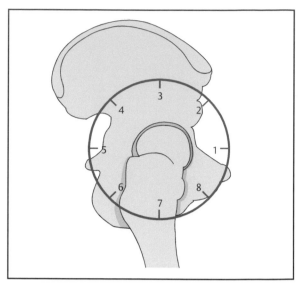

Fig. 2.43 Radial reconstructions around the femoral neck axis. Planes 1–3 are most crucial in the diagnosis of femoroacetabular impingement.

! Determination of the α angle is currently the best-established method for quantifying the abnormal shape of the femoral head (asphericity of the head with a bony bump at the femoral head–neck junction). It should be noted that only anterior bulges in the head–neck contour can be analyzed using the method of measurement described above. In many cases the maximum deviation from a spherical shape is anterosuperior, and in rare cases the bony bump is directed exclusively superiorly ("pistol-grip" deformity). These changes cannot be evaluated with the method described above.

Analysis of the femoral neck contour in additional planes requires radial reconstructions around the femoral neck axis, preferably based on an acquired three-dimensional data set. Changes involving the anterior, anterosuperior, and superior portions of the femoral head contour are relevant in the diagnosis of FAI (**Fig. 2.43**). For initial orientation purposes, an α angle of 55° on these extra planes can provide a useful cutoff value for diagnosing a predisposition to deformity.

Nötzli HP, Wyss TF, Stoecklin CH, Schmid MR, Treiber K, Hodler J. The contour of the femoral head-neck junction as a predictor for the risk of anterior impingement. J Bone Joint Surg Br 2002;84(4):556–560
Pfirrmann CW, Mengiardi B, Dora C, Kalberer F, Zanetti M, Hodler J. Cam and pincer femoroacetabular impingement: characteristic MR arthrographic findings in 50 patients. Radiology 2006;240(3):778–785

Fig. 2.44 Positioning technique for the cross-table radiograph.

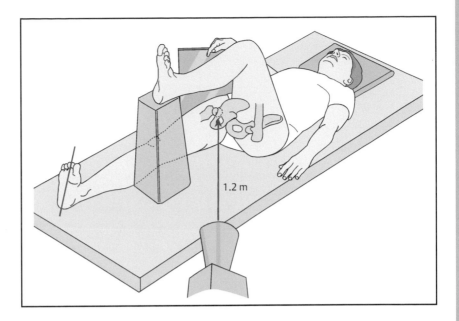

Conventional Radiographs

The α angle can also be measured on conventional radiographs, though with less precision than on MR images. The angle can be calculated on the cross-table view or the Rippstein view (Dunn–Rippstein–Müller view; see p. 12). The cross-table view is a horizontal projection taken with the beam directed upward toward the inguinal ligament. The cassette is mounted at an ~ 30° angle to the hip joint. The examined leg is placed in ~10–15° of internal rotation, and the opposite leg is elevated (**Fig. 2.44**).

As in the MRI method described above, the α angle is formed by the femoral neck axis and a second line drawn from the center of the femoral head to the point where the head first becomes aspherical (**Fig. 2.45**). The normal values and cutoff values for FAI are the same as in the MRI method (see above).

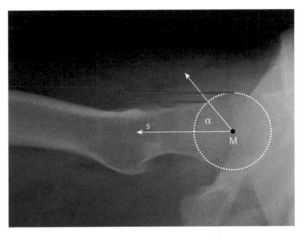

Fig. 2.45 Alpha angle and femoral head–neck offset measured on a cross-table radiograph.
M = Center of the femoral head
OS = Femoral head–neck offset
s = Femoral neck axis

Meyer DC, Beck M, Ellis T, Ganz R, Leunig M. Comparison of six radiographic projections to assess femoral head/neck asphericity. Clin Orthop Relat Res 2006;445:181–185

Tannast M, Siebenrock KA, Anderson SE. Femoroacetabular impingement: radiographic diagnosis—what the radiologist should know. AJR Am J Roentgenol 2007;188(6):1540–1552

Femoral Head–Neck Offset

Femoral head–neck offset is defined as the distance between the most prominent portions of the anterior contours of the femoral head and femoral neck.

The head–neck offset is determined by drawing two lines parallel to the femoral neck axis. One is tangent to the anterior femoral head contour, and the second is drawn through the point where the head–neck contour leaves the spherical part of the femoral head (see also α angle). The distance between the two parallel lines equals the femoral head–neck offset (see **Fig. 2.45**).

Femoral head–neck offset

- *Offset:*
  - Normal value: offset = 11.6 mm ± 0.7 mm
  - Indicator of FAI: offset < 10 mm
- *Offset ratio:* ratio of anterior femoral head–neck offset to femoral head diameter
  - Normal value: offset ratio = 0.21 ± 0.03
  - Patients with FAI: offset ratio = 0.13 ± 0.03
  - Indicator of FAI: offset ratio < 0.18

Eijer H, Leunig M, Mahomed MN, Ganz R. Cross-table lateral radiograph for screening of anterior femoral head-neck offset in patients with femoroacetabular impingement. Hip Int 2001;11:37–41

Tannast M, Siebenrock KA, Anderson SE. Femoroacetabular impingement: radiographic diagnosis—what the radiologist should know. AJR Am J Roentgenol 2007;188(6):1540–1552

Pincer Impingement

Pincer impingement is caused by linear contact between an "overcovering" acetabular rim and the femoral head–neck junction. It may be local, caused, for example, by an abnormal orientation of the acetabulum, or it may be circumferential because the acetabular fossa is too deep (coxa profunda). The head–neck junction is initially normal with pincer impingement alone, but over time the persistent abutment causes osseous changes to develop at the head–neck junction with subchondral edema and sclerosis, and may even incite the formation of a broad-based hump.

Pincer impingement can occur in various types of acetabular deformity, some congenital and some acquired, including:

- Coxa profunda (see p. 18)
- Protrusio acetabuli (see p. 19)
- Acetabular retroversion (see pp. 15–18)

Tannast M, Siebenrock KA, Anderson SE. Femoroacetabular impingement: radiographic diagnosis—what the radiologist should know. AJR Am J Roentgenol 2007;188(6):1540–1552

Class	Heterotopic ossification	
1	Islands of bone within the soft tissues about the hip	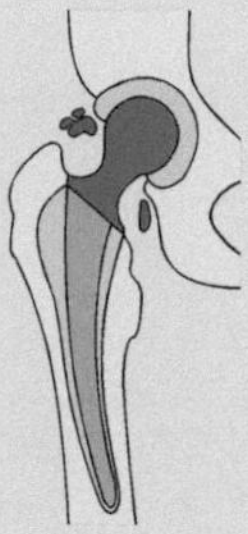
2	Bone spurs in the pelvis or proximal end of the femur, leaving at least 1 cm between the opposing bone surfaces	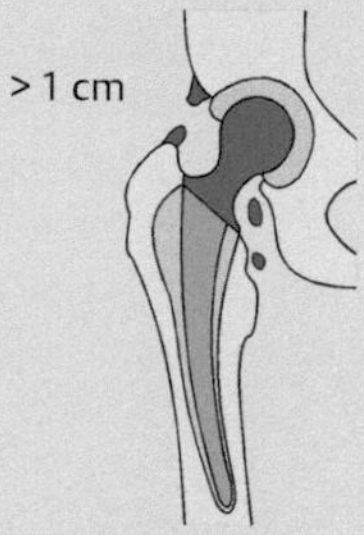 > 1 cm
3	Bone spurs extending from the pelvis or proximal end of the femur, reducing the space between opposing bone surfaces to less than 1 cm	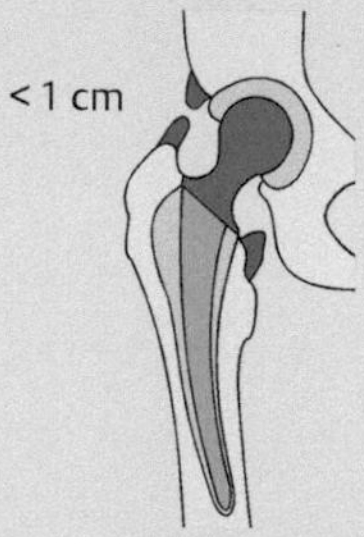 < 1 cm
4	Radiographic ankylosis of the hip	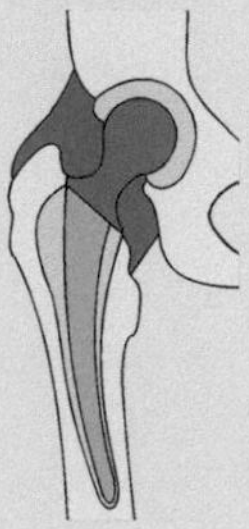

Fig. 2.46 Brooker classification of heterotopic ossification.

Classification of Heterotopic Ossification

Heterotopic ossification may occur about the hip joint following a total hip arthroplasty. The Brooker classification may be used (**Fig. 2.46**).

Brooker AF, Bowerman JW, Robinson RA, Riley LH Jr. Ectopic ossification following total hip replacement. Incidence and a method of classification. J Bone Joint Surg Am 1973;55(8):1629–1632

Appendix

Listed below are a set of age-adjusted nomograms for determining the summarized hip factor (**Fig. 2.47**).

Tönnis D. Die angeborene Hüftdysplasie und Hüftluxation im Kindes- und Erwachsenenalter. Chapter 9: Allgemeine Röntgendiagnostik des Hüftgelenks. Berlin: Springer; 1984; 129–134

Hip

2

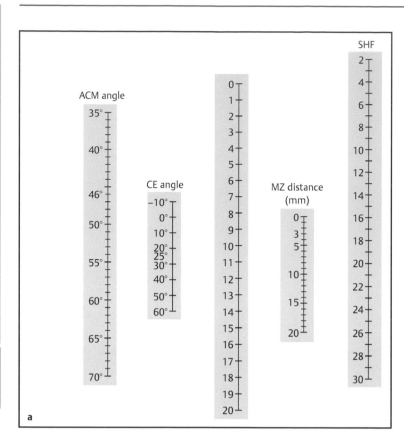

Fig. 2.47a–d Age-adjusted nomograms for determining the summarized hip factor (after Tönnis).
a Children 5–8 years of age.
b Children/adolescents 9–12 years of age.
c Adolescents 13–16 years of age.
d Adolescents/adults 17–20 years of age.

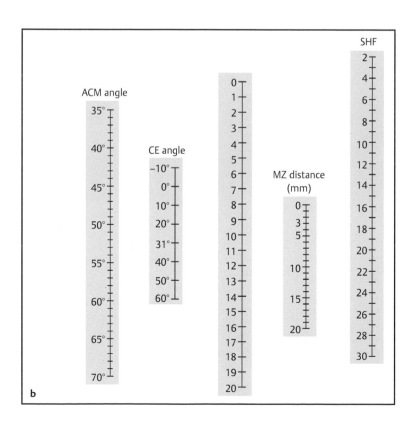

Hip

2

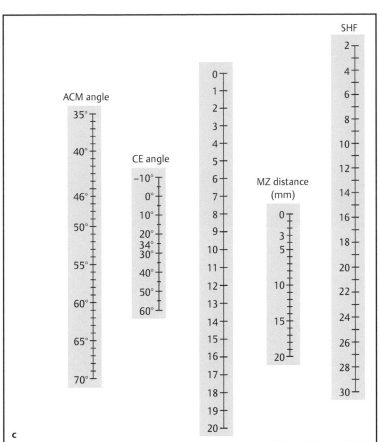

3 Knee

Patellofemoral Joint

Vertical Position of the Patella, Patellar Dystopia

■ Insall–Salvati Index

The Insall–Salvati index is perhaps the most widely used method for measuring the vertical position of the patella. On a lateral radiograph of the knee, the greatest diagonal length of the patella (LP) is measured from its posterosuperior corner to the apex. The length of the patellar tendon (LT) is measured from the patellar apex to the tibial tuberosity. The ratio of these two measurements (LP/LT) is the Insall–Salvati index (**Fig. 3.1**).

Insall–Salvati index	
• *Normal range:*	LP/LT = 0.8–1.2
• *High-riding patella (patella alta):*	LP/LT < 0.8
• *Low-riding patella (patella baja, patella infera):*	LP/LT > 1.2

Since the measurement is largely independent of joint position, it can be performed on routine X-ray films. The radiographs used by Insall and Salvati were obtained between 20° and 70° of knee flexion.

Insall J, Salvati E. Patella position in the normal knee joint. Radiology 1971;101(1):101–104

Insall J, Goldberg V, Salvati E. Recurrent dislocation and the high-riding patella. Clin Orthop Relat Res 1972;88:67–69

■ Caton–Deschamps Index

In the Caton or Caton–Deschamps method, the vertical position of the patella is defined by the ratio of the distance from the inferior border of the patellar articular surface to the anterior border of the upper tibia (B) and the length of the patellar articular surface (A) (**Fig. 3.2**). The measurements are made on a lateral radiograph of the knee, which may be flexed between 10° and 80°.

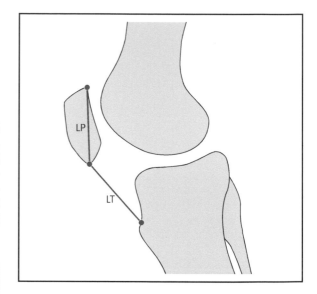

Fig. 3.1 Length measurements for calculating the Insall–Salvati index (LP/LT).
LP = Greatest diagonal length of the patella
LT = Length of the patellar tendon

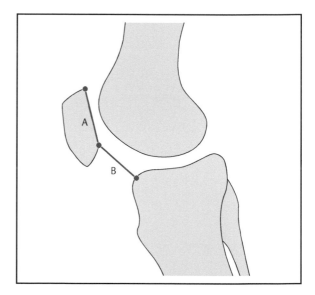

Fig. 3.2 Length measurements for calculating the Caton–Deschamps index (B/A).
A = Length of the patellar articular surface
B = Distance from the inferior border of the patellar articular surface to the anterosuperior bony margin of the tibia

Caton–Deschamps index

- *Normal range: B/A = 0.6 or 0.8–1.2*
- *High-riding patella (patella alta): B/A ≥ 1.2*
- *Low-riding patella (patella baja, patella infera): B/A ≤ 0.6*

Caton J, Deschamps G, Chambat P, Lerat JL, Dejour H. Patella infera. Apropos of 128 cases. [Article in French] Rev Chir Orthop Repar Appar Mot 1982;68(5):317–325
Caton J. Method of measuring the height of the patella. [Article in French] Acta Orthop Belg 1989;55(3):385–386

■ Blackburne–Peel Index

The method proposed by Blackburne and Peel for measuring patellar height differs from the two previous methods by its more precise definition of the distal reference point. First a line is drawn along the tibial plateau, and the perpendicular height of the lower edge of the patellar articular surface from the tibial plateau line is determined (A). The length of the patellar articular surface (B) is then measured, and the ratio A/B gives the Blackburne–Peel index (**Fig. 3.3**). The measurements are made on a lateral radiograph of the knee flexed at least 30° to tighten the patellar tendon.

Blackburne–Peel index

- *Normal values:*   A/B = 0.8 (0.6–1)
- *High-riding patella (patella alta):*   A/B > 1

!

The reproducibility of the Insall–Salvati index is limited by inaccuracies in identifying the insertion of the patellar tendon. Because the index is not changed by surgical advancement of the tibial tuberosity, this method is not very useful for preoperative planning. The Caton–Deschamps and Blackburne–Peel indices are advantageous in this respect.

Blackburne JS, Peel TE. A new method of measuring patellar height. J Bone Joint Surg Br 1977;59(2):241–242

Horizontal Position of the Patella, Patellar Dystopia

■ Congruence Angle

The congruence angle of the patellofemoral joint describes the relationship between the patella and the trochlear articular surface of the femur. It is influenced by the shape of the patella and trochlea (dysplasia) and especially by the mediolateral position of the patella (lateral patellar shift). The congruence angle is measured on an axial "sunrise" view of the patella. First, the deepest

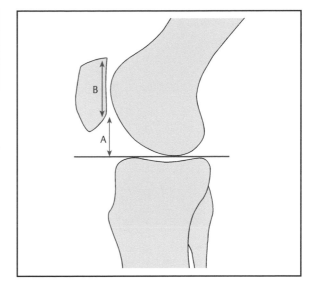

Fig. 3.3 Length measurements for calculating the Blackburne–Peel index.
A = Distance from inferior edge of patellar articular surface to a line along the tibial plateau
B = Length of the patellar articular surface

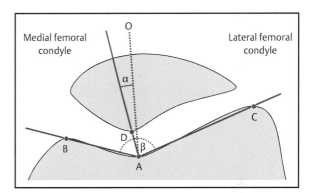

Fig. 3.4 Anatomic landmarks and lines for measuring the patellofemoral congruence angle.
A = Deepest point of the trochlea
B = Highest point on the medial femoral condyle
C = Highest point on the lateral femoral condyle
D = Lowest point of the patellar ridge
β = Sulcus angle
AO = Line bisecting the sulcus angle
α = Angle formed by an extension of AD and reference line AO

point of the trochlea is identified (A), and the highest points on the medial (B) and lateral femoral condyles (C) are marked. The angle formed by lines AB and AC is the *sulcus angle* (see below). The bisector of that angle is drawn as reference line AO. Next the lowest point on the articular ridge of the patella (D) is determined. The angle between an extension of line AD and reference line AO is the patellofemoral congruence angle (α, **Fig. 3.4**). If line AD is medial to AO, the angle has a negative value; if AD is lateral to AO, the angle is positive.

Knee

3

Knee

3

Patellofemoral congruence angle

- *Mean value: α = − 6°*
- *Standard deviation: 11°*
- *Abnormal: α > + 16°*

Merchant AC, Mercer RL, Jacobsen RH, Cool CR. Roentgenographic analysis of patellofemoral congruence. J Bone Joint Surg Am 1974;56(7):1391–1396

■ Axial Linear Patellar Displacement

Axial linear patellar displacement provides a simple, reproducible alternative to the patellofemoral congruence angle. On a sunrise view of the patella, a line is drawn between the highest points on the medial (M) and lateral (L) femoral condyles, and a perpendicular is dropped from that line through the deepest point of the trochlear sulcus (S). Another perpendicular is dropped from the lowest point on the patellar ridge (P). The distance between the two perpendicular lines equals the axial linear patellar displacement (**Fig. 3.5**). Its value is expressed in mm.

Axial linear patellar displacement

- *Normal range: ≤ 2 mm*
- *Abnormal lateralization: > 2 mm*

!

The absolute value of the measured axial linear patellar displacement depends on the magnification factor of the radiograph. This limits the value of comparative measurements, especially between different institutions and in scientific studies. The patellofemoral congruence angle appears to be a more reproducible measurement.

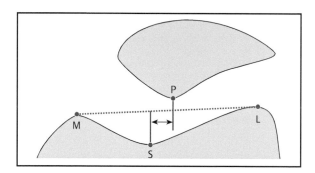

Fig. 3.5 Anatomic landmarks and lines for measuring axial linear patellar displacement.
M = Highest point on the medial femoral condyle
L = Highest point on the lateral femoral condyle
S = Deepest point of the trochlear sulcus
P = Lowest point of the patellar ridge
↔ = Axial linear patellar displacement

Urch SE, Tritle BA, Shelbourne KD, Gray T. Axial linear patellar displacement: a new measurement of patellofemoral congruence. Am J Sports Med 2009;37(5):970–973

■ Patellar Tilt

Patellar tilt refers to an abnormal angulation of the patella in the horizontal plane. The degree of tilt can be quantified in various ways. Common tools are the lateral patellofemoral angle of Laurin and the patellar tilt angle of Grelsamer.

Lateral Patellofemoral Angle of Laurin

The lateral patellofemoral angle is determined on the patellar sunrise view by drawing a line tangent to the highest points on the medial and lateral femoral condyles (A) and drawing a second line (B) across the lateral patellar facet (**Fig. 3.6**). In a normal joint, these lines will typically form an acute angle that opens on the lateral side. In patients with patellar instability, the lines will often be parallel or may even form an angle that opens on the medial side.

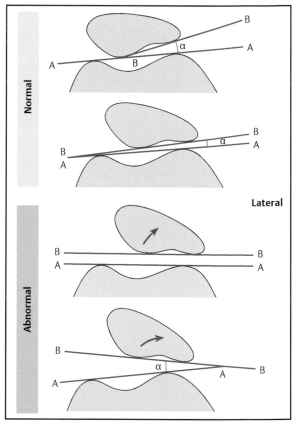

Fig. 3.6 Normal and abnormal lateral patellofemoral angles.
A = Line tangent to the highest points on the medial and lateral femoral condyles
B = Line across the lateral patellar facet
α = Lateral patellofemoral angle of Laurin

Laurin CA, Lévesque HP, Dussault R, Labelle H, Peides JP. The abnormal lateral patellofemoral angle: a diagnostic roentgenographic sign of recurrent patellar subluxation. J Bone Joint Surg Am 1978;60(1):55–60

Patellar Tilt Angle of Grelsamer

The patellar tilt angle (α) is measured on a patellar sunrise view between a line through the borders of the patella (medial and lateral edges of the subchondral bone) and a horizontal line (**Fig. 3.7**).

Patellar tilt angle of Grelsamer	
• *Normal range:*	2° ± 2°
• *Abnormal tilt:*	> 5°

! The lateral patellofemoral angle of Laurin is influenced by the shape and size of the patella and the configuration of the femoral condyles, and therefore some authors consider it less reliable. The tilt angle of Grelsamer is largely unaffected by these factors. On the other hand, measuring relative to the horizontal plane requires very precise radiographic positioning, and any rotation of the leg can distort the measurements.

Grelsamer RP, Bazos AN, Proctor CS. Radiographic analysis of patellar tilt. J Bone Joint Surg Br 1993;75(5):822–824

Trochlear Dysplasia

■ Sulcus Angle

The sulcus angle (β; synonym: trochlear angle) is the angle formed by the medial and lateral articular surfaces of the femoral trochlea. The lines forming the angle are found by connecting the deepest point of the trochlea to the highest points on the medial and lateral femoral condyles on a patellar sunrise view (**Fig. 3.8**). Trochlear dysplasia is characterized by a large sulcus angle, meaning that the groove is too shallow.

Sulcus angle	
• *Normal range:*	$\beta \le 145°$
• *Trochlear dysplasia:*	$\beta > 145°$

Brattstroem H. Shape of the intercondylar groove normally and in recurrent dislocation of patella. A clinical and X-ray-anatomical investigation. Acta Orthop Scand Suppl 1964;68(Suppl. 68):1–148

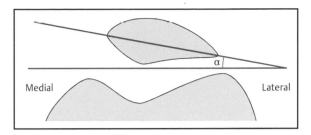

Fig. 3.7 Patellar tilt angle (α).

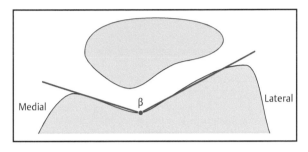

Fig. 3.8 Sulcus angle (β).

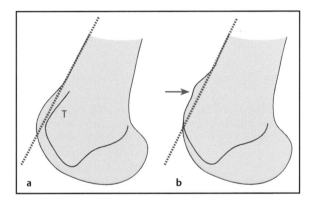

Fig. 3.9a,b Trochlear bump and crossing sign.
a Normal findings (explanation in text).
 T = floor of the trochlea
b Trochlear dysplasia: crossing sign and anterior "bump" in the upper portion of the trochlea (arrow).

■ Trochlear Bump and Crossing Sign

In a true lateral projection of the knee joint, the floor of the trochlea should normally be posterior to the anterior borders of the medial and lateral femoral condyles, and its anterior portion should not cross a line drawn along the anterior cortex of the distal femur (**Fig. 3.9a**). Extension past the anterior borders of the condyles (crossing sign) and the presence of a "trochlear bump" (**Fig. 3.9b**) are indicators of trochlear dysplasia. The trochlear bump can be quantified by measuring the distance between the trochlear floor and the line tangent to the anterior cortex.

Trochlear bump

- *Normal range:*   – 0.8 mm ± 2.9 mm
- *Abnormal trochlear bump:*   ≥ 3 mm

! According to a recent meta-analysis, published data are insufficient to support the reliability, validity, sensitivity, or specificity of various radiographic measuring techniques used in patients with patellar instability. These include the congruence angle, axial linear patellar displacement, lateral patellofemoral angle, and the trochlear bump and crossing sign.

Dejour H, Walch G, Nove-Josserand L, Guier C. Factors of patellar instability: an anatomic radiographic study. Knee Surg Sports Traumatol Arthrosc 1994;2(1):19–26

Grelsamer RP, Tedder JL. The lateral trochlear sign. Femoral trochlear dysplasia as seen on a lateral view roentgenograph. Clin Orthop Relat Res 1992;281(281):159–162

Malghem J, Maldague B. Depth insufficiency of the proximal trochlear groove on lateral radiographs of the knee: relation to patellar dislocation. Radiology 1989;170(2):507–510

Smith TO, Davies L, Toms AP, Hing CB, Donell ST. The reliability and validity of radiological assessment for patellar instability. A systematic review and meta-analysis. Skeletal Radiol 2011;40(4):399–414

Tibial Tuberosity to Trochlear Groove Distance

Measured from the trochlear sulcus (groove) to the tibial tuberosity, the tibial tuberosity to trochlear groove (TTTG) distance may be increased laterally in patients with patellar instability. The distance should be measured on axial computed tomography (CT) scans or magnetic resonance (MR) images of the knee. It represents the distance between a line perpendicular to the condylar line through the deepest point of the trochlea and a second line perpendicular to the condylar line through the center of the tibial tuberosity (**Fig. 3.10**).

TTTG distance

- *Normal range:* < 20 mm
- *Abnormal:* ≥ 20 mm

! The TTTG distance is considered an important parameter in patients with patellar instability. It is measured more accurately on CT or MR images than on radiographs and has an acceptable degree of inter-reader and intra-reader reliability.

Dejour H, Walch G, Nove-Josserand L, Guier C. Factors of patellar instability: an anatomic radiographic study. Knee Surg Sports Traumatol Arthrosc 1994;2(1):19–26

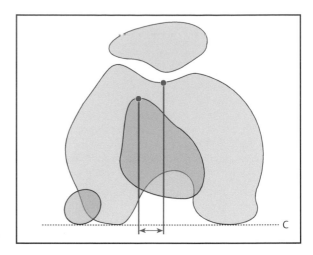

Fig. 3.10 Tibial tuberosity to trochlear groove (TTTG) distance. Measurements of the trochlea and tibial tuberosity are superimposed.
C = Condylar line

Goutallier D, Bernageau J, Lecudonnec B. The measurement of the tibial tuberosity. Patella groove distanced technique and results (author's transl). [Article in French] Rev Chir Orthop Reparatrice Appar Mot 1978;64(5):423–428

Schoettle PB, Zanetti M, Seifert B, Pfirrmann CW, Fucentese SF, Romero J. The tibial tuberosity–trochlear groove distance; a comparative study between CT and MRI scanning. Knee 2006;13(1):26–31

Wagenaar FCBM, Koëter S, Anderson PG, Wymenga AB. Conventional radiography cannot replace CT scanning in detecting tibial tubercle lateralisation. Knee 2007;14(1): 51–54

Tibial Plateau

Posterior Tibial Slope

! The posterior slope of the tibial plateau is an osseous factor contributing to the anteroposterior stability of the knee. The slope angle is important in cruciate ligament surgery, corrective osteotomies, and knee replacements.

The posterior tibial slope is measured on a lateral radiograph of the lower leg. The first step is to draw the axis of the tibial shaft. On radiographs that do not display the lower portion of the tibia, this line can be constructed by bisecting the distance between the anterior and posterior tibial margins at two points: just below the tibial tuberosity, and 10 cm distal to that level. The straight line connecting those two points is the tibial shaft axis. The posterior tibial slope is the angle formed by a line tangent to the tibial plateau and by a reference line drawn perpendicular to the tibial shaft axis (**Fig. 3.11**).

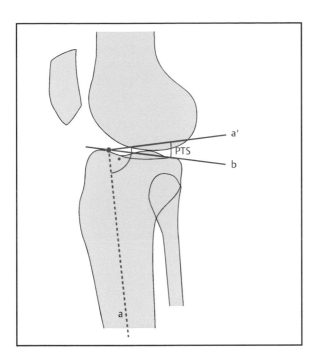

Fig. 3.11 Measurement of the posterior tibial slope (PTS).
a = Tibial shaft axis
a′ = Line perpendicular to a
b = Tangent to the tibial plateau

Various errors may arise when determining the posterior tibial slope on a conventional radiograph. Any rotation of the tibia relative to the image plane can significantly distort the measurement. Moreover, the tibial shaft axis and the line tangent to the tibial plateau can be difficult to determine even on a correctly positioned film, especially if degenerative joint changes are present or the medial and lateral condyles of the tibial plateau have different slope angles. This has led various authors to suggest determining the posterior tibial slope on CT or MR images and stating the angles separately for the medial and lateral condyles of the upper tibia.

Posterior tibial slope
Normal range: 0–18° (mean value: 7°)

Dejour H, Bonnin M. Tibial translation after anterior cruciate ligament rupture. Two radiological tests compared. J Bone Joint Surg Br 1994;76(5):745–749

Genin P, Weill G, Julliard R. The tibial slope. Proposal for a measurement method. [Article in French] J Radiol 1993;74(1):27–33

Hudek R, Schmutz S, Regenfelder F, Fuchs B, Koch PP. Novel measurement technique of the tibial slope on conventional MRI. Clin Orthop Relat Res 2009;467(8):2066–2072

Julliard R, Genin P, Weil G, Palmkrantz P. The median functional slope of the tibia. Principle. Technique of measurement.

Value. Interest. [Article in French] Rev Chir Orthop Repar Appar Mot 1993;79(8):625–634

Kessler MA, Burkart A, Martinek V, Beer A, Imhoff AB. Development of a 3-dimensional method to determine the tibial slope with multislice-CT. [Article in German] Z Orthop Ihre Grenzgeb 2003;141(2):143–147

Menisci

Classification of Meniscal Tears

Meniscal tears are classified by their orientation as follows (**Fig. 3.12**):
- Relative to the longitudinal axis of the meniscus:
  - Longitudinal tear
  - Radial tear
  - Flap tear (parrot beak tear, oblique tear)
- Relative to spatial (orthogonal) planes:
  - Vertical tear
  - Horizontal tear

!

> While *primary traumatic* meniscal tears tend to have a vertical orientation, *primary degenerative* tears are usually horizontal. In the case of vertical tears, the examiner should state whether the tear is located in the peripheral ("red") zone of the meniscus or in the central zone, because only tears in the vascularized peripheral zone can be successfully repaired in adults.

The following special types of meniscal tears are distinguished:
- *Complex tears* have elements of two or more of the basic tear patterns (see above).
- *Displaced flap tears* occur predominantly in the middle third of the medial meniscus. Typically the torn fragment is displaced inferiorly.
- *Bucket-handle tears* are vertical tears that run longitudinally through the meniscal tissue. The free edge of the meniscus is displaced medially, creating

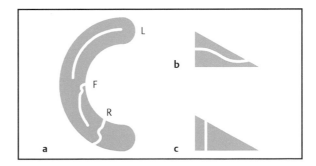

Fig. 3.12a–c Classification of meniscal tears.
a Horizontal section: orientation of longitudinal tears (L), flap tears (F), and radial tears (R).
b Vertical section: orientation of a horizontal tear.
c Vertical section: orientation of a vertical tear.

Knee

3

a bucket-handle fragment. This type of tear is more common in the medial meniscus than the lateral meniscus.

- A *meniscal root tear* is an avulsion of the meniscus from its tibial attachment (root), leading to meniscal instability. The posterior meniscal roots are most commonly affected. Not infrequently, root tears of the medial meniscus are found in association with degenerative joint changes.
- *Meniscocapsular separation* denotes a peripheral avulsion of the medial meniscus from its medial and/or posterior capsular attachment. This lesion may lead to hypermobility of the affected meniscus.

Wörtler K. MR imaging of the knee. [Article in German] Radiologe 2007;47(12):1131–1143

Treatment Options

While even small meniscal tears were routinely treated by partial or complete meniscectomy in the past, surgeons now try to preserve as much meniscal tissue for as long as possible. The specific treatment depends on the stability, location, and morphology of the meniscal tear and, to a degree, on the opinion and attitude of the operating surgeon. **Table 3.1** lists widely accepted criteria relating to the stability of meniscal tears and preferred treatment options.

Watanabe Classification of Discoid Meniscus

The discoid meniscus is a normal variant of the lateral meniscus that presents a range of morphologic features. Watanabe performed the first arthroscopic repair of a discoid meniscus in 1964 and later developed a three-part classification based on the arthroscopic appearance of the meniscus (**Fig. 3.13**).

Table 3.1 Treatment recommendations for meniscal tears

Treatment	Type of tear
Conservative treatment (stable tears)	Vertical (longitudinal) and flap tears ≤ 1 cm Radial tears ≤ 5 mm Partial vertical (longitudinal) tears (≤ 50% of craniocaudal diameter)
Surgical repair	Vertical (longitudinal) and flap tears > 1 cm
Partial meniscectomy (in symptomatic patients)	Radial tears > 5 mm Horizontal tears Complex tears

Types 1 and 2 are disk-shaped, but the type 3 lateral meniscus (Wrisberg-ligament type) often appears relatively normal. In the type 3, the posterior horn, which usually appears somewhat thickened, lacks its normal attachment by coronary and meniscocapsular ligaments and posterior meniscal root, and its sole posterior attachment consists of the posterior meniscofemoral ligament (of Wrisberg). As a result, the lateral meniscus is hypermobile and prone to subluxation with associated clinical symptoms.

Dickhaut SC, DeLee JC. The discoid lateral-meniscus syndrome. J Bone Joint Surg Am 1982;64(7):1068–1073
Neuschwander DC. Discoid meniscus. Oper Tech Orthop 1995;5:78–87
Watanabe M. Arthroscopy of the knee joint. In: Helfet AJ, ed. Disorders of the Knee. Philadelphia: Lippincott; 1974: 45

Cruciate and Collateral Ligaments

Anterior Tibial Translation

Anterior translation of the tibia relative to the femur provides indirect evidence of a torn anterior cruciate ligament on MRI. Two lines parallel to the longitudinal tibial axis are drawn on a midsagittal image through the lateral femoral condyle. One line is tangent to the posterior border of the tibial plateau, and one is tangent to the posterior cortical margin of the lateral femoral condyle. The distance between the two lines equals the anterior tibial translation (**Fig. 3.14**).

Anterior tibial translation
• *Normal range:* < 5 mm
• *Abnormal:* ≥ 5 mm

When described in the original publication, this sign was considered to have high specificity but relatively low sensitivity. More than 7 mm of anterior tibial translation was invariably associated with an anterior cruciate ligament rupture in that study.

Vahey TN, Hunt JE, Shelbourne KD. Anterior translocation of the tibia at MR imaging: a secondary sign of anterior cruciate ligament tear. Radiology 1993;187(3):817–819

Type	Designation	Diagnostic criteria	Arthroscopic appearance
1	Complete discoid meniscus	• Lateral meniscus abnormally thick • Complete coverage of tibial plateau by meniscal tissue • Normal meniscal attachments	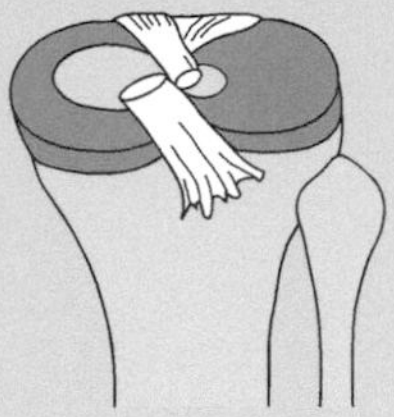
2	Incomplete discoid meniscus	• Lateral meniscus abnormally thick • > 80% but < 100% coverage of tibial plateau by meniscal tissue • Normal meniscal attachments	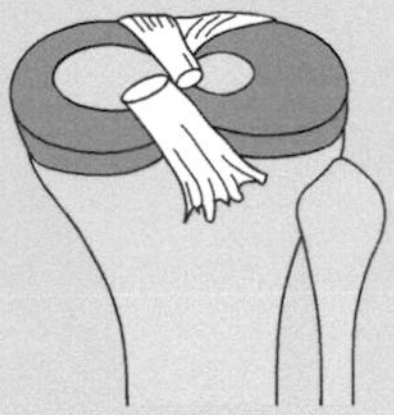
3	Wrisberg ligament type	• Posterior horn of lateral meniscus usually thickened • Only posterior meniscal attachment is to the Wrisberg ligament (posterior meniscofemoral ligament)	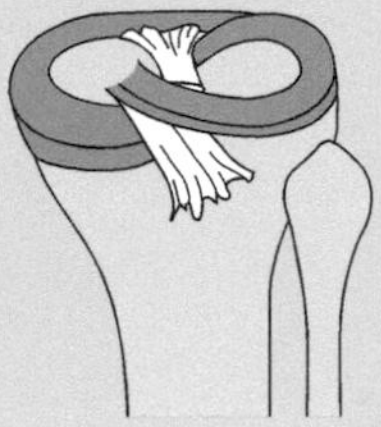

Fig. 3.13 Watanabe classification of discoid lateral meniscus.

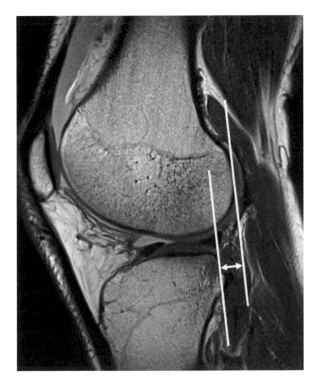

Fig. 3.14 Measurement of anterior tibial translation on a sagittal magnetic resonance image.

Anterior Cruciate Ligament Reconstruction

Today the most widely used technique for stabilizing the knee with a ruptured anterior cruciate ligament is a single-bundle reconstruction using autologous patellar tendon or semitendinosus-gracilis tendon grafts passed through tunnels drilled in the femur and tibia. The patellar tendon is harvested with attached bone plugs while semitendinosus-gracilis tendons are used without bone plugs. A variety of techniques have been described for this type of reconstruction. Correct positioning of the bone tunnels and the graft critically affects the prognosis of the reconstruction and is most accurately assessed by postoperative MRI.

To evaluate the tunnel position on a midsagittal image, the roof of the intercondylar notch and the tibial plateau are each divided into four equal-length segments (**Fig. 3.15**).

The opening of the femoral tunnel, or the site where the graft exits the femur, should be placed in segment 4 or even posterior to it. The opening of the tibial tunnel, or the site where the graft enters the tibia, should begin in segment 2. The graft should be posterior to the Blumensaat line (tangent to the roof of the intercondylar notch) and should have a smooth, straight orientation.

Viewed in the axial plane, the graft should exit the intercondylar notch at the 10 to 11 o'clock position in the

Knee

3

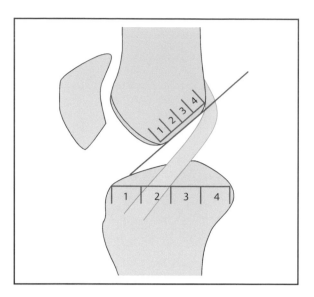

Fig. 3.15 Tunnel positions for a single-bundle reconstruction of the anterior cruciate ligament. Diagram shows the correct placement of an anterior cruciate ligament graft in the femur and tibia and its position relative to the Blumensaat line in a midsagittal section.

right knee, or at the 1 to 2 o'clock position in the left knee (**Fig. 3.16**).

Placing the femoral tunnel too far anteriorly or placing the tibial tunnel too far posteriorly can result in a vertical graft orientation that may cause instability. Conversely, placing the tibial tunnel too far anteriorly yields a more horizontal graft that may impinge against the roof or wall of the intercondylar notch during extension of the knee.

Wörtler K. MRT des Kniegelenks nach Kreuzband- und Meniskusoperationen. Radiologie up2date 2009;9:67–81

Classification of Medial Collateral Ligament Injuries

Injuries of the medial collateral ligament can be classified by their severity on MRI as shown in **Table 3.2**.

Schweitzer ME, Tran D, Deely DM, Hume EL. Medial collateral ligament injuries: evaluation of multiple signs, prevalence and location of associated bone bruises, and assessment with MR imaging. Radiology 1995;194(3):825–829

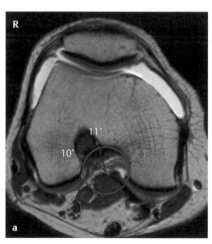
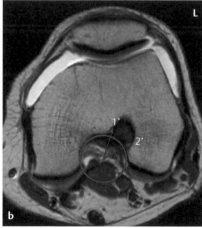

Fig. 3.16a,b Correct position of the femoral tunnel outlet for an anterior cruciate ligament graft in axial magnetic resonance images through the intercondylar notch of each knee. The correct position is between the 10 and 11 o'clock positions on the right side (**a**) and between the 1 and 2 o'clock positions on the left side (**b**).

Table 3.2 Classification of medial collateral ligament injuries on magnetic resonance imaging

Grade	Type of lesion	Magnetic resonance image findings
1	Overstretching or microtears	Increased periligamentous signal intensity with intact ligament fibers
2	Partial tear	Partial discontinuity, intrinsic hyperintensity, expansion, separation from bone
3	Complete tear	Complete discontinuity affecting all portions of the ligament

4 Foot

Foot Shapes

Three classic foot shapes are distinguished based on the relative lengths of the first and second toes (**Fig. 4.1**):
- *Egyptian foot:* The big toe is longer than the second toe.
- *Greek foot:* The big toe is shorter than the second toe.
- *Roman foot* (synonym: square foot): The big toe and second toe are equal in length.

> ! The shape of the foot can be assessed by visual inspection or by viewing an anteroposterior radiograph of the foot.

Alignment of the Foot

- *Anatomic axis* (**Fig. 4.2**): The anatomic axis of the foot runs through the center of the head of the second metatarsal and through the center of the calcaneal tuberosity.
- *Mechanical axis* (**Fig. 4.2**): The mechanical axis of the foot passes through the center of the head of the first metatarsal and through the center of the calcaneal tuberosity.

> ! The weight-bearing platform of the foot is shaped like a triangle. One side is formed by the mechanical axis of the foot. The axis through the center of the fifth metatarsal head and calcaneal tuberosity forms the second side, and a line connecting the heads of the first and fifth metatarsals forms the third side.

Radiographic Measurements of Foot Deformities

Longitudinal Arch of the Foot

Calcaneal Inclination Angle

The calcaneal inclination angle (**Fig. 4.3**) is measured on a standing lateral radiograph of the foot. The angle is formed by a line tangent to the inferior cortex of the calcaneus and a horizontal reference line (or the plantar plane).

The tangent to the inferior cortical border is most accurately defined by the following two points:
- Point 1: anterior extension of the calcaneal tuberosity on the plantar side.

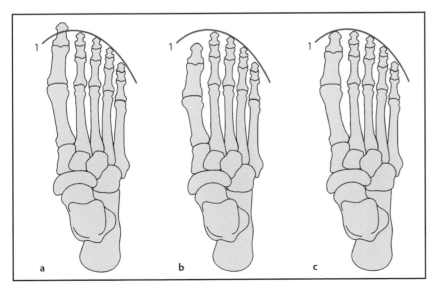

Fig. 4.1a–c Foot shapes. Schematic representation.
1 = Arc across the ends of the second through fifth distal phalanges
a Egyptian type.
b Greek type.
c Roman (square) type.

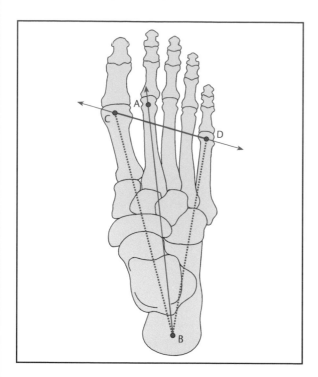

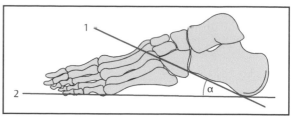

Fig. 4.3 Calcaneal inclination angle.
1 = Line tangent to inferior calcaneal border
2 = Plantar plane
α = Calcaneal inclination angle

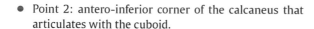

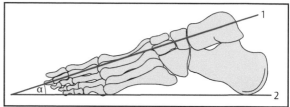

Fig. 4.2 Alignment of the foot in the dorsoplantar projection.
A–B = Anatomic axis
C–B = Mechanical axis
B–C–D = Weight-bearing triangle of the foot

Fig. 4.4 Talar declination angle.
1 = Longitudinal axis of talus
2 = Plantar plane
α = Talar declination angle

- Point 2: antero-inferior corner of the calcaneus that articulates with the cuboid.

The horizontal reference line passes between the lowest point of the calcaneus and the lowest point of the fifth metatarsal. Some authors suggest using the floor as the horizontal line.

Calcaneal inclination angle	
• *Normal range:*	α = 20–30°
• *Flatfoot (pes planovalgus):*	α < 20°
• *Pes cavus:*	α > 30°

Talar Declination Angle

Measured on a standing lateral radiograph, the talar declination angle (**Fig. 4.4**) is defined by the longitudinal axis of the talus and a horizontal reference line (or the plantar plane). The longitudinal talar axis is constructed by drawing a perpendicular line through the midpoint of a line through the upper and lower borders of the talar articular surface with the navicular. The angle of that axis is measured relative to a horizontal line tangent to the inferior borders of the calcaneus and fifth metatarsal.

Talar declination angle	
• *Normal range:*	α = 14–36°
• *Mean value:*	α = 21°
• *Flatfoot (pes planovalgus):*	α > 35°
• *Pes cavus:*	α < 14°

Talar–First Metatarsal Angle

The talar–first metatarsal angle (**Fig. 4.5**) is measured on a true lateral radiographic projection of the foot. It is formed by the longitudinal axis of the first metatarsal shaft and the longitudinal axis of the talus. In a normal pedal arch, the two axes are parallel or congruent so that the talar–first metatarsal angle is ~ 0°.

Talar–first metatarsal angle	
• *Normal range:*	α = + 4 to – 4°
• *Flatfoot (pes planovalgus):*	α < – 4°
• *Pes cavus:*	α > 4°

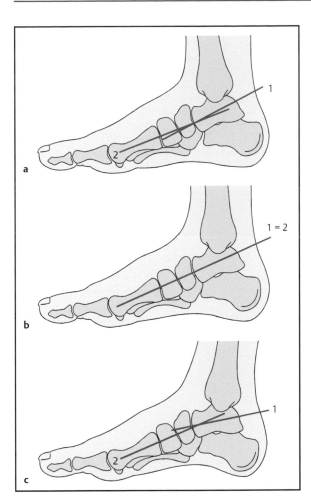

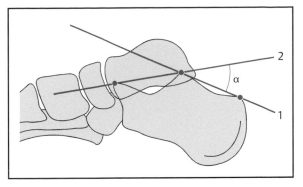

Fig. 4.6 Boehler angle.
1 = Line tangent to posterosuperior calcaneal border
2 = Line tangent to anterosuperior calcaneal border
α = Boehler angle

Boehler angle
Normal range: α = 20–40°

! The Boehler angle is used to evaluate calcaneal deformity resulting from a fracture. With fractures involving the anterior process of the calcaneus, the angle is decreased and may assume negative values.

Fig. 4.5a–c Talar–first metatarsal angle in the lateral projection.
1 = Longitudinal axis of talus
2 = Longitudinal axis of first metatarsal
a Pes planovalgus (α is negative and less than – 4°).
b Normal foot.
c Pes cavus (α is positive and more than + 4°).

! The talar–first metatarsal angle is used in the diagnosis of flatfoot and pes cavus. It can also be measured to evaluate the flexibility of the foot. More than an 8° change in the angle from weight-bearing to non-weight-bearing suggests hyperflexibility of the foot.

Boehler L. Diagnosis, pathology and treatment of fractures of the os calcis. J Bone Joint Surg Am 1931;13(1):75–89
Hauser ML, Kroeker RO. Boehler's angle: a review and study. J Am Podiatry Assoc 1975;65(6):517–521

Hindfoot Geometry

Tuber Joint Angle (Boehler Angle)

Boehler angle (**Fig. 4.6**) is determined on a lateral radiograph of the ankle joint. It is measured between lines tangent to the posterosuperior and anterosuperior borders of the calcaneus.

Longitudinal Axis of the Calcaneus, Longitudinal Axis of the Hindfoot (Dorsoplantar View)

The longitudinal axis of the hindfoot corresponds to the longitudinal axis of the calcaneus (**Fig. 4.7**). This axis is defined by the anteromedial corner of the calcaneus and by the midpoint of the posterior calcaneal border. Since the posterior border of the calcaneus is often obscured by overlying structures on the dorsoplantar radiograph, another option is to use the tangent to the lateral calcaneal border as a reference line. Because the lateral process of the calcaneal tuberosity and the peroneal trochlea may create an apparent bulge in the lateral outline of the calcaneus, the anterior third of that border is the most favorable site for drawing the tangent. A parallel line drawn through the anteromedial corner of the calcaneus will correspond closely to the longitudinal axis of the calcaneus, and a forward extension of that line will approximate the longitudinal axis of the fourth metatarsal.

Christman R. Foot and Ankle Radiology. St. Louis: Elsevier; 2003
Gamble FO, Yle I. Clinical Foot Roentgenology. 2nd ed. Huntington NY: Krieger Publishing; 1975

Foot

4

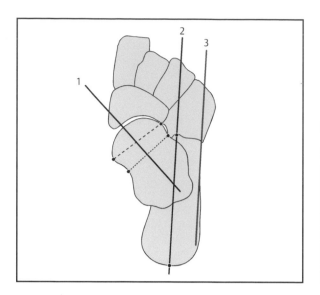

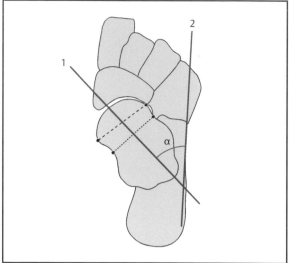

Fig. 4.7 Longitudinal axis of the hindfoot (calcaneus) and longitudinal axis of the talus.
1 = Longitudinal axis of talus
2 = Longitudinal axis of calcaneus
3 = Alternative longitudinal axis of calcaneus drawn tangent to lateral calcaneal border (anterior third)

Fig. 4.9 Talocalcaneal angle (dorsoplantar view).
1 = Longitudinal axis of talus
2 = Longitudinal axis of calcaneus
α = Talocalcaneal angle

Longitudinal Axis of the Talus (Dorsoplantar View)

The longitudinal axis of the talus or talar neck is defined by the midpoints of two lines drawn through opposite points on the talar margins at the widest and narrowest parts of the neck and head of the talus (see **Fig. 4.7**). Normally this axis will correspond closely to the longitudinal axis of the first metatarsal.

Talocalcaneal Angle

Lateral Radiograph

The lateral talocalcaneal angle is formed by the longitudinal axes of the talus and calcaneus on a standing lateral radiograph of the foot (**Fig. 4.8**). The longitudinal axis of the calcaneus is given by a tangent to the inferior calcaneal border. This line is defined by the anterior plantar

extension of the calcaneal tuberosity and the antero-inferior corner of the calcaneus at its articulation with the cuboid. In newborns and small children, who still have an oval-shaped talus and calcaneus, the longitudinal axes are simply drawn along the midlines of the bones.

Talar declination angle
• *Normal range:*
• Newborns: α = 25–55°
• Adults: α = 30–50° (mean value: 35°)
• *Hindfoot valgus:*   α > 55°
• *Hindfoot varus:*   α < 30°

Dorsoplantar Radiograph

The talocalcaneal angle (**Fig. 4.8**) is measured between the longitudinal axes of the talus and the calcaneus on the standing dorsoplantar radiograph of the foot (**Fig. 4.9**). While the axes in older patients are located as described above, they can be identified in small children by drawing midlines through the oval-shaped tarsal bones. In a normal foot the longitudinal axis of the talus points approximately toward the head of the first metatarsal while the longitudinal axis of the calcaneus points toward the head of the fourth metatarsal. The talocalcaneal angle normally decreases somewhat during growth.

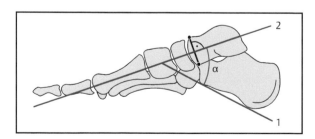

Fig. 4.8 Talocalcaneal angle (lateral view).
1 = Line tangent to inferior calcaneal border
2 = Longitudinal axis of talus
α = Talocalcaneal angle

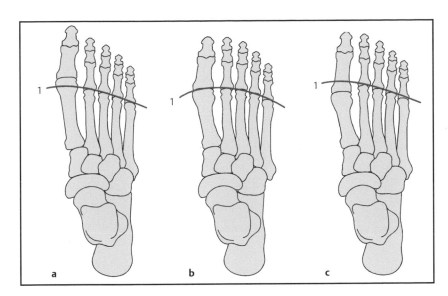

Fig. 4.10a–c Metatarsal index.
1 = Arc across ends of second
through fifth metatarsals
a Plus index.
b Plus–minus index.
c Minus index.

Talocalcaneal angle (dorsoplantar view)
• *Normal range:*
• Newborns: α = 25–55°
• Adults: α = 20–45° (mean value: 35°)
• *Hindfoot valgus:* α > 45°
• *Hindfoot varus:* α < 20°

!

The talocalcaneal angle is an indicator of hindfoot alignment. In deformities where the hindfoot is in varus, the talocalcaneal angle is decreased in both the dorsoplantar and lateral views (clubfoot, pes cavus). When the hindfoot is in valgus, however, the talocalcaneal angle is increased in both the dorsoplantar and lateral projections (pes planovalgus, vertical talus).

The talocalcaneal angles are important in the diagnosis of congenital foot deformities in clubfoot. The talocalcaneal angles are typically small, and the longitudinal axes of the tarsus and calcaneus may even be parallel in some cases. Congenital vertical talus is marked by increased angles as well as medial angulation of the first metatarsal in the dorsoplantar view.

Midfoot and Forefoot Geometry

■ Relative Metatarsal Lengths

Metatarsal Index

The metatarsal index describes the length relationship between the first metatarsal and the second through fifth metatarsals (**Fig. 4.10**). It is of clinical importance because different positions of the metatarsal heads, especially of the first metatarsal head relative to the other metatarsal heads, can alter the pressure loads acting on the forefoot.

The length relationship of the first metatarsal to the other metatarsals is determined on a standing dorsoplantar radiograph by drawing a uniform arc across the distal ends of the second through fifth metatarsals.

- *Plus index:* The head of the first metatarsal is distal to the arc.
- *Plus–minus index:* The distal end of the first metatarsal head touches the arc.
- *Minus index:* The first metatarsal head is proximal to the arc.

!

A minus index indicates a certain predisposition to hallux valgus and (associated) metatarsalgia because of increased loads on the second and third metatarsal heads. From a therapeutic standpoint, hallux valgus deformities with a minus index of the metatarsals should not be treated by an osteotomy that shortens the first metatarsal.

Morton Method

The Morton method evaluates the relative lengths of the first and second metatarsals (**Fig. 4.11**). The distance is measured between two lines drawn perpendicular to the longitudinal axis of the second metatarsal at the heads of the first and second metatarsals.

- *Plus index:* The line at the first metatarsal head is more than 2 mm distal to the second line.
- *Minus index:* The line at the first metatarsal head is more than 2 mm proximal to the second line.

!

One disadvantage of this method is that a valgus or varus deformity of the first ray can distort the measurements.

Karasick D, Wapner KL. Hallux valgus deformity: preoperative radiologic assessment. AJR Am J Roentgenol 1990;155(1):119–123

Foot

4

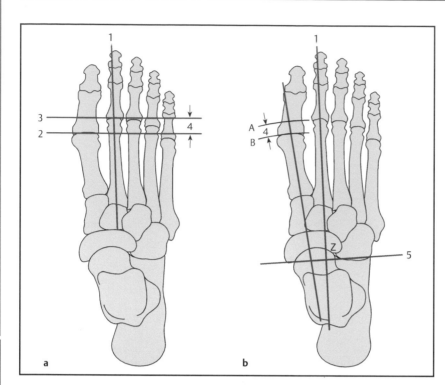

Fig. 4.11a,b Alternative methods of evaluating the relative lengths of the first and second metatarsals.

1 = Longitudinal axis of second metatarsal
2 = Line perpendicular to 1 at distal end of first metatarsal
3 = Line perpendicular to 1 at distal end of second metatarsal
4 = Distance evaluated for plus or minus index
5 = Line through posteromedial corner of navicular and lateral corner of calcaneocuboid joint
Z = Center of arcs A and B, constructed as intersection point between 1 and 5
A = Arc, centered on Z, through distal end of second metatarsal head
B = Arc, centered on Z, through distal end of first metatarsal head
a Morton method.
b Hardy and Clapham method.

Hardy and Clapham Method

The Hardy and Clapham method (**Fig. 4.11**) is widely used for evaluating the relative lengths of the first and second metatarsals. First a point (Z) is established in the talar head as the center of two circular arcs. Z is defined as the point where the longitudinal axis of the second metatarsal shaft intersects a straight line passing through the posteromedial corner of the navicular and through the lateral corner of the calcaneocuboid joint. Then two arcs, centered on Z, are drawn through the distal ends of the first and second metatarsal heads. The distance between the two arcs indicates the distance between the two metatarsals.

- *Plus index:* The arc at the first metatarsal head is more than 2 mm distal to the second arc.
- *Minus index:* The arc at the first metatarsal head is more than 2 mm proximal to the second arc.

> **!** Hardy and Clapham did not state normal values for the interarc distance, but it is widely accepted that values > 2 mm are interpreted as abnormal, as in the Morton method.

Hardy RH, Clapham JC. Observations on hallux valgus; based on a controlled series. J Bone Joint Surg Br 1951;33-B(3): 376–391

Metatarsal Depth Angle

The metatarsal depth angle (of Meschan) is formed by a line tangent to the heads of the first and second metatarsals and a second line tangent to the heads of the second and fifth metatarsals. The angle is used to diagnose shortening of the first metatarsal relative to the second metatarsal (**Fig. 4.12**).

> **Metatarsal depth angle**
> - *Normal range: α = 142.5°*
> - *Minus index (relative shortening of the first metatarsal): α < 135°*

Gamble FO, Yle I. Clinical Foot Roentgenology. 2nd ed. Huntington NY: Krieger Publishing; 1975

■ Tarsal Joint Surface Angles

These angles are used to evaluate the alignment of the tarsal joints (**Fig. 4.13**). They are formed by a line parallel to the plantar plane and straight lines drawn through the tarsal articular surfaces on a lateral radiograph.

Physiologically, the articular surfaces of the talonavicular, naviculocuneiform and first tarsometatarsal joints should show an approximately parallel alignment. The following normal ranges of tarsal joint surface angles have been reported in the literature:

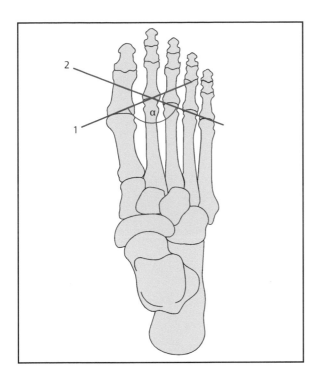

Fig. 4.12 Metatarsal depth angle.
1 = Line tangent to heads of first and second metatarsals
2 = Line tangent to heads of second and fifth metatarsals
α = Metatarsal depth angle

Tarsal joint surface angles	
• Talonavicular joint:	54–74°
• Naviculocuneiform joint:	51–68°
• First tarsometatarsal joint:	55–72°

Foot Deformities in Adults

Pes Transversus

Pes transversus (splayfoot) refers to abnormal widening of the forefoot with a fan-shaped splaying of the first and fifth metatarsals. The deformity can be diagnosed on dorsoplantar radiographs by measuring the intermetatarsal angles between the first and fifth, first and second, and fourth and fifth metatarsal bones.

- *First–fifth intermetatarsal angle* (**Fig. 4.14**): angle measured between the longitudinal axes of the first and fifth metatarsals.
- *First–second intermetatarsal angle* (**Fig. 4.15**): angle measured between the longitudinal axes of the first and second metatarsals.
- *Fourth–fifth intermetatarsal angle* (see **Fig. 4.15**): angle measured between the longitudinal axes of the fourth and fifth metatarsals.

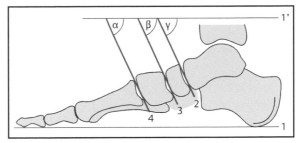

Fig. 4.13 Tarsal joint surface angles.
1   = Plantar plane
1'   = Line parallel to plantar plane
2   = Line through talonavicular joint
3   = Line through naviculocuneiform joint
4   = Line through first tarsometatarsal joint
α, β, γ = Tarsal joint surface angles

Intermetatarsal angles in splayfoot	
• *First–fifth intermetatarsal angle:*	
• Normal range:	α = 14–35°
• Splayfoot:	α > 35°
• *First–second intermetatarsal angle:*	
• Normal range:	α < 10°
• Metatarsus primus varus:	α ≥ 10°
• *Fourth–fifth intermetatarsal angle:*	
• Normal range:	β < 10°

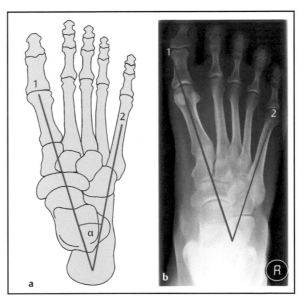

Fig. 4.14a,b First–fifth intermetatarsal angle.
1 = Longitudinal axis of first metatarsal
2 = Longitudinal axis of fifth metatarsal
α = First–fifth intermetatarsal angle
a Schematic drawing.
b Splayfoot deformity (dorsoplantar radiograph).

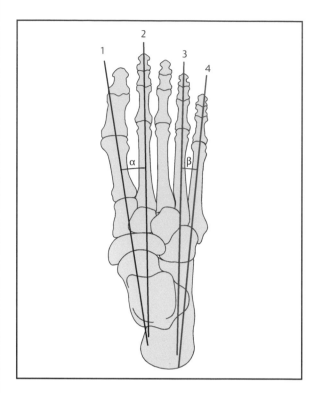

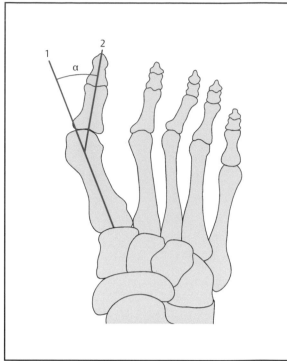

Fig. 4.15 First–second and fourth–fifth intermetatarsal angles.
1 = Longitudinal axis of first metatarsal
2 = Longitudinal axis of second metatarsal
3 = Longitudinal axis of fourth metatarsal
4 = Longitudinal axis of fifth metatarsal
α = First–second intermetatarsal angle
β = Fourth–fifth intermetatarsal angle

Fig. 4.16 Hallux valgus angle.
1 = Longitudinal axis of first metatarsal
2 = Longitudinal axis of proximal phalanx
α = Hallux valgus angle

 Hallux valgus as well as lesser toe deformities develop secondarily to an underlying splayfoot. One main cause of hallux valgus is an inability of muscular stabilizers to follow the medial deviation of the first metatarsal in splayfoot deformity. This leads to a (lateral) muscular predominance that increasingly forces the big toe into a valgus position. Deformities of the lesser toes result from crowding of the centrally converging toe rays and less pressure transfer to the first metatarsal head due to hallux valgus.

Hallux Valgus

Hallux valgus is a deformity characterized by lateral (valgus) deviation of the big toe at the metatarsophalangeal joint with concomitant medial (varus) deviation of the first metatarsal. Preoperative planning requires a weight-bearing (standing) dorsoplantar radiograph of the foot with the beam centered on the midfoot. The following quantitative parameters are evaluated on this view:

■ Parameters

Hallux Valgus Angle

The hallux valgus angle (**Fig. 4.16**) is measured on a dorsoplantar radiograph of the forefoot between the longitudinal axes of the first metatarsal and proximal phalanx.

Hallux valgus angle	
• *Normal value:*	α ≤ 15°
• *Hallux valgus:*	α > 15°

First–Second Intermetatarsal Angle

The first–second intermetatarsal angle (**Fig. 4.15**; see above) is measured between the longitudinal axes of the first and second metatarsal bones.

First–second intermetatarsal angle	
• *Normal value:*	α < 10°
• *Metatarsus primus varus:*	α ≥ 10°

Metatarsus primus varus is a foot deformity characterized by varus deviation of the first metatarsal. In hallux valgus, the first–second intermetatarsal angle is almost always increased due to the underlying splayfoot deformity.

> ! The first–second intermetatarsal angle is of key importance in the treatment of hallux valgus, as the size of the angle determines the choice of osteotomy technique to correct the varus deformity of the first metatarsal. Angles > 15° require a basal osteotomy of the first metatarsal or an arthrodesis of the tarsometatarsal joint, whereas smaller angles ($\alpha \leq 15°$) can be corrected by a retrocapital or diaphyseal osteotomy.

Distal Metatarsal Articular Angle

The distal metatarsal articular angle (DMAA) is measured between a line perpendicular to the long axis of the first metatarsal and a line along the articular surface of the first metatarsal head (**Fig. 4.17**).

Distal metatarsal articular angle (DMAA)
Normal value: $\alpha < 10°$

> ! If the distal articular surface of the first metatarsal head has more than a 10° lateral slope relative to the long axis of the bone, it should be corrected by a retrocapital or proximal osteotomy. If there is a large increase in the first–second intermetatarsal angle as well, a basal osteotomy should be combined with a retrocapital or diaphyseal osteotomy (two-level osteotomies).

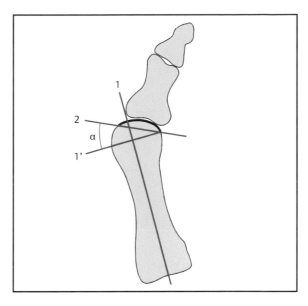

Fig. 4.17 Distal metatarsal articular angle.
1 = Longitudinal axis of first metatarsal
1' = Line perpendicular to longitudinal axis of first metatarsal
2 = Line connecting medial and lateral margins of articular surface
α = Distal metatarsal articular angle (DMAA)

Evaluation of First Metatarsophalangeal Joint Congruence

The congruence of the first metatarsophalangeal joint is evaluated by measuring the angle between reference lines drawn across the articular surface of the first metatarsal head and the base of the proximal phalanx (**Fig. 4.18**).
- *Congruent:* the reference lines are parallel
- *Deviated:* the reference lines are not parallel, forming an angle < 20°

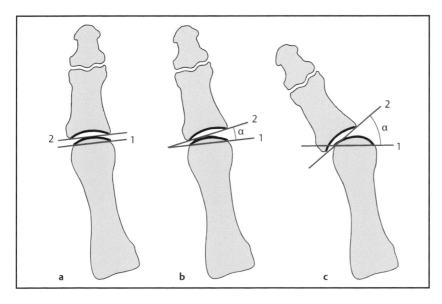

Fig. 4.18a–c First metatarsophalangeal joint congruence. Schematic drawing.
1 = Line connecting medial and lateral margins of first metatarsal articular surface
2 = Line connecting medial and lateral margins of proximal phalangeal articular surface
α = Angle between metatarsophalangeal articular surfaces
a Congruent.
b Deviated.
c Subluxated.

Foot

4

- *Subluxated:* angle > 20°

> !
>
> Congruence of the first metatarsophalangeal joint should always be restored or preserved in the treatment of hallux valgus. Hence, an incongruent metatarsophalangeal joint always requires a corrective distal soft-tissue procedure, whereas a congruent joint would contraindicate a soft-tissue procedure, which could result in loss of congruence.

■ Mann Grading of Hallux Valgus Deformity

Hallux valgus can be classified into three grades of severity based on measurable parameters, as shown in **Table 4.1**.

Measurements performed on a dorsoplantar radiograph of the foot are of key importance in published algorithms dealing with the treatment of hallux valgus. A somewhat simplified algorithm is shown in **Fig. 4.19**.

Fuhrmann RA. Degenerative Erkrankungen des Vorfusses—Hallux valgus und Kleinzehendeformitäten. Orthopädie und Unfallchirurgie up2date 2006; 1: 143–166

Mann RA. Decision-making in bunion surgery. Instr Course Lect 1990;39:3–13

Mann RA, Coughlin MJ. Hallux valgus—etiology, anatomy, treatment and surgical considerations. Clin Orthop Relat Res 1981;157(157):31–41

Mann RA, Coughlin MJ. Surgery of the Foot and Ankle. 6th ed. St. Louis: Mosby Year Book; 1993

Table 4.1 Grades of severity of hallux valgus (Mann classification)

Grade	Description
1 (mild)	• Hallux valgus angle ≤ 20°
	• First–second intermetatarsal angle ≤ 11°
	• Anatomic position of sesamoids or < 50% subluxation of lateral sesamoid
2 (moderate)	• Hallux valgus angle > 20–40°
	• First–second intermetatarsal angle ≤ 11–18°
	• 50–75% subluxation of lateral sesamoid
3 (severe)	• Hallux valgus angle > 40°
	• First–second intermetatarsal angle > 18°
	• Dislocation of lateral sesamoid

Lesser Toe Deformities

Deformities of the lesser toes (**Fig. 4.20**) most commonly involve the second and third toes and are generally secondary to a splayfoot deformity with hallux valgus. An exception is the isolated, usually congenital, varus deformity of the fifth toe, which rarely develops as a result of splayfoot.

Lesser toe deformities typically involve flexion deformities at the proximal interphalangeal joint and extension deformities at the metatarsophalangeal joint. The following deformities are distinguished based on their flexion/extension components:

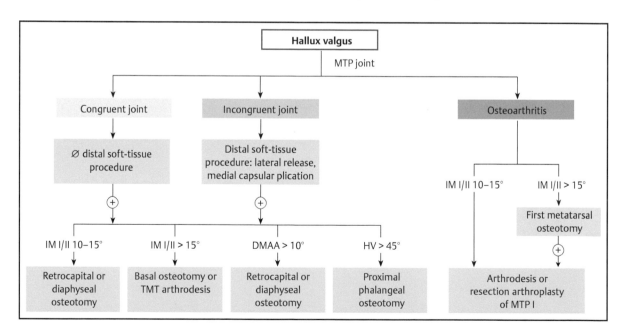

Fig. 4.19 Algorithm for the treatment of hallux valgus based on radiographic measurements.

IM I/II = First–second intermetatarsal angle
DMAA = Distal metatarsal articular angle
HV = Hallux valgus angle

MTP = Metatarsophalangeal joint
TMT = Tarsometatarsal joint

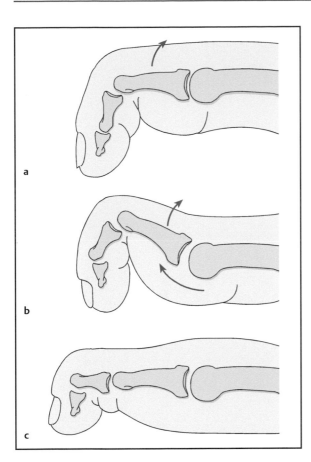

Fig. 4.20a–c Lesser toe deformities.
a Hammer toe.
b Claw toe.
c Mallet toe.

- *Hammer toe:* an isolated flexion deformity of the toe at the proximal interphalangeal joint.
- *Claw toe:* an extension deformity at the metatarsophalangeal joint combined with a flexion deformity at the proximal interphalangeal joint. Unlike hammer toe, the ball of the clawed toe loses contact with the ground at an early stage.
- *Mallet toe:* an isolated flexion deformity (contracture) of the toe at the distal interphalangeal joint.
- *Varus deformity of the fifth toe:* medial deviation and supination of the fifth toe at the metatarsophalangeal joint.

Overview of Pediatric and Congenital Foot Deformities

Descriptions of congenital and pediatric foot deformities vary widely in the literature, and varying techniques have been used in their radiographic measurement. **Figs. 4.21 and 4.22** review the diagnostic work-up of pediatric foot deformities based on three studies conducted in patients 0–12 years of age. A common feature of all the studies is that the authors placed key emphasis on the evaluation of the hindfoot.

Specific deformities, measurements, and diagnostic techniques are described more fully in the sections below.

Davis LA, Hatt WS. Congenital abnormalities of the feet. Radiology 1955;64(6):818–825

Gamble FO, Yle I. Clinical Foot Roentgenology. 2nd ed. Huntington NY: Krieger Publishing; 1975

Ritchie GW, Keim HA. A radiographic analysis of major foot deformities. Can Med Assoc J 1964;91:840–844

Templeton AW, McAlister WH, Zim ID. Standardization of terminology and evaluation of osseous relationships in congenitally abnormal feet. Am J Roentgenol Radium Ther Nucl Med 1965;93:374–381

Foot Deformities in Children and Adults

■ Flatfoot (Pes Planovalgus)

Because the components of flexible flatfoot deformity in children and adolescents are basically the same as in acquired flatfoot in adults (usually caused by tibialis posterior tendon dysfunction), radiographic examination and interpretation are identical. Flattening of the longitudinal pedal arch is typically accompanied by valgus deviation of the hindfoot and abduction of the forefoot (**Figs. 4.23 and 4.24**).

The components of the deformity can be diagnosed and quantified on standard radiographs of the foot based on the parameters listed in **Table 4.2**.

> While the calcaneal inclination angle is used to evaluate the flattening of the longitudinal arch, the talar declination angle and talar–first metatarsal angle describe the inferomedial angulation of the talus. The talocalcaneal angles evaluate the valgus position of the hindfoot whereas the talar–first metatarsal angle (dorsoplantar view) quantifies the degree of forefoot abduction.

■ Pes Cavus

Pes cavus is a foot deformity in which the forefoot is fixed in plantar flexion, creating an abnormally high longitudinal arch. Subtypes are identified on the basis of clinical findings and the position of the hindfoot (**Figs. 4.25 and 4.26**). If the dominant features are inclination of the forefoot and associated toe deformities, the condition is classified as pes cavovarus. Pes calcaneocavus is characterized by an increased vertical position of the heel. Measuring techniques can be used to evaluate the different components of the deformity (**Table 4.3**).

Lateral view	Talocalcaneal angle	Talar–first metatarsal angle	Tibiocalcaneal angle	Angle between inferior border of calcaneus and fifth metatarsal	Schematic drawing
Normal foot	25–55° (acute angle)	No angle; lines coincide after age 5	Normal; 60–80°	Obtuse angle (150–175°), apex upward	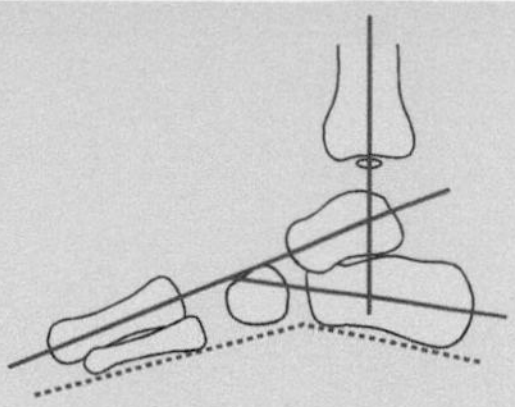
Pes equinovarus (clubfoot)	Angle decreased ($\alpha < 25°$), may equal 0°	Obtuse angle; apex downward	Obtuse angle	Obtuse angle; apex downward	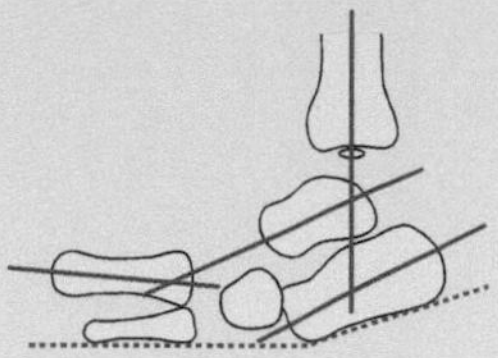
Overcorrected clubfoot (rocker-bottom deformity)	Angle decreased ($\alpha < 25°$), may equal 0°	Obtuse angle; apex downward	Obtuse angle	Obtuse angle; apex downward	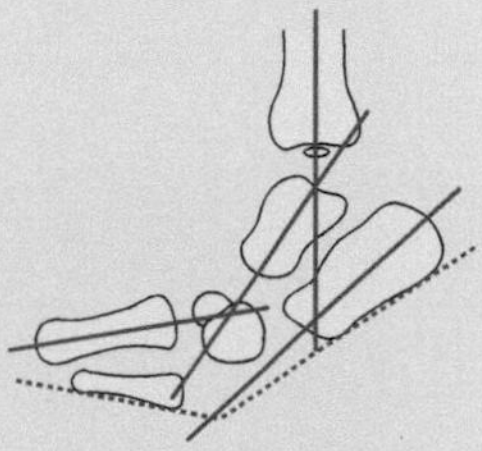
Pes planovalgus (flatfoot)	Angle increased ($\alpha > 55°$)	Obtuse angle; apex downward	Slightly increased	Obtuse angle; apex upward; may be slightly increased	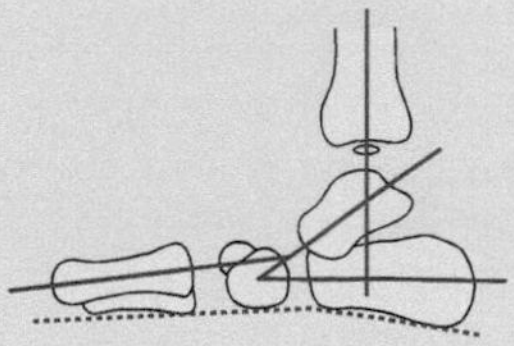
Metatarsus adductus	May be slightly increased	Obtuse angle; apex downward			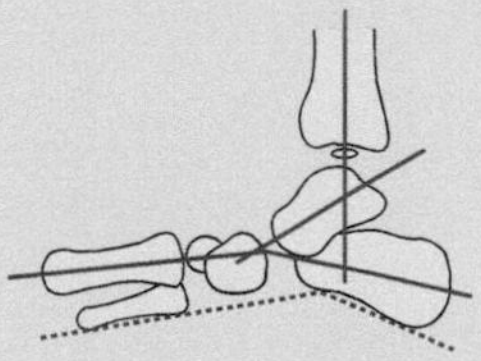
Pes cavus	Variable position of hindfoot; angle may be slightly increased	Obtuse angle; apex upward	Decreased	Decreased angle ($\alpha < 150°$); apex upward	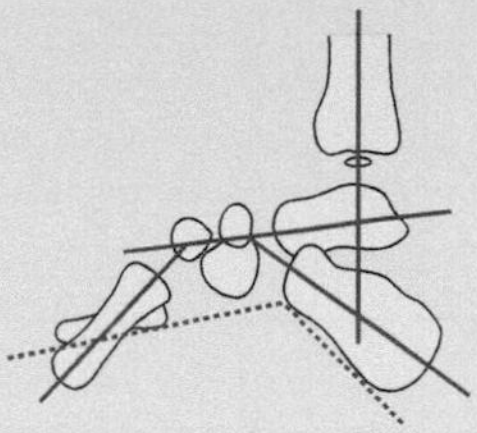

Fig. 4.21 Reference lines and angles used in evaluating pediatric foot deformities on lateral radiographs.

Dorsoplantar view	Talocalcaneal angle	Longitudinal axis of talus	Longitudinal axis of calcaneus	Metatarsal shafts	Schematic drawing
Normal foot	25–55° (acute angle)	Coincides with first metatarsal axis	Coincides with fourth metatarsal axis	Almost parallel	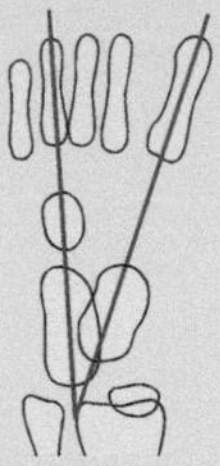
Pes equinovarus (clubfoot)	Angle decreased (α < 25°), may even be reversed	Runs lateral to first metatarsal; talar–first metatarsal angle: apex lateral (positive angle)	Runs lateral to fourth metatarsal	Shafts converge posteriorly, bases overlap	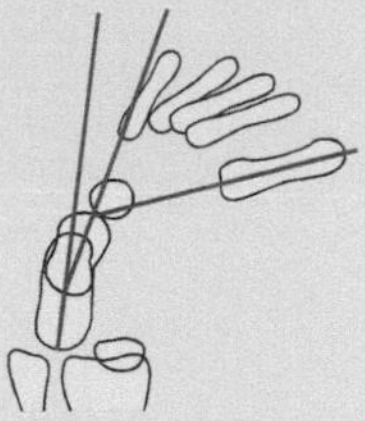
Overcorrected clubfoot (rocker-bottom deformity)	Angle decreased (α < 25°)				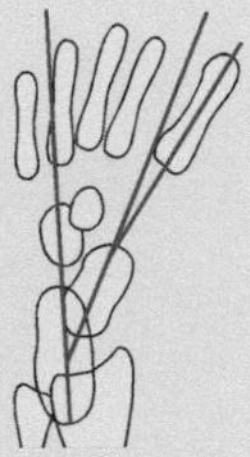
Pes planovalgus (flatfoot)	Angle increased (α > 55°)	Runs medial to first metatarsal; talar–first metatarsal angle: apex medial (negative angle)	Variable	Abducted forefoot	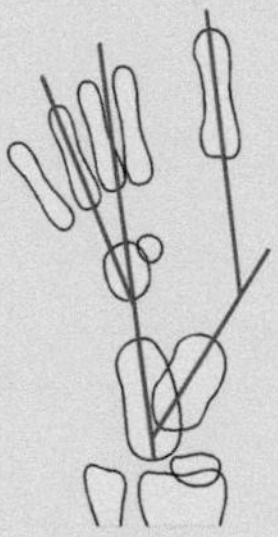
Metatarsus adductus		Crosses first metatarsal axis; talar–first metatarsal angle: apex lateral (positive angle)	Fourth metatarsal axis is farther lateral	Shafts converge posteriorly, bases overlap	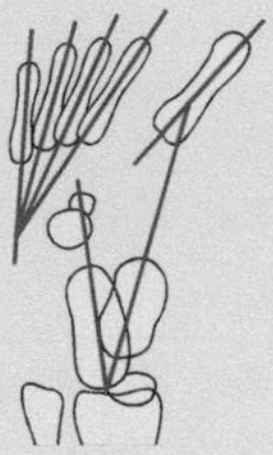
Pes cavus	Variable position of hindfoot; angle may be slightly increased	Normal findings unless associated with other abnormal components			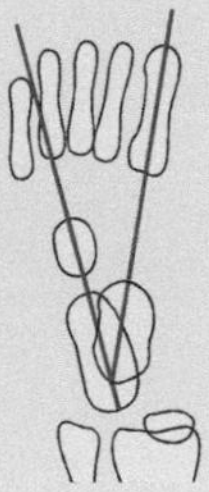

Fig. 4.22 Reference lines and angles used in evaluating pediatric foot deformities on dorsoplantar radiographs.

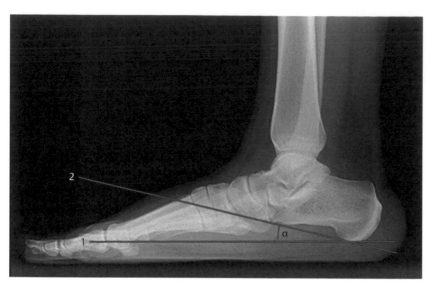

Fig. 4.23 Pes planovalgus with a decreased calcaneal inclination angle.
1 = Plantar plane
2 = Line tangent to inferior border of calcaneus
α = Calcaneal inclination angle (α = 15°)

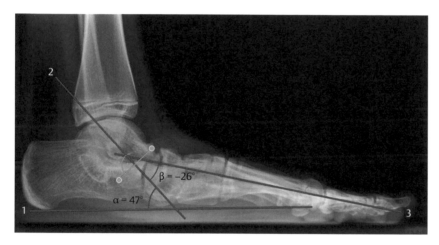

β = –26°

α = 47°

Fig. 4.24 Pes planovalgus with an increased talar declination angle and abnormal (negative) talar–first metatarsal angle.
1 = Plantar plane
2 = Longitudinal axis of talus
3 = Longitudinal axis of first metatarsal
α = Talar declination angle (α = 47°)
β = Talar–first metatarsal angle (β = – 26°)

Table 4.2 Radiographic measurements in pes planovalgus

	Normal range	Mean value	Value in pes planovalgus
Calcaneal inclination angle (see pp. 59–60)	20–30°		< 20°
Talar declination angle (see p. 60)	14–36°	21°	> 35°
Talar–first metatarsal angle			
• Lateral view (see p. 61)	+4 to – 4°		< – 4°
• Dorsoplantar view	0 to – 20°		Abducted forefoot: < 0°
Talocalcaneal angle			
• Lateral view (see p. 62)	Adults: 30–50°	35°	Hindfoot in valgus: > 50°
• Dorsoplantar view (see p. 62)	Adults: 20–45°	35°	Hindfoot in valgus: > 45°

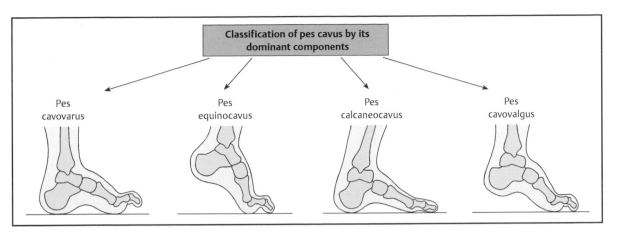

Fig. 4.25 Classification of pes cavus based on the dominant component of the deformity.

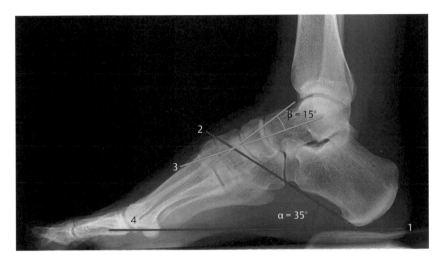

Fig. 4.26 Pes cavus with an increased calcaneal inclination angle and talar–first metatarsal angle.
1 = Plantar plane
2 = Line tangent to inferior border of calcaneus
3 = Longitudinal axis of talus
4 = Longitudinal axis of first metatarsal
α = Calcaneal inclination angle (α = 35°)
β = Talar–first metatarsal angle (β = 15°)

Table 4.3 Radiographic measurements in pes cavus

	Normal range	Mean value	Value in pes cavus
Calcaneal inclination angle (see pp. 59–60)	20–30°		> 30°
Talar declination angle (see p. 60)	14–36°	21°	< 14°
Talar–first metatarsal angle (lateral view; see pp. 60–61)	+4 to – 4°		> 4°
Talocalcaneal angle			
• Lateral view (see p. 62)	Adults: 30–50°	35°	
• Dorsoplantar view (see pp. 62–63)	Adults: 20–45°	35°	

! A vertical position of the calcaneus is the radiographic hallmark of pes calcaneocavus, in which markedly increased calcaneal inclination angles are typically found. The talar–first metatarsal angle is useful for quantifying the plantar flexion of the forefoot. Medial pes cavovarus is a relatively common form of pes cavus in which the inclination of the metastases decreases laterally to an almost normal alignment of the fifth metatarsal. The resulting crossed position of the first and fifth metatarsals is a characteristic feature of this deformity.

The position of the hindfoot is variable in pes cavus. In principle, the hindfoot may occupy a varus, neutral, or slightly valgus position. Varus is most common, however, and can be evaluated by measuring the talocalcaneal angles on dorsoplantar and lateral radiographs. Pes cavus is often accompanied by clawing of the lesser toes.

■ Metatarsus Adductus

Various terms have been used as synonyms for metatarsus adductus in the literature:
- Pes adductus
- Metatarsus varus
- Forefoot varus
- Sickle foot

The key feature of congenital metatarsus adductus is medial deviation of the forefoot at the level of the tarsometatarsal joints (Lisfranc joint). This differs somewhat from pes adductus, which is defined as a deviation the apex of which is located farther back at the level of the midtarsal joint (Chopart joint). In both deformities the hindfoot occupies a normal position or may be slightly everted.

As in other foot deformities, the radiographic analysis of metatarsus adductus is based on dorsoplantar and lateral radiographic views.

Metatarsal Convergence

The degree of medial deviation of the forefoot in metatarsus adductus decreases from the medial to lateral side. Viewed on a dorsoplantar radiograph of the foot, the longitudinal axes of the metatarsal shafts converge posteriorly and typically pass posterolateral to the tarsus. In a normal foot, the longitudinal axes of the metatarsals show only a slight degree of convergence and are directed posteriorly rather than posterolaterally (**Fig. 4.27**).

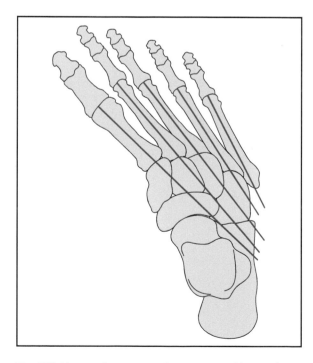

Fig. 4.27 Metatarsal convergence in metatarsus adductus. The longitudinal axes of the metatarsal shafts converge posterolateral to the tarsus.

Davis LA, Hatt WS. Congenital abnormalities of the foot. Radiology 1955;64(6):818–825

Metatarsus Adductus Angle

The metatarsus adductus angle, measured on a dorsoplantar radiograph of the foot, describes the angle formed by the longitudinal axis of the lesser tarsus and the longitudinal axis of the second metatarsal (**Fig. 4.28**). The metatarsals normally occupy a slightly adducted position relative to the lesser tarsus (10–20°). "Lesser tarsus" refers collectively to the cuneiform, cuboid and navicular bones.

> As it is somewhat tedious to construct the longitudinal axis of the lesser tarsus, Engel recommends using the longitudinal axis of the medial cuneiform as an alternative. That line is roughly parallel to the longitudinal axis of the lesser tarsus.

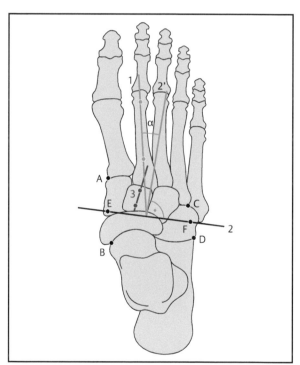

Fig. 4.28 Metatarsus adductus angle.
1 = Longitudinal axis of second metatarsal
2 = Line connecting points E and F
2' = Longitudinal axis of anterior tarsus (perpendicular to 2)
3 = Longitudinal axis of medial cuneiform (alternative to longitudinal axis of anterior tarsus)
A = Medial corner of first metatarsal
B = Medial border of talar articular surface
C = Lateral corner of fourth metatarsal
D = Anterolateral corner of calcaneus
E = Midpoint of line AB
F = Midpoint of line CD
α = Metatarsus adductus angle

The precise longitudinal axis of the lesser tarsus is constructed as follows: First, two straight lines are drawn on the medial and lateral sides of the tarsus. On the lateral side, a line is drawn from the anterolateral corner of the calcaneus to the lateral proximal corner of the fourth metatarsal. On the medial side, a line is drawn through the medial corner of the talar articular surface of the talonavicular joint and through the medial proximal corner of the first metatarsal. The line connecting the midpoints of the medial and lateral lines is the transverse axis of the lesser tarsus. The longitudinal axis of the lesser tarsus is then found by drawing a line perpendicular to the transverse axis.

The longitudinal axis of the medial cuneiform deviates from that axis by ~ 3°. Ranges of normal values are listed below:

Metatarsus adductus angle
• *Metatarsus adductus angle:*
• Normal range: α = 10–20°
• Metatarsus adductus: α > 20°
• *Simplified metatarsus adductus angle (Engel method):*
• Normal range: α = 13–23°
• Metatarsus adductus: α > 23°

> **!** The metatarsus adductus angle is useful only in children whose tarsal bones are mostly ossified and have well-defined radiographic margins. For this reason, the angle between the longitudinal axis of the calcaneus and the second metatarsal (see below) is used in newborns and small children to evaluate the relationship of the tarsus and metatarsals.

Engel E, Erlick N, Krems I. A simplified metatarsus adductus angle. J Am Podiatry Assoc 1983;73(12):620–628

Angle Between Longitudinal Axes of Calcaneus and Second Metatarsal

This angle is measured between the longitudinal axis of the calcaneus and the longitudinal axis of the second metatarsal viewed on a dorsoplantar radiograph (**Fig. 4.29**).

Angle between long axes of calcaneus and second metatarsal	
• *Normal value:*	α ≤ 22° (mean value: 10°)
• *Metatarsus adductus:*	α > 23°

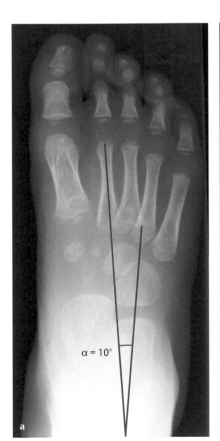
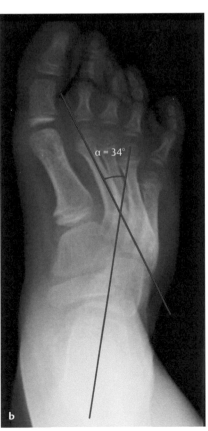

α = 10°

α = 34°

Fig. 4.29a,b Angle between longitudinal axes of calcaneus and second metatarsal.
a Normal foot.
b Increased angle in clubfoot deformity with adducted forefoot.

Foot

> **!** Because metatarsus adductus is often on a continuum with skew foot, which is characterized by concomitant medial deviation of the longitudinal talar axis, the talar–second metatarsal angle is less rewarding and can mimic normal findings in patients with coexisting deviation of the talus.

■ Pes Calcaneus

Pes calcaneus (**Fig. 4.30**) is characterized by a dorsiflexed position of the foot. It is common in newborns due to intrauterine pressure and is usually reversible in the absence of osseous deformity. Acquired pes cavus deformity is characterized by an abnormally high longitudinal arch with fixed plantar flexion of the forefoot typically associated with a pes calcaneus deformity.

Radiographic parameters for evaluating pes calcaneus are the calcaneal inclination angle and lateral tibiocalcaneal angle. The latter is measured between the longitudinal axes of the tibia and calcaneus on a lateral radiograph. Typically this angle is decreased in pes calcaneus.

> **Pes calcaneus**
> - *Calcaneal inclination angle:*
>   - Normal range: α = 20–30°
>   - Pes calcaneus: α > 30°
> - *Lateral tibiocalcaneal angle:*
>   - Normal values:
>   - Adults: α ≈ 70°
>   - Children age 6 years: α ≈ 65°
>   - Newborns: α ≈ 75°
>   - Pes calcaneus: α < 65°

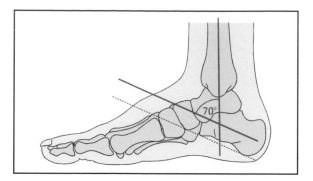

Fig. 4.30 Radiographic measurements in pes calcaneus. Lateral tibiocalcaneal angle.

may be lower than the calcaneus. As a rule, the lateral radiograph also shows a significant increase in the talocalcaneal angle.

> **!** The longitudinal axis of the calcaneus is horizontal in vertical talus, but sometimes it may be tilted upward, making the talocalcaneal angle a less useful indicator in the lateral radiograph.

> **Talocalcaneal angles in vertical talus**
> - *Dorsoplantar radiograph (newborns):*
>   - Normal range: α = 25–55°
>   - Vertical talus: α > 55°
> - *Lateral radiograph (newborns):*
>   - Normal range: α = 25–55°
>   - Vertical talus: α > 55° (often ≈ 90°)

Congenital Foot Deformities

■ Vertical Talus

Congenital vertical talus (**Fig. 4.31**) is a rare, mostly unilateral foot deformity that is often associated with other congenital anomalies (e.g., myelomeningocele, arthrogryposis). Its morphologic hallmarks are a downward-directed (vertical) talus and a dislocated talonavicular joint with posterolateral dislocation of the navicular.

Talocalcaneal Angles

Typically the talocalcaneal angle is markedly increased in the dorsoplantar view as the result of significant hindfoot valgus and forefoot abduction.

The lateral radiograph shows an almost vertically oriented talus that is displaced downward and whose head

Functional Examination in Plantar Flexion

Vertical talus can be distinguished from flexible flatfoot (pes planovalgus) by comparing the standard lateral radiograph with a radiograph taken in maximum plantar flexion and assessing the reducibility of the talus and navicular (**Fig. 4.32**):
- *Vertical talus:* The navicular in vertical talus is not reduced by maximum plantar flexion, so that the longitudinal axis of the talus is roughly parallel to the tibial axis in both the standard and flexion views. The talus and first metatarsal are not parallel.
- *Pes planovalgus (flexible flatfoot):* Plantar flexion reduces the navicular and realigns the talus and first metatarsal, lining up their longitudinal axes.

Drennan JC. Congenital vertical talus. J Bone Joint Surg Am 1995;77:1916–1923

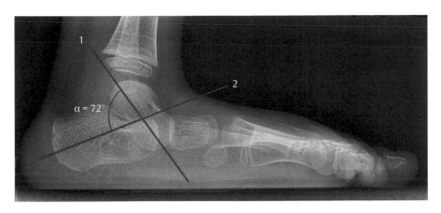

Fig. 4.31 Pediatric flatfoot deformity with a markedly increased talocalcaneal angle.
1 = Longitudinal axis of talus
2 = Longitudinal axis of calcaneus
α = Talocalcaneal angle (α = 72°)

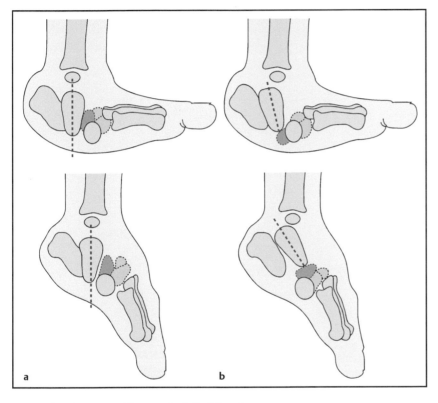

Fig. 4.32a,b Functional examination of pediatric flatfoot to distinguish between vertical talus and flexible flatfoot (pes planovalgus). Dashed lines indicate the tarsal bones preformed in cartilage. Upper drawing shows each foot in a plantigrade position, lower drawing in maximum plantar flexion.
a Vertical talus.
b Flexible flatfoot.

■ Pes Equinovarus (Congenital Clubfoot)

Pes equinovarus (**Fig. 4.33**) is a complex congenital foot deformity made up of the following components, which are not fully correctable:

- *Pes equinus:* plantar flexion of the foot
- *Pes varus:* varus position of the hindfoot
- *Metatarsus adductus:* adducted position of the forefoot and midfoot relative to the hindfoot
- *Pes supinatus:* supination of the forefoot and midfoot relative to the hindfoot
- *Pes cavus*

Clubfoot is evaluated on dorsoplantar and lateral radiographs of the foot. The dorsoplantar view is obtained with the beam angled 30° to the horizontal and centered on the talar neck.

> **!** In small children, an assistant should hold the foot in a position of maximum correction during the exposure.

Talocalcaneal Angles

The radiographic analysis of congenital clubfoot is focused on the talocalcaneal complex. Most important are the talocalcaneal angles, which are measured on dorsolantar and lateral radiographs. In newborns, whose tarsal bones still have an elliptical shape, the talocalcaneal angles are

4

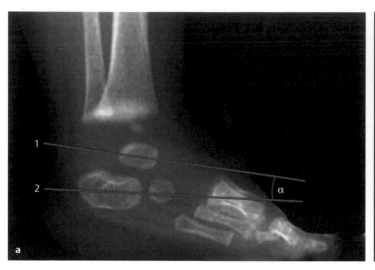
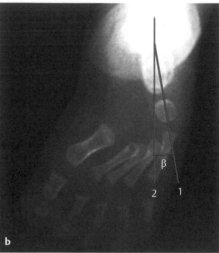

Fig. 4.33a,b Clubfoot deformity with abnormal talocalcaneal angles.

1 = Longitudinal axis of talus
2 = Longitudinal axis of calcaneus

a Lateral view. Talocalcaneal angle α = 5°.
b Dorsoplantar view. Talocalcaneal angle β = 9°.

defined by the longitudinal axes of the talus and calcaneus. Clubfoot deformity is marked by a decrease in the talocalcaneal angles on dorsoplantar and lateral radiographs; the longitudinal axes of the talus and calcaneus may even be parallel.

Talocalcaneal angles in pes equinovarus	
• *Dorsoplantar radiograph (newborns):*	
• Normal range:	α = 25–55°
• Clubfoot:	α < 25°
• *Lateral radiograph (newborns):*	
• Normal range:	α = 25–55°
• Clubfoot:	α < 25°

Talar–First Metatarsal Angle (Dorsoplantar View)

The talar–first metatarsal angle can be measured on the dorsoplantar radiograph to evaluate the increased adduction of the forefoot in pes equinovarus.

The angle is measured between the longitudinal axis of the talus and the longitudinal axis of the first metatarsal. Normally the longitudinal axes of the talus and first metatarsal are approximately parallel or the long axis of the talus is directed somewhat more medially (resulting in a negative measured angle). But if the long axis of the talus is directed more laterally than that of the first metatarsal, the radiograph will show a positive, abnormal angle signifying increased adduction of the forefoot.

Talar–first metatarsal angle
• *Normal range:* α = 0 to – 20°
• *Clubfoot:* increased forefoot adduction: α > 0°

! Because radiographs in newborns show only the ossification centers of the talus, calcaneus and metatarsals, they are of limited use for evaluating the foot deformity in three dimensions. In particular, the prognostically important talonavicular joint cannot be directly evaluated because the navicular is not ossified until the second or third year of life. A combined assessment of the dorsoplantar talonavicular angle and talar–first metatarsal angle is helpful in evaluating the talonavicular joint. If the talar–first metatarsal angle is > 15° and the talonavicular angle is < 15°, talonavicular subluxation should be diagnosed.

Simons GW. Analytical radiography of club feet. J Bone Joint Surg Br 1977;59-B(4):485–489

Plantar Soft-Tissue Thickness

The generalized soft-tissue enlargement that occurs in acromegaly can be measured at certain sites of predilection. This includes thickening of the plantar soft tissues (**Fig. 4.34**).

The thickness of the plantar soft tissues is measured as the distance between the lowest point of the calcaneus and the skin line and also between the inferior margin of the proximal fifth metatarsal head and the skin line.

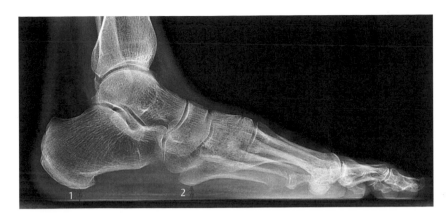

Fig. 4.34 Plantar soft-tissue thickness.
1 = Measurement of soft-tissue thickness at the lowest point of the calcaneus
2 = Measurement of soft-tissue thickness below the proximal head of the fifth metatarsal

Plantar soft-tissue thickness

- *Normal values:*
  - Calcaneal fat pad: ≤ 25 mm
  - Metatarsal fat pad: 5 to ≤ 16 mm
- *Values in acromegaly:*
  - Calcaneal fat pad: > 25 mm
  - Metatarsal fat pad: > 16 mm

! Thickening of the plantar fat pad may also occur in other diseases associated with diffuse soft-tissue swelling in the foot (myxedema, reflex sympathetic dystrophy, lymphedema, traumatic edema), so this sign should always be interpreted within the overall context. A thickened fat pad should be interpreted only as a sign suggestive of acromegaly or as a characteristic feature of the disease.

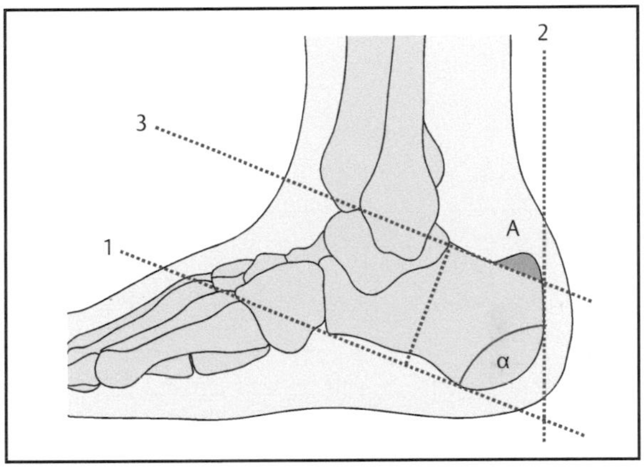

Fig. 4.35 Radiographic measurement of Haglund deformity.
1 = Line tangent to inferior border of calcaneus
2 = Line tangent to calcaneal tuberosity and posterosuperior border of calcaneus
3 = Line parallel to 1 through posterior margin of subtalar joint
A = Portion that extends beyond parallel pitch line 3 is interpreted as Haglund exostosis
α = Philip–Fowler angle

Haglund Deformity

Haglund deformity (**Fig. 4.35**) is a circumscribed, painful swelling at the Achilles tendon insertion caused by an abnormal prominence or projection of the posterosuperior calcaneus along with repetitive stresses and mechanical irritation. Adjacent soft-tissue structures show variable involvement by reactive inflammatory changes (Achilles tendon enthesopathy or retrocalcaneal bursitis).

The calcaneus is evaluated on a standing lateral radiograph of the foot and ankle. The film typically shows a prominent right-angled or acute-angled bump projecting upward from the posterior border of the calcaneus.

Various methods have been described for detecting and quantifying the bony prominence (see below).

Philip–Fowler Angle

The calcaneal angle of Philip–Fowler is constructed by drawing a line tangent to the posterosuperior border of the calcaneus and the calcaneal tuberosity. The Philip–Fowler angle is formed by that line and a line tangent to the inferior border of the calcaneus (longitudinal axis of the calcaneus).

Philip–Fowler angle

- *Normal range:* α = 44–69°
- *Prominence of superior calcaneal tuberosity:* α > 75°

Fowler A, Philip JF. Abnormality of calcaneus as a cause of painful heel: its diagnosis and operative treatment. Br J Surg 1945;32:494–498

Parallel Pitch Lines of Pavlov

Evaluation of the parallel pitch lines (PPL) is a method for detecting a bony prominence or projection on the posterosuperior border of the calcaneus. First a reference line is drawn along the inferior border of the calcaneus. It passes through the anterior projection of the calcaneal tuberosity on the plantar side and the inferior corner of the calcaneus, which articulates with the cuboid. This line corresponds to the tangent to the inferior calcaneal border (longitudinal axis of the calcaneus) used in the other methods. Next a line parallel to that line is constructed through the posterior edge of the subtalar joint. If the posterosuperior border of the calcaneus extends above that line, it is considered to be prominent and a predisposing factor for Haglund deformity.

- – *PPL*: normal finding; the posterosuperior border of the calcaneus is below the line through the posterior edge of the subtalar joint.
- + *PPL*: abnormal finding; prominent posterosuperior border of the calcaneus.

!

Both methods used to evaluate the shape of the posterosuperior border of the calcaneus are deemed controversial in the orthopedic literature. One large study found no significant difference in the prevalence of osseous changes between a group of patients with clinically diagnosed Haglund deformity and a control group. Besides the shape of the calcaneus, it is clear that the position of the calcaneus and other factors play a role in the pathogenesis of Haglund deformity.

Lu CC, Cheng YM, Fu YC, Tien YC, Chen SK, Huang PJ. Angle analysis of Haglund syndrome and its relationship with osseous variations and Achilles tendon calcification. Foot Ankle Int 2007;28(2):181–185

Pavlov H, Heneghan MA, Hersh A, Goldman AB, Vigorita V. The Haglund syndrome: initial and differential diagnosis. Radiology 1982;144(1):83–88

Radiographic Evaluation of the Syndesmosis

Before the distal tibiofibular syndesmosis could be directly assessed by magnetic resonance imaging (MRI), diagnostic imaging had to rely on indirect signs of syndesmotic insufficiency. Traditionally the syndesmosis was evaluated on radiographs taken in a (true) anteroposterior (AP) and lateral projection and supplemented by an oblique mortise view. The mortise view is an AP projection of the ankle joint with the foot in ~ 20° of internal rotation. The parameters measured in the AP view are described below.

!

A common practice in many European countries is to obtain the "standard" AP view with the foot in 15–20° of internal rotation. This gives a clear projection of the ankle mortise and eliminates the need for a third view.

The parameters listed in **Table 4.4** and **Fig. 4.36** have traditionally been used to asses the integrity of the syndesmosis. The cutoff values listed in **Table 4.4** refer to the AP radiograph with the foot internally rotated (15–20°).

In a true AP projection of the ankle joint, the anterior tubercle, which gives attachment to the anterior syndesmosis, forms the lateral border of the tibia (overlapped by the fibula) and the total clear space (TCS) is bounded by the posterior tubercle, or the posterior aspect of the tibia (**Fig. 4.38**). With increasing internal rotation of the foot, the anterior tubercle moves farther medially. On radiographs with more than 20° of internal foot rotation, the anterior tubercle forms the boundary of the TCS. On radiographs with moderate internal rotation, the posterior tubercle borders on the TCS, but the anterior and posterior tubercles cannot be reliably differentiated.

The normal values for a true AP projection of the ankle mortise are a TCS < 5 mm and a tibiofibular overlap

Table 4.4 Indicators of the integrity of the distal tibiofibular syndesmosis on conventional radiographs (anteroposterior view, foot in 10–20° internal rotation)

Parameter	Technique	Normal value	Suggestive of syndesmotic injury
Total clear space (TCS)	Distance between the medial margin of fibular groove (posterior border of the tibia) and the medial border of the fibula, measured 1 cm above the tibial plafond	< 5 mm	≥ 5 mm
Tibiofibular overlap (TFO)	Distance between the lateral border of the distal tibia and the medial border of the fibula, also measured 1 cm above the tibial plafond	> 1 mm	≤ 1 mm
Medial clear space (MCS)	Distance between the lateral border of the medial malleolus and the medial border of the talus, measured 0.5 cm below the tibial plafond	≤ 4 mm	> 4 mm
Talocrural angle (Fig. 4.37)	Formed by a line perpendicular to the distal tibial articular surface and a line connecting the distal ends of the malleoli	83° ± 4°	> 87°

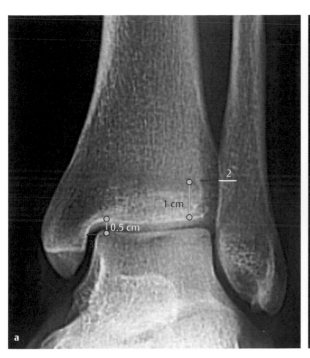 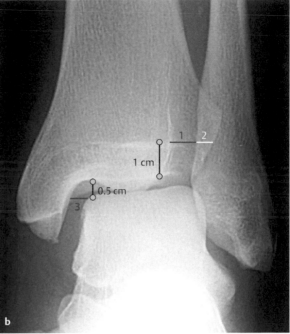

Fig. 4.36 Measurement of TCS, TFO and MCS on anteroposterior radiograph of the ankle joint (foot in 10–20° of internal rotation, standard projection).

1 = Total clear space (TCS)
2 = Tibiofibular overlap (TFO)
3 = Medial clear space (MCS)

a Normal ankle joint (TCS = 0.4 cm, TFO = 0.3 cm, MCS = 0.2 mm).
b Isolated tear of the tibiofibular syndesmosis (TCS = 0.7 cm, TFO = 0.25 cm, MCS = 0.5 cm).

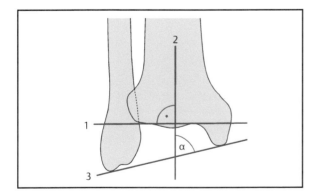

Fig. 4.37 Talocrural angle.
1 = Line tangent to tibial articular surface of ankle joint
2 = Line perpendicular to 1
3 = Line connecting the tips of the malleoli
α = Talocrural angle

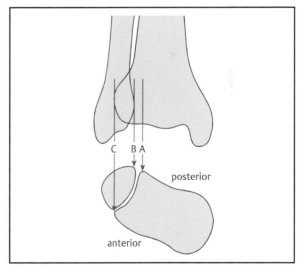

Fig. 4.38 Projection of the anterior and posterior tubercles on an anteroposterior radiograph of the ankle joint (true anteroposterior view, no internal rotation of the foot).
A = Posterior tubercle (gives attachment to posterior syndesmosis)
B = Medial border of fibula
C = Anterior tubercle (gives attachment to anterior syndesmosis)

Foot

4

> 10 mm. The dependence of the reference values on joint position is a weakness of this method.

!

> These parameters have a very low sensitivity for detecting syndesmotic injuries. Sensitivities reported in the literature are no higher than 65%. All syndesmotic tears that do not present with a pathologic joint alignment are missed. Consequently, MRI should always be the imaging modality of choice when there is clinical suspicion of a syndesmotic tear. As false-positive findings are rare on conventional radiographs, however, abnormal measurements warrant investigation by MRI because the likelihood of a syndesmotic injury is high.

Sclafani SJ. Ligamentous injury of the lower tibiofibular syndesmosis: radiographic evidence. Radiology 1985;156(1):21–27

Types of Accessory Navicular Described by Lawson

The accessory navicular (synonym: os tibiale externum) is an accessory ossicle located posteromedial to the navicular tuberosity. It is present in 15–20% of the population. Lawson described three types of accessory navicular (**Fig. 4.39**).

Whereas type 1 is a normal variant with no pathologic significance, type 2 is a relatively common source of medial foot pain and is often associated with disorders at the insertion of the tibialis posterior tendon. In type 2 cases the tibialis posterior tendon usually inserts (atypically) on the accessory navicular. Reactive, microtrauma-induced changes about the synchondrosis and tendon insufficiency leading to flatfoot are typical secondary findings. Type 3, also called a "cornuate navicular," is associated with similar findings related to a prominent bony margin at the tendon attachment.

Lawson JP, Ogden JA, Sella E, Barwick KW. The painful accessory navicular. Skeletal Radiol 1984;12(4):250–262

Type	Description	
1	Appears on radiographs as an oval, well-circumscribed ossicle just separate from the navicular; a sesamoid in the tibialis posterior tendon	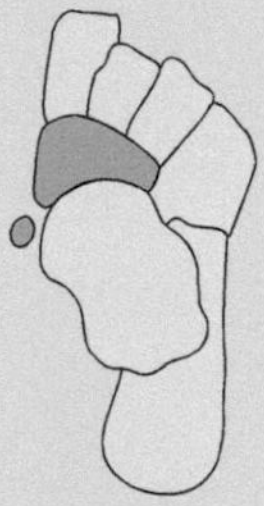
2	Represents an accessory ossification center for the navicular. The triangular or heart-shaped ossicle is broadly attached to the navicular by a synchondrosis, reflected radiographically by slightly irregular margins at the interface and by the shape of the accessory navicular	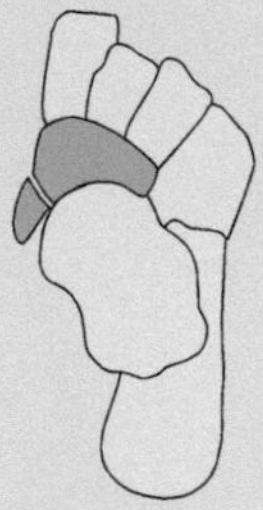
3	Cornuate navicular. The accessory ossification center is fused to the navicular, creating a prominent medial extension	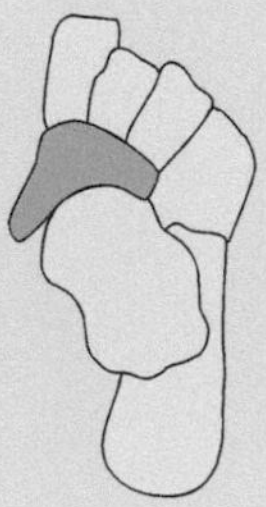

Fig. 4.39 Lawson classification of accessory navicular types.

Foot

4

Classification of Peroneal Tendon Dislocation

Dislocations of the peroneal tendons, which may result from sudden, jarring movements of the ankle joint in pronation and abduction, lead to injuries of the peroneal retinacula. At the level of the distal fibula, the bony tendon groove is reinforced laterally by a fibrocartilage ridge to which the superior retinaculum is attached.

The fibrocartilage ridge and superior retinaculum are important anatomic stabilizers of the peroneal tendons on the posterolateral side. Eckert and Davis published a classification of peroneal tendon dislocations describing the various grades of injury (**Fig. 4.40**).

Eckert WR, Davis EA Jr. Acute rupture of the peroneal retinaculum. J Bone Joint Surg Am 1976;58(5):670–672

Type	Description	
1	Separation of the superior retinaculum from the lateral malleolus and fibrocartilage ridge	
2	Separation of the superior retinaculum and fibrocartilage ridge from the lateral malleolus	
3	Bony avulsion of the superior retinaculum and fibrocartilage ridge from the lateral malleolus	

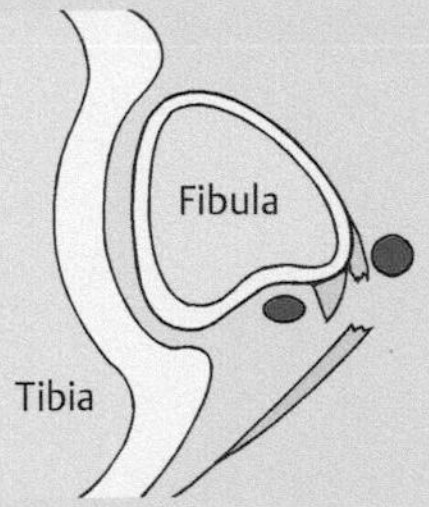

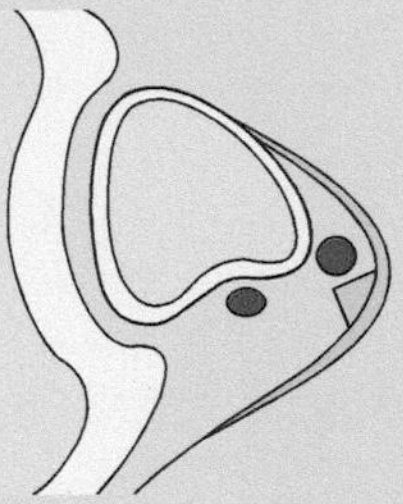

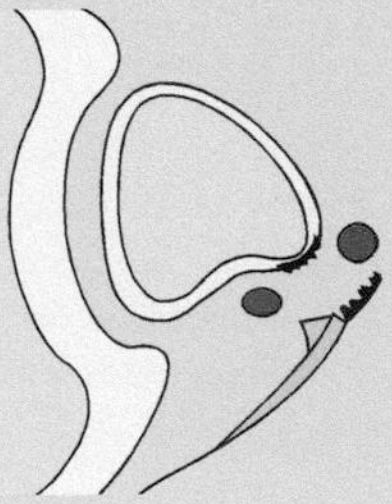

Fig. 4.40 Eckert and Davis classification of peroneal tendon dislocation.

Foot

4

5 Shoulder Joint

Bigliani Classification of Acromial Morphology

Bigliani et al (1986) identified three anatomic variants of acromial morphology in cadaver specimens based on radiographic outlet views of the shoulder joint (**Fig. 5.1**):

- Type 1: flat
- Type 2: curved
- Type 3: hooked

Moreover, a correlation was found between the type 3 acromion (and, to a lesser degree, type 2) and the development of rotator cuff tears.

Following the technique of Bigliani et al, acromial shape is evaluated on the outlet view radiograph (Y view).

If magnetic resonance imaging (MRI) is used, acromial shape is evaluated on sagittal oblique images perpendicular to the supraspinatus muscle belly. The accuracy of this method is limited by the fact that the appearance of acromial shape varies somewhat with the position of the MRI plane. Mayerhofer et al performed a comparative study to determine the slice position that is most representative for depicting acromial shape (**Fig. 5.2**). When just one sagittal MRI slice is used to evaluate acromial shape, the slice position S1 should be just lateral to the acromioclavicular joint. The image plane should not cut the joint capsule or acromioclavicular ligament. Accuracy

can be increased by evaluating a second slice at a more lateral position, S2 (~ 4 mm lateral to the acromial margin). The shape of the acromion is assessed on slice S1. If a type 3 acromion is suspected, then the S2 slice is additionally evaluated because it is more specific for a type 3 morphology. This means that if S2 does not confirm type 3, a type 2 acromion is present.

A quantitative method is also available for determining acromial type. First a sagittal oblique slice is acquired, and a line tangent to the undersurface of the acromion is drawn and divided into thirds with two orthogonal lines as shown in **Fig. 5.2**. Then the angle α between the anterior third and the posterior two-thirds of the acromion is measured. If $\alpha > 20°$, then the angle between the anterior two-thirds and the posterior third (β) is also measured. The findings are interpreted as follows:

Acromial types	
• *Type 1 (flat acromion):*	$\alpha \leq 10°$
• *Type 2 (curved acromion):*	$10 < \alpha \leq 20°$ or
	$\alpha > 20°$ and $\beta > 10°$
• *Type 3 (hooked acromion):*	$\alpha > 20°$ and $\beta \leq 10°$

The analysis is most accurate when the arithmetic means of the angles measured in S1 and S2 are calculated.

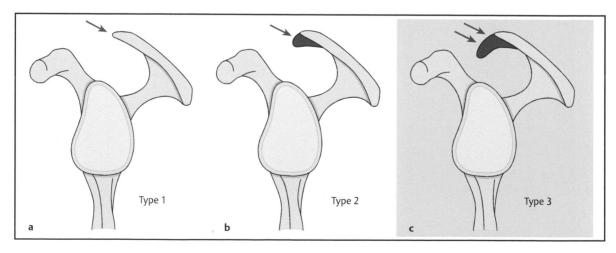

Fig. 5.1a–c Bigliani classification of acromial morphology. Type 3 is considered a predisposing factor for subacromial impingement.

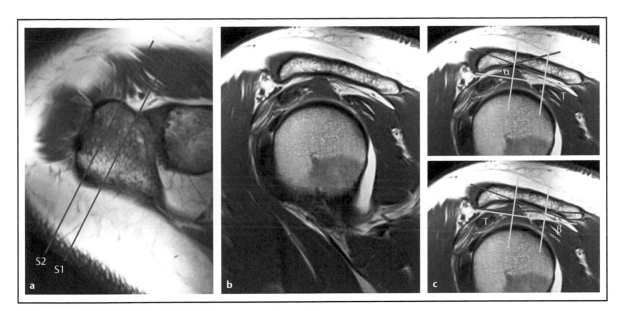

Fig. 5.2a–c Evaluation of acromial shape on sagittal oblique magnetic resonance images.

a Transverse magnetic resonance image for locating the sagittal oblique slices S1 and S2, which will be used to assess acromial morphology.

b The sagittal oblique slice just lateral to the acromioclavicular joint (S1) is the most important position for evaluating acromial shape.

c Acromial shape can be assessed on S1 or calculated by determining angles α and β.

T = Line tangent to the acromial undersurface, divided into thirds
α = Angle or slope between the anterior third and posterior two-thirds of the acromion
β = Angle or slope between the two anterior thirds and posterior third of the acromion

Bigliani et al also found a slight correlation between the type 2 acromion and rotator cuff tears, but subsequent studies were unable to confirm this finding. At present, only type 3 is considered a predisposing factor for subacromial impingement and rotator cuff tears. It appears, however, that the type 3 acromion is acquired rather than congenital, i.e., that the downward bony prominence results from age-related degenerative processes, usually involving the presence of enthesophytes at the attachment of the coracoacromial ligament.

Bigliani LU, Morrison DS, April EW. The morphology of the acromion and its relationship to rotator cuff tears. Orthop Trans 1986;10:228

Mayerhoefer ME, Breitenseher MJ, Roposch A, Treitl C, Wurnig C. Comparison of MRI and conventional radiography for assessment of acromial shape. AJR Am J Roentgenol 2005;184(2):671–675

Types of Os Acromiale

The acromion is preformed in cartilage. Three ossification centers appear in the acromion between 10 and 18 years of age and fuse by age 25 (**Fig. 5.3**). A persistent ossification center (with a corresponding unfused growth plate) is called an os acromiale. The three acromial ossification centers are named as follows:

- Preacromion
- Mesoacromion
- Meta-acromion

Park et al distinguished seven types of os acromiale based on the location of the fusion defect (**Fig. 5.3**). Type I, caused by failure of fusion between the mesoacromion and meta-acromion, is by far the most common form. With conventional radiography, an os acromiale is most clearly depicted on axial views of the shoulder joint. With MRI and computed tomography (CT), transverse and coronal oblique images can be used to classify the type of os acromiale.

Os acromiale is important because it might be a predisposing factor for subacromial impingement.

Liberson F. Os acromiale: a contested anomaly. J Bone Joint Surg 1937;19:683–689

Park JG, Lee JK, Phelps CT. Os acromiale associated with rotator cuff impingement: MR imaging of the shoulder. Radiology 1994;193(1):255–257

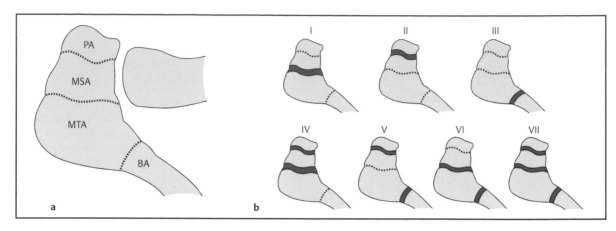

Fig. 5.3a,b Development of the acromion.

a Ossification centers of the acromion.

b Possible configurations of the os acromiale due to nonfusion of one or two growth plates (after Park et al).

PA = Preacromion

MSA = Mesoacromion
MTA = Meta-acromion
BA = Basiacromion

Glenoid Version

Glenoid version or inclination is described by the scapuloglenoid angle, which is formed by the glenohumeral articular surface and a plane perpendicular to the body of the scapula (**Fig. 5.4**). The scapuloglenoid angle can be measured on a transverse CT or MRI section that is perpendicular to the glenohumeral joint or glenoid articular surface and passes through the center of the glenoid fossa.

First the following reference lines are drawn: The first line (a) is tangent to the anterior and posterior glenoid rims. The second line (b) runs through the center of the glenoid and through the posterior margin of the scapular body. Glenoid version is then measured between line a and line b', which is perpendicular to b.

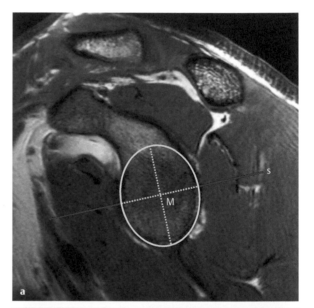

Glenoid version	
• *Normal range:*	0–9° of retroversion
• *Decreased posterior stability:*	Retroversion > 15°
• *Decreased anterior stability:*	Anteversion > 5°

Note: These reference values have been determined in an experimental setting.

Fig. 5.4a,b Measurement of glenoid version (scapuloglenoid angle).

a The measurement is performed on a transverse section s through the center M of the glenoid.

  M = Center of glenoid

  s = Transverse section through M

b The scapuloglenoid angle is formed by a and b'.

  a = Line connecting the anterior and posterior glenoid rims

  b = Line through the glenoid center and the posterior scapular margin

  b'= Line perpendicular to b

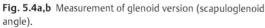

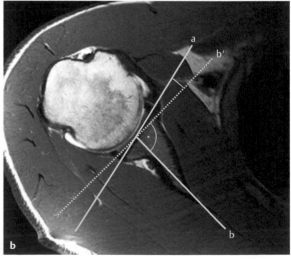

! Abnormally increased retroversion is a significant causal factor in posterior instability. With glenoid dysplasia, retroversion is increased as the result of hypoplasia of the posteroinferior glenoid. The presence of 15° or more retroversion signifies at least an incomplete form of glenoid dysplasia. Increased anteversion (rare) may promote anterior instability of the glenohumeral joint.

Churchill RS, Brems JJ, Kotschi H. Glenoid size, inclination, and version: an anatomic study. J Shoulder Elbow Surg 2001;10(4):327–332

Kikuchi K, Itoi E, Yamamoto N, et al Scapular inclination and glenohumeral joint stability: a cadaveric study. J Orthop Sci 2008;13(1):72–77

Weishaupt D, Zanetti M, Nyffeler RW, Gerber C, Hodler J. Posterior glenoid rim deficiency in recurrent (atraumatic) posterior shoulder instability. Skeletal Radiol 2000;29(4):204–210

Acromiohumeral Distance

Large rotator cuff tears and fatty degeneration of the constituent muscles may lead to secondary superior migration of the humeral head. The degree of this upward migration can be quantified on conventional radiographs by measuring the acromiohumeral distance (AHD; **Fig. 5.5**).

The AHD can be measured on an anteroposterior (AP) radiograph of the shoulder joint in neutral rotation, the Rockwood view, or the outlet view (Y-view). The advantage of the Rockwood view is that the central ray is tangent to the slope of the acromion. Nevertheless, an AP radiograph in neutral rotation is still the most widely recommended view in the literature. The patient's back is angled 30–45° to the film plane to give a tangential projection of the glenohumeral joint. The AHD is measured as the distance between the superior margin of the humeral head and the undersurface of the acromion. The reference values are as follows:

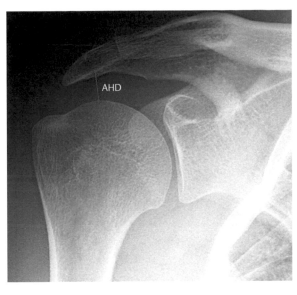

Fig. 5.5 Measurement of the acromiohumeral distance (AHD) on an anteroposterior radiograph of the shoulder joint in neutral rotation.

Acromiohumeral distance	
• *Mean value (in healthy subjects):*	AHD = 1.05 cm
• *Abnormal:*	AHD ≤ 7 mm

! If the acromiohumeral distance is at or below the cutoff value of 7 mm, it should be assumed that a complete rotator cuff tear is present. In a study by Saupe et al, the size of the rotator cuff tear and the degree of fatty degeneration of the infraspinatus muscle were found to have the greatest influence on acromiohumeral distance.

Cotty P, Proust F, Bertrand P, et al. Rupture of the rotator cuff. Quantification of indirect signs in standard radiology and the Leclercq maneuver. [Article in French] J Radiol 1988;69(11):633–638

Saupe N, Pfirrmann CW, Schmid MR, Jost B, Werner CM, Zanetti M. Association between rotator cuff abnormalities and reduced acromiohumeral distance. AJR Am J Roentgenol 2006;187(2):376–382

Shoulder Joint

5

Rotator Cuff Tears

General Classification

Rotator cuff tears are classified as complete or partial (**Fig. 5.6**):

- *Complete tear:* A complete tear is defined as one that extends through the full thickness of the tendon (from the articular to the bursal surface). It is sufficient for the tear to involve the entire thickness of the tendon at a single site. Thus, "complete" does not necessarily mean that the tendon is completely severed over its entire width.
- *Partial tear:* Partial tears are partial-thickness lesions. They are further classified by their location as bursal-sided tears, articular-sided tears, and intratendinous tears. These types are most easily identified on oblique coronal MRI images angled parallel to the supraspinatus muscle.

Specific Types of Rotator Cuff Tears

Recent discoveries on the location, pathogenic mechanism, and treatment implications of rotator cuff tears have led to subclassifications that stress the importance of specific lesion types. Because a uniform classification does not exist, lesions that are the same or very similar are sometimes described with different terms and are often designated by acronyms.

Several types of tear are described and illustrated in **Fig. 5.7**.

Ellman Classification of Rotator Cuff Tears

Partial rotator cuff tears can be classified by the depth of the tear (**Fig. 5.8**). The diameter of an intact tendon is 1.0–1.2 cm. The Ellman classification also indicates which side of the tendon is affected (A = Articular side, B = Bursal side).

Ellman H. Diagnosis and treatment of incomplete rotator cuff tears. Clin Orthop Relat Res 1990;254(254):64–74

Snyder Classification of Rotator Cuff Tears

The Snyder or SCOI (Southern California Orthopedic Institute) classification of rotator cuff tears is widely used in orthopedics. The initial letter of the designation indicates whether the lesion is an articular-sided partial tear (A), a bursal-sided partial tear (B), or a complete tear (C). The letter is followed by a number indicating the degree of tendon damage visible at arthroscopy.

Table 5.1 shows the numerical designations used for partial tears, and **Table 5.2** shows the designations used for complete tears.

> Since the evaluation of tendon damage in this classification is based on arthroscopic appearance, the designations are not fully applicable to radiologic findings.

Snyder SJ. Arthroscopic classification of rotator cuff lesions and surgical decision making. In: Snyder SJ. Shoulder arthroscopy. 2ed. Philadelphia: Lippincott Williams & Wilkens; 2003: 201–207

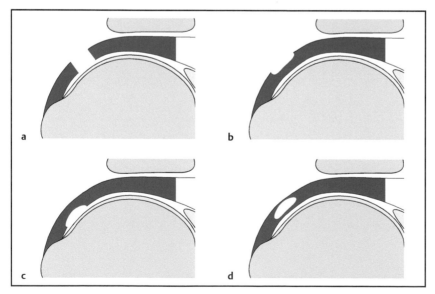

Fig. 5.6a–d General classification of rotator cuff tears on coronal oblique magnetic resonance images. Schematic representation.
a Complete (full-thickness) tear.
b Bursal-sided partial tear.
c Articular-sided partial tear.
d Intratendinous partial tear.

Type	Description	
PASTA lesion	Partial articular-sided supraspinatus tendon avulsion lesion. Articular-sided partial tear of the supraspinatus tendon with involvement of the tendo-osseous junction (= footprint lesion). Tension and shear forces cause an avulsion at the footprint attachment with variable delamination of deep tendon components	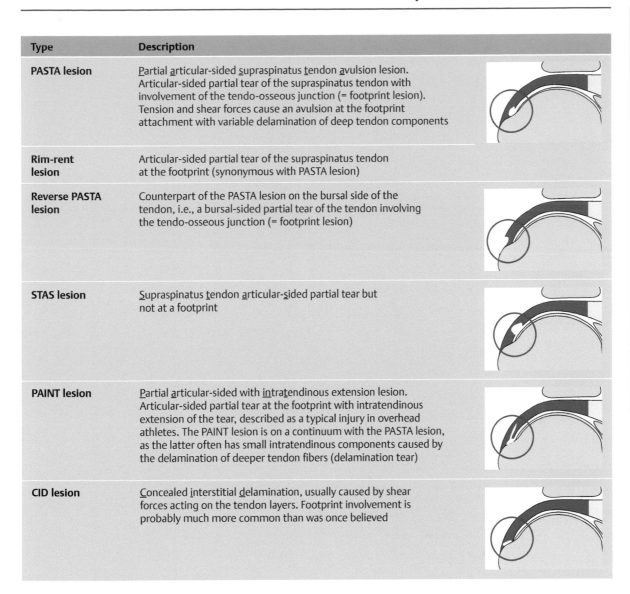
Rim-rent lesion	Articular-sided partial tear of the supraspinatus tendon at the footprint (synonymous with PASTA lesion)	
Reverse PASTA lesion	Counterpart of the PASTA lesion on the bursal side of the tendon, i.e., a bursal-sided partial tear of the tendon involving the tendo-osseous junction (= footprint lesion)	
STAS lesion	Supraspinatus tendon articular-sided partial tear but not at a footprint	
PAINT lesion	Partial articular-sided with intratendinous extension lesion. Articular-sided partial tear at the footprint with intratendinous extension of the tear, described as a typical injury in overhead athletes. The PAINT lesion is on a continuum with the PASTA lesion, as the latter often has small intratendinous components caused by the delamination of deeper tendon fibers (delamination tear)	
CID lesion	Concealed interstitial delamination, usually caused by shear forces acting on the tendon layers. Footprint involvement is probably much more common than was once believed	

Fig. 5.7 Common types of rotator cuff lesions.

Table 5.1 Snyder classification of partial rotator cuff tears (A = Articular-sided, B = Bursal-sided)

Type	Description
0	Normal tendon with smooth coverings of synovium and bursa
1	Minimal, superficial bursal or synovial irritation or slight capsular fraying in a small localized area; usually < 1 cm
2	Actually fraying and failure of some rotator cuff fibers in addition to synovial, bursal or capsular injury; usually < 2 cm
3	More severe rotator cuff injury that includes fraying and fragmentation of tendon fibers, often involving the whole surface of a cuff tendon (most often the supraspinatus); usually < 3 cm
4	Very severe partial tear that usually contains, in addition to fraying and fragmentation of tendon tissue, a sizeable flap tear and often involves more than one tendon

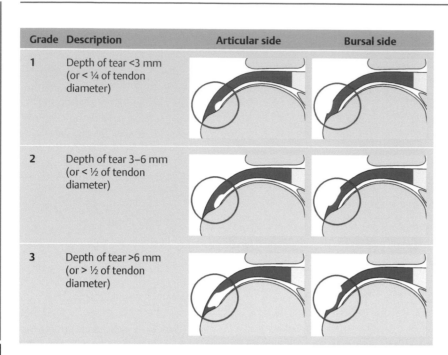

Grade	Description	Articular side	Bursal side
1	Depth of tear <3 mm (or < ¼ of tendon diameter)		
2	Depth of tear 3–6 mm (or < ½ of tendon diameter)		
3	Depth of tear >6 mm (or > ½ of tendon diameter)		

Fig. 5.8 Ellman classification of partial rotator cuff tears.

Table 5.2 Snyder classification of complete rotator cuff tears (C)

Type	Description
1	Small, complete tear such as a puncture wound
2	Complete tear of moderate size (usually < 2 cm) that involves only one rotator cuff tendon with no retraction of the tendon end
3	Large, complete tear (usually 3–4 cm) involving an entire tendon with minimal retraction of torn edge
4	Massive rotator cuff tear involving at least two tendons, often associated with marked retraction of the torn ends and scarring of the tendon stumps; often L-shaped tear; irreparable tear, indicating that there is no possibility of direct repair

Patte Classification of Tendon Retraction

In patients with large, complete rotator cuff tears, the proximal tendon stump may undergo considerable medial retraction over time (depending on the size and age of the tear). Patte defined criteria for quantifying the degree of tendon retraction on coronal oblique MR images (**Table 5.3** and **Fig. 5.9**).

> **!**
> While most torn tendons with grade 1 retraction are relatively easy to reattach, the defect caused by a grade 3 retraction usually requires a tendon transfer for repair. In the preoperative assessment of tears with grade 2 retraction it is difficult to predict the mobility of tendon stumps and the proportion of viable tendon components.

Patte D. Classification of rotator cuff lesions. Clin Orthop Relat Res 1990;254(254):81–86

Table 5.3 Patte classification of tendon retraction

Grade	Description
1	Proximal tendon end is close to the bony insertion. The retracted tendon stump does not extend to the apex of the humeral head
2	Proximal tendon stump is between the humeral head apex and glenoid
3	Proximal tendon stump has retracted to or past the level of the glenoid

Tangent Sign of Zanetti

Significant atrophy of the supraspinatus muscle belly can be detected by making a semiquantitative evaluation of that muscle on sagittal oblique MR images (**Fig. 5.10**). The "tangent sign" is assessed by drawing a line tangent to the superior borders of the scapular spine and coracoid and determining whether the muscle belly crosses the

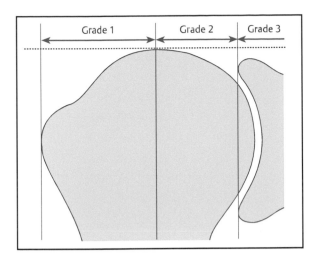

Fig. 5.9 Patte classification of tendon retraction (coronal oblique magnetic resonance image).

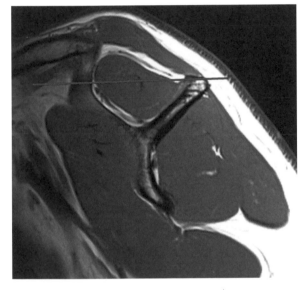

Fig. 5.10 Tangent sign of Zanetti. A line drawn tangent to the superior border of the scapular spine and the superior margin of the coracoid will normally pass through the supraspinatus muscle belly (negative tangent sign).

line (negative tangent sign) or passes below it (positive tangent sign). This determination should be made on the first lateral sagittal oblique MRI section that shows a Y-shaped appearance of the scapula.

> **!** While supraspinatus atrophy involves a decrease in the volume or cross-sectional area of the muscle (reversible), fatty degeneration describes an increase in the fatty tissue content of the muscle (irreversible).

Zanetti M, Gerber C, Hodler J. Quantitative assessment of the muscles of the rotator cuff with magnetic resonance imaging. Invest Radiol 1998;33(3):163–170

Goutallier Classification of Fatty Degeneration of the Rotator Cuff

Goutallier et al developed a scale for grading muscular fatty degeneration in the rotator cuff. The classification was established for CT examinations of the shoulder joint. The rotator cuff muscles are evaluated for the presence of interposed fatty tissue on noncontrast CT scans (**Table 5.4**).

Table 5.4 Goutallier scale for grading fatty degeneration

Grade	Description
0	Normal muscle, no fat
1	Muscle contains some streaks of fat
2	Marked fatty degeneration with still more muscle than fat
3	Advanced fatty degeneration with muscle equal to fat
4	Advanced fatty degeneration with more fat than muscle

> **!** Owing to its superior soft-tissue contrast, the Goutallier scale can also be used on MR images. MRI allows for a more accurate assessment resulting in an underestimation of relative fat content when using CT.
>
> If the grade of fatty degeneration is two or more, surgical cuff repair is no longer indicated.

Goutallier D, Postel JM, Bernageau J, Lavau L, Voisin MC. Fatty muscle degeneration in cuff ruptures. Pre- and post-operative evaluation by CT scan. Clin Orthop Relat Res 1994;304(304):78–83

Anterior Shoulder Instability

Dislocation of the shoulder joint exerts strong traction on the antero-inferior labroligamentous and capsular structures, causing injuries of the labroligamentous complex at the glenoid attachment, in the course of the inferior glenohumeral ligament, or at the humeral attachment. These injuries are best demonstrated by transverse MR or CT arthrography and are classified as shown in **Fig. 5.11**.

Shoulder Joint

5

Type of lesion	Description	
Normal findings		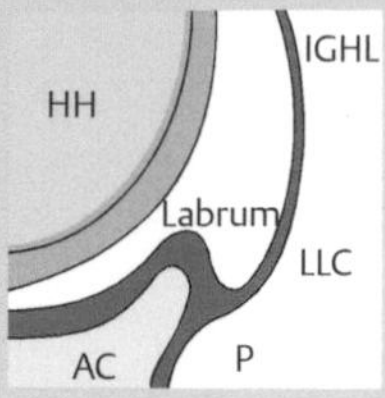
Injuries at the glenoid insertion		
Bankart lesion	Complete detachment of the antero-inferior labroligamentous complex from the glenoid rim with disruption of the adjacent scapular periosteum. The labrum is completely separated from the glenoid rim and displaced into the joint space. MR/CT arthrography shows contrast extension between the labrum and glenoid	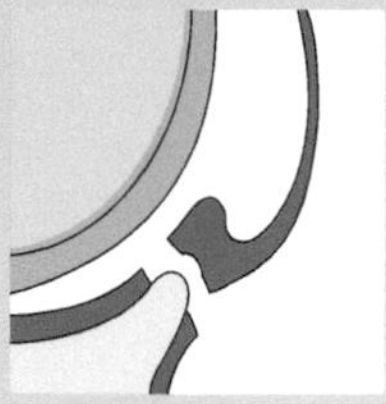
Bony Bankart lesion	Avulsion fracture of the antero-inferior glenoid rim. The labroligamentous complex is attached to the avulsed fragment	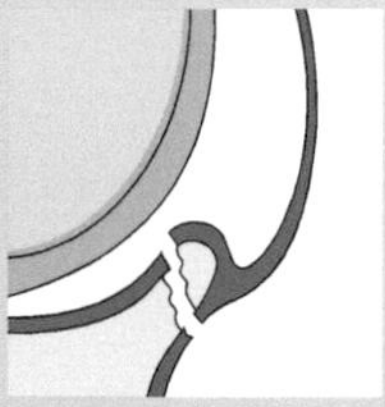
Perthes lesion	Avulsion of the antero-inferior labrum from the glenoid rim with intact periosteum that prevents labral displacement. MR/CT arthrography may show the intact periosteum as a linear structure attached to bone and labrum	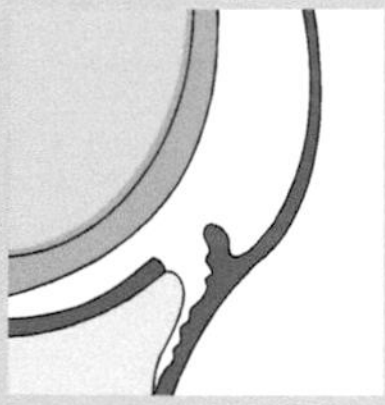
ALPSA lesion	Anterior labro-ligamentous periosteal sleeve avulsion lesion. Avulsion of the antero-inferior labrum from the glenoid rim with peeling back of the periosteum and displacement of the entire inferior glenohumeral ligament complex onto the scapular neck. MR/CT arthrography typically shows medial displacement of the deformed labroligamentous complex (anterior and/or inferior to the glenoid). ALPSA lesions occur in chronic instability because the displaced labro-ligamentous complex may become fixed to the scapular neck by scarring and resynovialization	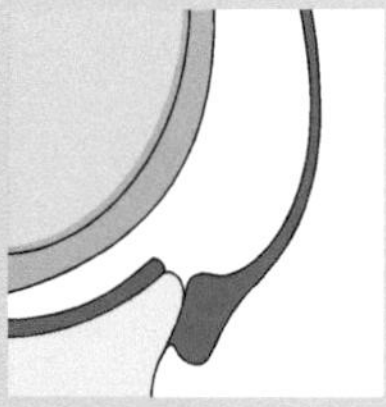
GLAD lesion	Glenolabral articular disruption lesion. Superficial tear of the antero-inferior labrum with an associated articular cartilage lesion of the glenoid. Labral tear and chondral lesions (of variable degrees) are demarcated by contrast on MR/CT arthrography. In most cases the causal mechanism of the injury is not a dislocation of the shoulder but a forced adduction injury from an abducted and externally rotated position. As the continuity of the inferior glenohumeral ligament complex is preserved, this is a stable lesion, unlike the others listed above	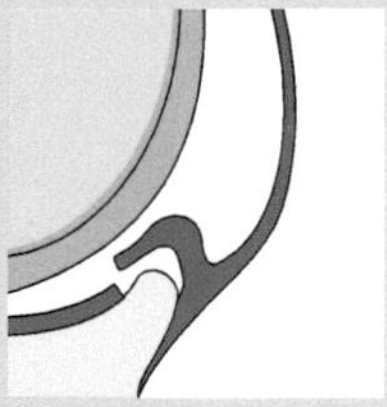

Fig. 5.11 Classification of injuries to the labroligamentous complex.

AC = Articular cartilage
HH = Humeral head
IGHL = Inferior glenohumeral ligament

LLC = Labroligamentous complex
P = Scapular periosteum

▶

Type of lesion	Description
Injuries at the humeral insertion	
HAGL lesion	Humeral avulsion of glenohumeral ligaments lesion. Avulsion of the inferior glenohumeral ligament from its humeral attachment. MR/CT arthrography shows the torn inferior glenohumeral ligament as J-shaped structure on coronal oblique images ("J sign") and contrast extravasation at the humeral insertion of the inferior glenohumeral ligament 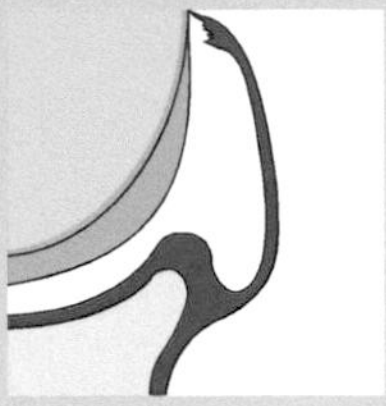
BHAGL lesion	Bony HAGL lesion. Avulsion fracture of the inferior glenohumeral ligament at its humeral insertion

Fig. 5.11 *Continued*

Neviaser TJ. The GLAD lesion: another cause of anterior shoulder pain. Arthroscopy 1993;9(1):22–23

Neviaser TJ. The anterior labroligamentous periosteal sleeve avulsion lesion: a cause of anterior instability of the shoulder. Arthroscopy 1993;9(1):17–21

Wörtler K, Waldt S. MR imaging in sports-related glenohumeral instability. Eur Radiol 2006;16(12):2622–2636

Normal Variants of the Superior Labrum and Labral–Bicipital Complex

Normal variants of the superior labrum and labral–bicipital complex are relatively common and require differentiation from injuries of the labral–bicipital complex. The following variants have been identified:

Sublabral Recess

The sublabral recess is a synovium-lined sulcus of variable depth located between the superior labrum and the glenoid margin. Smith classified the sublabral recess into three types based on its depth (**Fig. 5.12**). The sublabral recess can be most accurately evaluated on coronal oblique MR or CT arthrograms.

Sublabral Foramen

The sublabral foramen is a circumscribed area in which anterosuperior labrum is congenitally unattached to the glenoid (**Fig. 5.13a**).

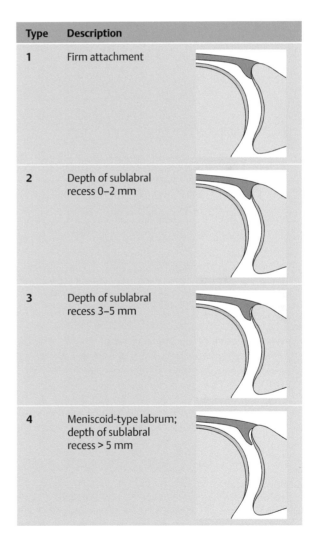

Type	Description
1	Firm attachment
2	Depth of sublabral recess 0–2 mm
3	Depth of sublabral recess 3–5 mm
4	Meniscoid-type labrum; depth of sublabral recess > 5 mm

Fig. 5.12 Smith classification of the sublabral recess.

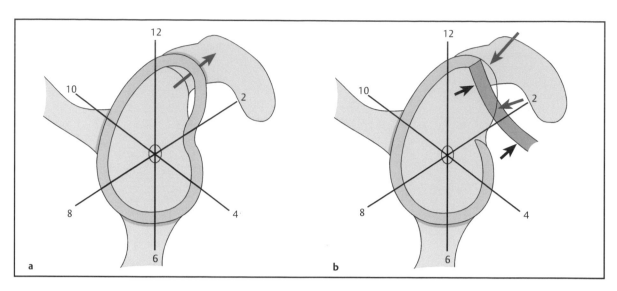

Fig. 5.13a,b Normal variants of the superior labrum and labral–bicipital complex.

a Sublabral foramen: absence of attachment of the anterosuperior labrum to the glenoid.

b Buford complex: congenital absence of the anterosuperior labrum and a thick, cordlike middle glenohumeral ligament.

Buford Complex

The Buford complex has the following characteristics (**Fig. 5.13b**):

- Congenital absence of the anterosuperior labrum
- A thick, cordlike middle glenohumeral ligament
- Middle glenohumeral ligament arising directly from the superior labrum anterior to the attachment of the biceps tendon

Smith DK, Chopp TM, Aufdemorte TB, Witkowski EG, Jones RC. Sublabral recess of the superior glenoid labrum: study of cadavers with conventional nonenhanced MR imaging, MR arthrography, anatomic dissection, and limited histologic examination. Radiology 1996;201(1):251–256

Williams MM, Snyder SJ, Buford D Jr. The Buford complex—the "cord-like" middle glenohumeral ligament and absent anterosuperior labrum complex: a normal anatomic capsulolabral variant. Arthroscopy 1994;10(3):241–247

Types of Long Biceps Tendon Attachment

The long biceps tendon most commonly arises by a Y-shaped expansion from the supraglenoid tubercle and from the superior (usually posterosuperior) part of the glenoid labrum. Variations in this origin are relatively common. Vangsness et al studied the variability of the labral origin and identified the types of biceps tendon attachment shown in **Fig. 5.14**.

> **!**
> In the study performed by Vangsness et al (100 cadaveric shoulders), type 1 was present in 22% of cases, type 2 in 33%, type 3 in 37%, and type 4 in 8%.
>
> More recent evidence suggests, however, that the fibers contributing most to stability attach to the supraglenoid tubercle.

Vangsness CT Jr, Jorgenson SS, Watson T, Johnson DL. The origin of the long head of the biceps from the scapula and glenoid labrum. An anatomical study of 100 shoulders. J Bone Joint Surg Br 1994;76(6):951–954

Lesions of the Labral–Bicipital Complex and Long Biceps Tendon

SLAP Lesions

A SLAP (superior labral anterior to posterior) lesion is an injury to the labral–bicipital complex consisting of the superior labrum and biceps tendon attachment. The superior labrum is torn in an anterior-to-posterior direction relative to the biceps anchor, and there may be variable involvement of the tendon attachment itself.

■ Snyder Classification

SLAP lesions were first described and classified into four subtypes by Snyder et al (**Table 5.5** and **Fig. 5.15**).

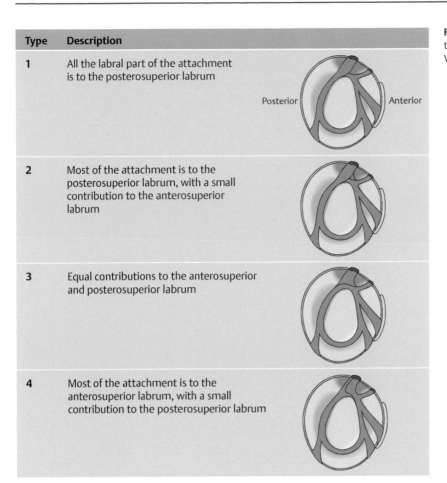

Type	Description
1	All the labral part of the attachment is to the posterosuperior labrum
2	Most of the attachment is to the posterosuperior labrum, with a small contribution to the anterosuperior labrum
3	Equal contributions to the anterosuperior and posterosuperior labrum
4	Most of the attachment is to the anterosuperior labrum, with a small contribution to the posterosuperior labrum

Fig. 5.14 Types of long biceps tendon attachment described by Vangsness.

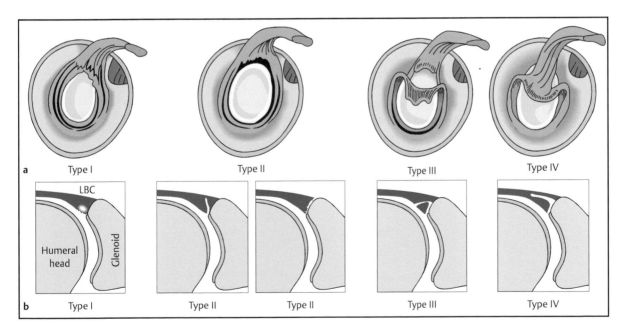

Fig. 5.15a,b Snyder classification of superior labral anterior to posterior (SLAP) lesions.

a Arthroscopic appearance.

b Magnetic resonance arthrographic appearance on coronal oblique images.

LBC = Labral–bicipital complex

Table 5.5 Snyder classification of SLAP lesions

Type	Description
I	Degenerative fraying of the superior labrum with a stable biceps tendon attachment. A normal degenerative process in older patients. No treatment is indicated, except for possible debridement.
II	Detachment of the labral–bicipital complex from the glenoid. The lesion is unstable. Surgical treatment (arthroscopic reattachment/tenodesis) is indicated.
III	Displaced bucket-handle tear of the superior labrum. The biceps tendon attachment is stable. Debridement is required.
IV	Bucket-handle tear of the superior labrum with involvement of the biceps tendon attachment. The lesion is unstable. Surgical treatment (arthroscopic reattachment/tenodesis) is indicated.

SLAP = superior labral anterior to posterior

!

Surgical repair is appropriate for SLAP lesions causing instability of the biceps tendon attachment (type II and type IV lesions). Surgery may consist of arthroscopic reattachment of the labrum or biceps tenodesis. The treatment of choice depends on the extent of the lesion (and on the surgeon). A good rule of thumb is that lesions involving > 50% of the biceps tendon diameter should be treated by tenodesis. Arthroscopic repair is recommended for lesser degrees of tendon involvement.

Type III lesions are commonly treated by debridement.

Snyder SJ, Karzel RP, Del Pizzo W, Ferkel RD, Friedman MJ. SLAP lesions of the shoulder. Arthroscopy 1990;6(4):274–279

Snyder SJ. Labral lesions (non-instability) and SLAP lesions. In: Snyder SJ, ed. Shoulder Arthroscopy. New York, NY: McGraw-Hill 1994: 115–131

Snyder SJ. Superior labrum, anterior to posterior lesions of the shoulder. In: Snyder SJ. Shoulder arthroscopy. 2ed. Philadelphia: Lippincott Williams & Wilkens; 2003: 147–165

■ Expanded Classification of SLAP Lesions

The Snyder classification has been expanded several times, and a total of 10 types of SLAP lesion have been described to date (**Table 5.6**).

Table 5.6 Expanded classification of SLAP lesions

Type	Description
Snyder et al 1990	
I	Degenerative fraying of the superior labrum at the biceps tendon attachment
II	Detachment of the labral–bicipital complex from the glenoid
III	Bucket-handle tear of the superior labrum with preserved biceps anchor
IV	Bucket-handle tear of the superior labrum with involvement of the biceps tendon attachment
Maffet et al 1995	
V	Bankart lesion, on a continuum with detachment of the labral–bicipital complex from the glenoid (SLAP type II)
VI	Unstable radial tear (flap tear) of the anterosuperior or posterosuperior labrum with separation of the labrum from the biceps tendon attachment ("bucket handle avulsed on one side")
VII	Detachment of the labral–bicipital complex from the glenoid (SLAP type II) with antero-inferior extension of the labral tear into the middle glenohumeral ligament
Resnick (unpublished data)	
VIII	Detachment of the labral–bicipital complex from the glenoid (SLAP type II) with extension of the labral tear into the posterior labrum
IX	Detachment of the labral–bicipital complex from the glenoid (SLAP type II) and complete detachment of the labrum from the glenoid circumference
Beltran (data presented at the RSNA, Chicago, 12/2000)	
X	Detachment of the labral–bicipital complex from the glenoid (SLAP type II) with extension of the lesion into the rotator interval (pulley lesion)

SLAP = superior labral anterior to posterior.

!

Because associated lesions (separate from lesions of the biceps tendon attachment) mainly determine the subclassification into types V–X, this expanded classification is of limited value and we recommend using the original Snyder classification. Types I–X are described here for completeness, however (**Table 5.6**).

Maffet MW, Gartsman GM, Moseley B. Superior labrum–biceps tendon complex lesions of the shoulder. Am J Sports Med 1995;23(1):93–98

Snyder SJ. Superior labrum, anterior to posterior lesions of the shoulder. In: Snyder SJ. Shoulder arthroscopy. 2ed. Philadelphia: Lippincott Williams & Wilkens; 2003: 147–165

Shoulder Joint

5

■ Subtypes of SLAP Type II Lesions

Morgan et al subclassified type II SLAP lesions according to their location:

- *Type IIA:* detachment of the anterosuperior labrum and adjacent biceps tendon attachment ("anterior SLAP lesion")
- *Type IIB:* detachment of the posterosuperior labrum and adjacent biceps tendon attachment ("posterior SLAP lesion")
- *Type IIC:* detachment of the anterosuperior and posterosuperior labrum and biceps tendon attachment ("combined SLAP lesion")

Morgan CD, Burkhart SS, Palmeri M, Gillespie M. Type II SLAP lesions: three subtypes and their relationships to superior instability and rotator cuff tears. Arthroscopy 1998;14(6):553–565

Pulley Lesions

The long head of the biceps tendon is stabilized by a fibrous sling before its entry into the intertubercular groove. The superficial (bursal-side) part of the sling is formed by portions of the joint capsule (oblique fascicle), the coracohumeral ligament, and portions of the superior glenohumeral ligament, which passes beneath the biceps tendon on entering the intertubercular groove and so forms the deep part of the pulley sling (**Fig. 5.16**). Injuries to the pulley sling may be isolated or may occur in the setting of rotator cuff tears.

Pulley lesions lead to instability of the long biceps tendon—a condition that is worsened by further extension of the lesion or the involvement of adjacent structures. Habermeyer et al classified pulley lesions into four groups (**Fig. 5.17**).

Habermeyer P, Magosch P, Pritsch M, Scheibel MT, Lichtenberg S. Anterosuperior impingement of the shoulder as a result of pulley lesions: a prospective arthroscopic study. J Shoulder Elbow Surg 2004;13(1):5–12

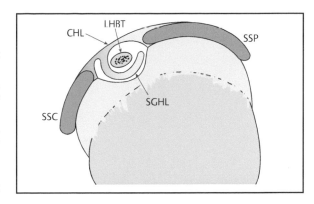

Fig. 5.16 Pulley system. Schematic representation of the pulley sling at the level above the intertubercular groove.
CHL = Coracohumeral ligament
LHBT = Long head biceps tendon
SGHL = Superior glenohumeral ligament
SSC = Subscapularis tendon
SSP = Supraspinatus tendon

Calcifying Tendinitis

Localization of Calcium Deposits on Conventional Radiographs

Radiographs of the shoulder joint in internal and external rotation are used to localize calcium deposits to a specific tendon on conventional radiographs (**Fig. 5.18**). The affected tendon can be identified by the apparent displacement of the calcium deposit between the two views and by its relation to the tubercles.

- *Supraspinatus insertion:* Calcification at the supraspinatus tendon insertion is nonsuperimposed in the external rotation view, presenting a clear outline next to the greater tubercle. The internal rotation view shows little apparent displacement of the calcification, which may still present a clear outline or may be superimposed by the greater tuberosity.
- *Infraspinatus insertion:* Calcification at the infraspinatus tendon insertion is projected posterior to the humeral head (or greater tuberosity) in the external rotation view. It is nonsuperimposed in the internal rotation view and presents a clear outline lateral to the greater tuberosity.
- *Subscapularis insertion:* Calcification at the subscapularis tendon insertion is superimposed by the humeral head (or lesser tuberosity) in the external rotation view. In the internal rotation view it presents a nonsuperimposed outline medial to the lesser tuberosity.

Group	Description	
1	Isolated lesion of the superior glenohumeral ligament	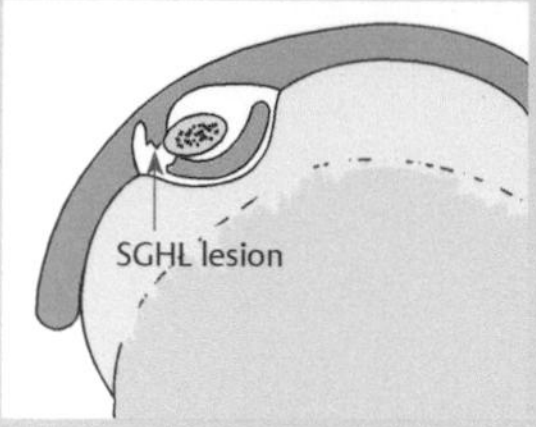
2	Lesion of the superior glenohumeral ligament and partial articular-sided supraspinatus tendon tear	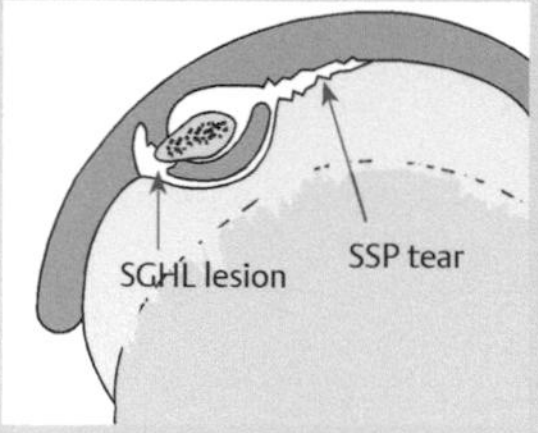
3	Lesion of the superior glenohumeral ligament and articular-sided (deep surface) tear of the subscapularis tendon	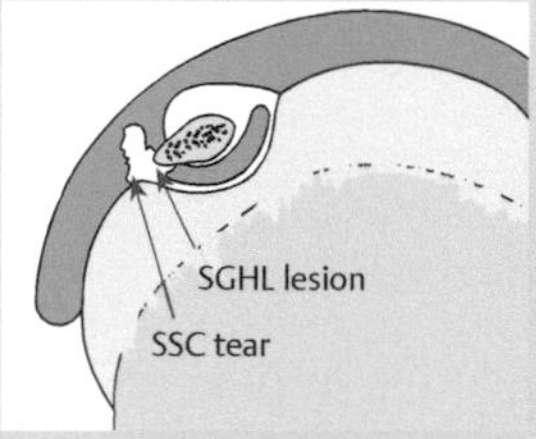
4	Lesion of the superior glenohumeral ligament combined with an articular-sided partial supraspinatus and subscapularis tendon tear	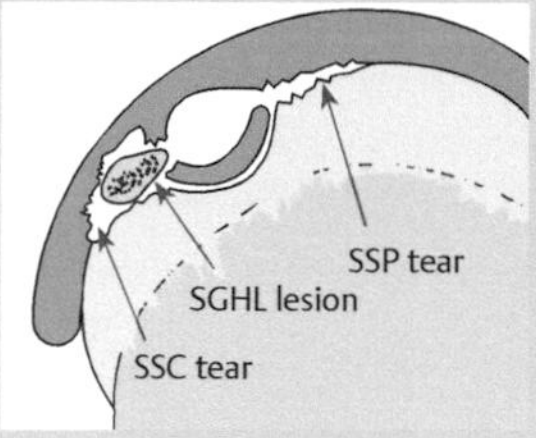

Fig. 5.17 Habermeyer classification of pulley lesions.
SGHL = Superior glenohumeral ligament
SSC = Subscapularis tendon
SSP = Supraspinatus tendon

Gärtner Classification of Calcium Deposits

Gärtner classified calcium deposits into three types based on their radiographic margins and lucency (**Table 5.7** and **Fig. 5.19**).

Gärtner believed that his classification mirrored the chronology of the natural history of calcium deposits (formative phase → resting phase → resorptive phase):

- *Type 1:* resting phase (hard, chalky appearance)
- *Type 2:* not assignable to a specific phase
- *Type 3:* resorptive phase (milky consistency)

!

More recent studies have shown that this correlation is uncertain and that, in routine clinical work, radiographic morphology is only one criterion for assigning a calcium deposit to a specific chronologic phase. Nevertheless, the Gärtner classification is still widely used especially in some European countries.

Gärtner J, Heyer A. Calcific tendinitis of the shoulder. [Article in German] Orthopade 1995;24(3):284–302

Table 5.7 Gärtner classification of calcium deposits

Type	Description
1	Dense deposit with sharp margins
2	Dense deposit with indistinct margins or radiolucent deposit with sharp margins
3	Radiolucent deposit with indistinct margins

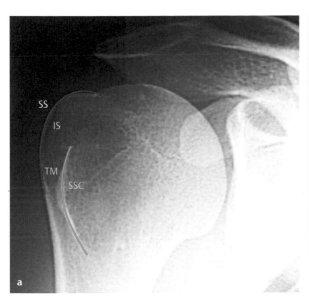

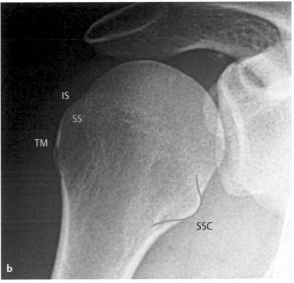

Fig. 5.18a,b Localization of calcium deposits on conventional shoulder radiographs in external and internal rotation. The affected tendon can be identified by noting the apparent displacement of calcification.

SS	= Supraspinatus tendon	Yellow labels	= Tendon insertions with superimposed bone
IS	= Infraspinatus tendon	Blue	= Outline of lesser tuberosity
TM	= Teres minor tendon	Red	= Outline of greater tuberosity
SSC	= Subscapularis tendon	**a**	Radiograph in external rotation.
White labels	= Nonsuperimposed tendon insertions	**b**	Radiograph in internal rotation.

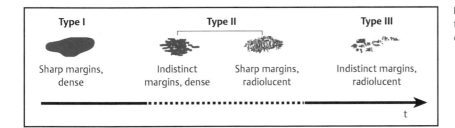

Type I	Type II		Type III
Sharp margins, dense	Indistinct margins, dense	Sharp margins, radiolucent	Indistinct margins, radiolucent

t

Fig. 5.19 Gärtner classification of the radiographic morphology of calcifying tendinitis.

Bosworth Classification of Calcium Deposits

Bosworth used the size of the deposit as a simple criterion for the classification of calcifying tendinitis (**Table 5.8**).

Bosworth B. Calcium deposits in the shoulder and subacromial deposits. J Am Med Assoc 1941;116:2477–2484

Table 5.8 Bosworth classification of calcium deposits

Size	Description
Large	Maximum diameter of deposit > 1.5 cm
Medium	0.5–1.5 cm
Small	< 0.5 cm, difficult to identify on radiographs

Injuries of the Acromioclavicular Joint

Tossy Classification

Tossy et al classified acromioclavicular joint injuries into three grades of severity (**Table 5.9**). The injury is evaluated on a panoramic radiograph of the acromioclavicular joints or a Zanca view of the acromioclavicular joint. The panoramic radiograph is an AP stress radiograph of both shoulder joints taken in a standing or sitting position with the arms hanging at the sides. Each arm bears a traction weight of 5 or 10 kg (different authors describe different weights), which should be suspended from the wrists rather than held in the hands. The Zanca view is an AP projection of the shoulder joint with the central ray angled 15° cephalad (**Fig. 5.20**). The Tossy classification evaluates the extent of ligamentous injury based on the vertical displacement of the lateral end of the clavicle.

Table 5.9 Tossy classification of acromioclavicular joint injuries

Type	Description	Radiographic findings
Tossy 1	Sprain of acromioclavicular ligaments	Conventional radiograph is normal. Stress radiograph may demonstrate slight widening of the acromioclavicular joint
Tossy 2	Disruption of acromioclavicular ligaments and sprain of coracoclavicular ligaments	Radiograph shows the clavicle displaced by approximately half the craniocaudal diameter of the acromioclavicular joint
Tossy 3	Complete disruption of acromioclavicular and coracoclavicular ligaments	The acromioclavicular joint is dislocated by more than half the craniocaudal diameter of the joint. The lateral end of the clavicle is markedly elevated, and there is increased distance between the coracoid process and clavicle

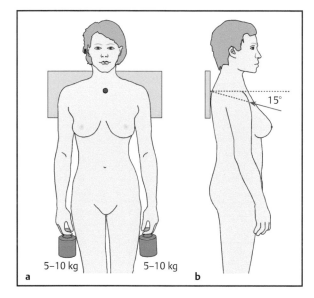

5–10 kg   5–10 kg

a   b

Fig. 5.20a,b Radiographs for evaluating acromioclavicular joint injuries.

a Panoramic stress radiograph of both shoulders in the anteroposterior projection.

b Zanca view with the central ray angled 15° cephalad.

Rockwood Classification

The Rockwood classification is an expansion of the Tossy classification. Tossy type 3 is further subclassified into types 3–6 (**Fig. 5.21** and **Table 5.10**). The injury is evaluated on conventional radiographs. Besides the Zanca or panoramic radiograph (AP view of both shoulders; see **Fig. 5.20**), the Rockwood classification requires a second projection, preferably an axial view, to detect horizontal instability with posterior displacement of the lateral clavicle.

> **!** The Rockwood classification is considered the standard system for classifying acromioclavicular joint injuries. Besides the injury patterns covered in the Tossy classification, the Rockwood classification also takes into account the integrity of the muscle attachments and includes less common injuries such as posterior and inferior dislocations, which are important for treatment planning. While type 1 and type 2 injuries are managed conservatively, type 4–6 injuries are definite indications for surgery. Type 3 injuries can be managed conservatively or surgically depending on the patient's age, general level of activity and athletic demands.

Tossy JD, Mead NC, Sigmond HM. Acromioclavicular separations: useful and practical classification for treatment. Clin Orthop Relat Res 1963;28:111–119

Rockwood CA, Wirth MA. Injuries to the acromioclavicular joint. In: Rockwood CA, Green DP, Bucholz RW, Heckmann JD, eds. Fractures in Adults. Philadelphia: Lippincott-Raven; 1996: 1341–1414

Rockwood CA. Fractures and dislocation of the shoulder in children. In: Rockwood CA, Frederick A, eds. The shoulder. Philadelphia: W-B Saunders; 1990: 991–1032

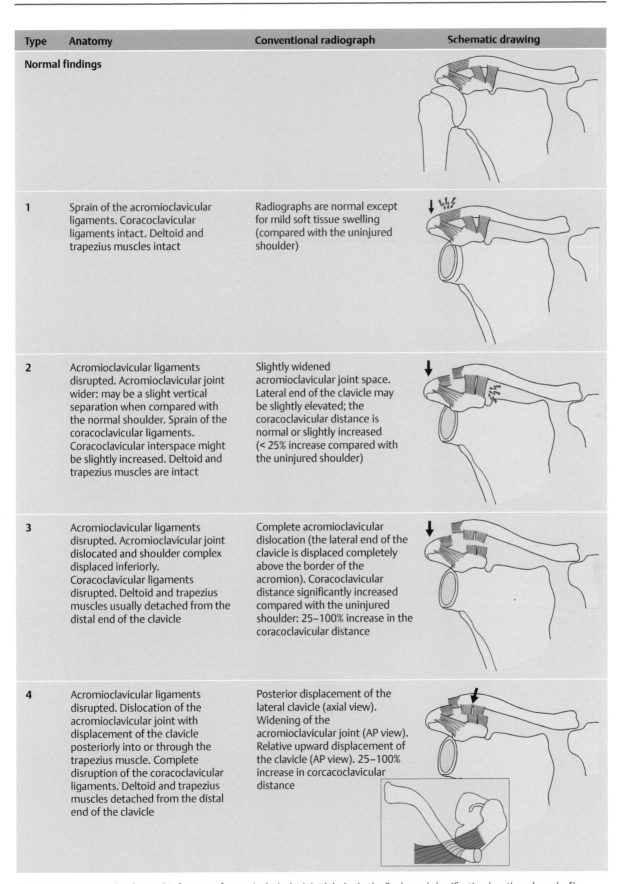

Type	Anatomy	Conventional radiograph	Schematic drawing
Normal findings			
1	Sprain of the acromioclavicular ligaments. Coracoclavicular ligaments intact. Deltoid and trapezius muscles intact	Radiographs are normal except for mild soft tissue swelling (compared with the uninjured shoulder)	
2	Acromioclavicular ligaments disrupted. Acromioclavicular joint wider: may be a slight vertical separation when compared with the normal shoulder. Sprain of the coracoclavicular ligaments. Coracoclavicular interspace might be slightly increased. Deltoid and trapezius muscles are intact	Slightly widened acromioclavicular joint space. Lateral end of the clavicle may be slightly elevated; the coracoclavicular distance is normal or slightly increased (< 25% increase compared with the uninjured shoulder)	
3	Acromioclavicular ligaments disrupted. Acromioclavicular joint dislocated and shoulder complex displaced inferiorly. Coracoclavicular ligaments disrupted. Deltoid and trapezius muscles usually detached from the distal end of the clavicle	Complete acromioclavicular dislocation (the lateral end of the clavicle is displaced completely above the border of the acromion). Coracoclavicular distance significantly increased compared with the uninjured shoulder: 25–100% increase in the coracoclavicular distance	
4	Acromioclavicular ligaments disrupted. Dislocation of the acromioclavicular joint with displacement of the clavicle posteriorly into or through the trapezius muscle. Complete disruption of the coracoclavicular ligaments. Deltoid and trapezius muscles detached from the distal end of the clavicle	Posterior displacement of the lateral clavicle (axial view). Widening of the acromioclavicular joint (AP view). Relative upward displacement of the clavicle (AP view). 25–100% increase in corcacoclavicular distance	

Fig. 5.21 Anatomy and radiographic features of acromioclavicular joint injuries in the Rockwood classification (continued overleaf).

Shoulder Joint

5

Type	Anatomy	Conventional radiograph	Schematic drawing
5	Acromioclavicular ligaments disrupted. Coracoclavicular ligaments disrupted. Dislocation of the acromioclavicular joint with gross disparity between the clavicle and the scapula. Deltoid and trapezius muscle attachments detached from the distal half of the clavicle	Complete acromioclavicular dislocation. The clavicle is grossly displaced superiorly away from the acromion... Marked, 100–300% increase in coracoclavicular distance	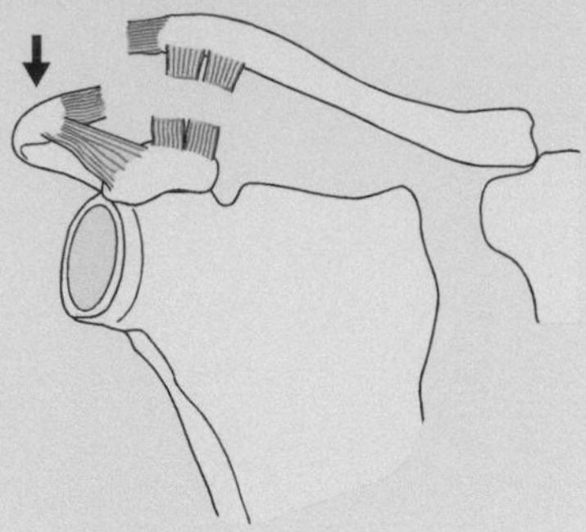
6	Acromioclavicular ligaments disrupted. Dislocation of the acromioclavicular joint with inferior displacement of the clavicle beneath the acromion or coracoid process. Coracoclavicular ligaments are disrupted in subcoracoid type and intact in subacromial type. The corcacoclavicular interspace is reversed in the subcoracoid type (i.e., clavicle inferior to the coracoid), or decreased in the cubacromial type (i.e., clavicle inferior to the acromion). Deltoid and trapezius muscles are detached from the distal clavicle	Complete dislocation of the acromioclavicular joint. Coracoclavicular distance reduced in the subacromial type and reversed in the subcoracoid type.	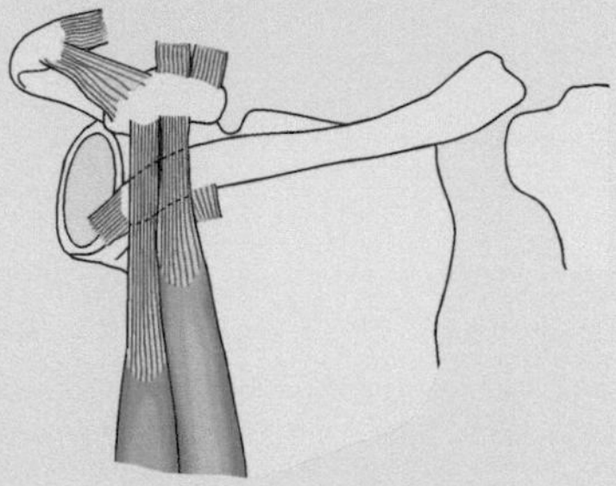

Fig. 5.21 *Continued*

Table 5.10 Rockwood classification of acromioclavicular joint injuries

Type	AC ligament	CC ligament	DT fascia	Direction and degree of dislocation
1	Sprain	Intact	Intact	No subluxation
2	Rupture	Sprain	Intact	Superior, with < 25% increase in CC distance
3	Rupture	Rupture	Intact	Superior, with 25–100% increase in CC distance
4	Rupture	Rupture	Injured	Clavicle displaced posteriorly into trapezius
5	Rupture	Rupture	Detached	Superior, with 100–300% increase in CC distance
6	Rupture	Rupture	Detached	Clavicle displaced inferior to acromion or coracoid

AC = Acromioclavicular
CC = Coracoclavicular
DT = Deltoid and trapezius

Cubital Angle (Carrying Angle of the Elbow)

Various techniques have been described for measuring the cubital angle (synonym: carrying angle) of the elbow joint. The humerus–elbow–wrist angle of Oppenheim, which is somewhat more accurate than the humeroulnar angle, has become well established in the planning of corrective osteotomies and as a follow-up parameter in clinical studies. The Baumann angle can be used in children to make an approximate, indirect measurement of the joint axis in cases where the joint cannot be examined in full extension because of injury or immobilization.

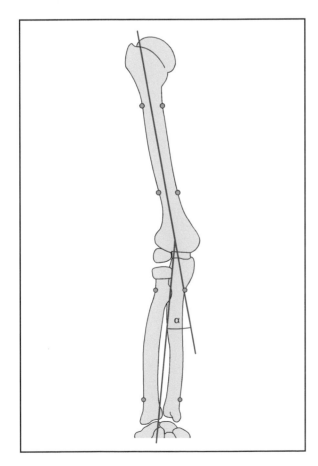

Fig. 6.1 Cubital angle: the humerus–elbow–wrist angle.

Humerus–Elbow–Wrist Angle of Oppenheim

The humerus–elbow–wrist (HEW) angle of Oppenheim (**Fig. 6.1**) is determined on an anteroposterior (AP) radiograph of the arm with full elbow extension (180°) and supination. The radiograph should cover the arm from the proximal humerus down to the wrist.

The angle is measured between the humeral shaft axis and the forearm axis. The humeral shaft axis is defined by the midpoints of two lines perpendicular to the shaft spaced as far apart as possible. The forearm axis is defined by the midpoints of two lines perpendicular to the forearm bones (lateral border of the radius and medial border of the ulna).

Humerus–elbow–wrist angle of Oppenheim	
• *Mean value:*	10°
• *Cubitus varus:*	< 5°
• *Cubitus valgus:*	> 15°

> **!**
> Because the cubital angle is highly variable, a radiograph of the healthy side should always be obtained for comparison when planning a corrective osteotomy. If the affected elbow cannot be fully extended, the radiograph should be taken in maximum possible extension and the comparison view taken with the healthy limb in the same position.

Oppenheim WL, Clader TJ, Smith C, Bayer M. Supracondylar humeral osteotomy for traumatic childhood cubitus varus deformity. Clin Orthop Relat Res 1984;188(188):34–39

Humeroulnar Angle

The humeroulnar angle (**Fig. 6.2**) is measured on the AP radiograph of the arm or elbow joint. As the ulna often has some degree of curvature, especially in children, the accuracy of the measurement can be increased by displaying the entire ulna and entire humerus on one radiograph. The radiograph should be taken with full elbow extension (180°) and supination.

The humeroulnar angle is measured between the axes of the humeral and ulnar shafts. Ideally, both axes are drawn through the midpoints of two lines perpendicular to the shaft that are spaced as far apart as possible.

Elbow Joint

6

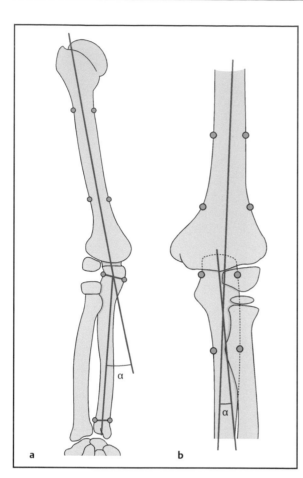

Fig. 6.2 a,b Cubital angle: the humeroulnar angle.
a Anteroposterior radiograph of the arm.
b Anteroposterior radiograph of the elbow joint.

If the radiograph displays only the bone segments close to the joint, the humeral axis can be defined by reference points placed at the level where the metaphysis begins to flare and at the distal diaphysis. The ulnar shaft axis is defined by two proximal reference points at the level of the proximal ulnar border and the radial tuberosity.

Humeroulnar angle	
• *Mean value in females (after Keats):*	13°
• *Mean value in males (after Keats):*	11°

!
The normal values stated in the literature vary considerably owing to differences in methodology, population size, and the variability of the carrying angle. Thus, comparison with the opposite side (= treatment goal) is essential for surgical planning. As a general rule, the angle is slightly greater in females than in males and also increases by a few degrees from childhood to adulthood.

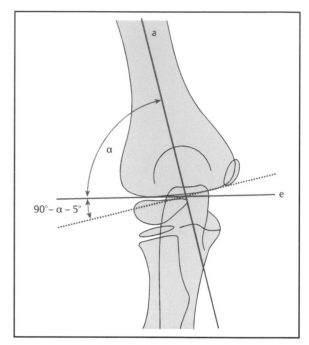

Fig. 6.3 Baumann angle.
a = Longitudinal axis of the humerus
e = Axis through the epiphyseal plate of the lateral epicondyle
α = Baumann angle
(90°–α–5°) = cubital angle of Baumann

Beals RK. The normal carrying angle of the elbow. A radiographic study of 422 patients. Clin Orthop Relat Res 1976;119(119):194–196
Keats TE, Teeslink R, Diamond AE, Williams JH. Normal axial relationships of the major joints. Radiology 1966;87(5):904–907

Baumann Angle

A true AP projection of the elbow joint is necessary for accurate determination of the Baumann angle (synonym: humerocapitellar angle; **Fig. 6.3**). In contrast to the other cubital angles, it is not necessary to obtain the image with full elbow extension. The AP view may be achieved with any degree of elbow extension.

The Baumann angle (α) is formed by the longitudinal axis of the humerus and a straight line through the epiphyseal plate of the lateral condyle (capitulum) of the humerus. Baumann equated the reciprocal angle (90°–α–5°) with the cubital angle and stated a normal range of 75–80°, which Williamson et al expanded to 64–81°.

Baumann angle
Normal range according to Williamson: 64–81°

The Baumann angle is an important aid for the accurate reduction of a supracondylar humeral fracture in children.

> **!**
> More recent studies have shown that the relationship of the α angle to the cubital angle is more complex than Baumann believed, and it would be incorrect to equate the cubital angle of Baumann (90°–α–5°) with the "real" cubital angle, especially when there is rotational malalignment of the distal fragment in supracondylar humeral fractures. Nevertheless, the Baumann angle can detect any displacement or malalignment of the fragment that would lead to axial deformity at the elbow. Hence, the angle can provide indirect but valuable information on the joint axis and is used most effectively in a side-to-side comparison for assessing the position of the distal fracture fragment. Discrepancies > 5° in comparison with the uninjured elbow joint should not be tolerated.

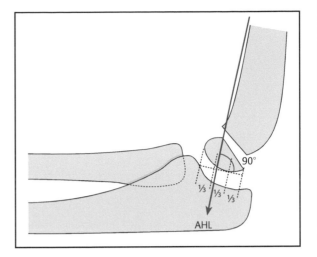

Fig. 6.4 Anterior humeral line (AHL) used in the diagnosis of supracondylar humeral fractures.

> **!**
> With pediatric fractures, deviation of the anterior humeral line may be the only evidence of a supracondylar humeral fracture. A true lateral projection is essential. Often the only way to achieve a true lateral projection in children (especially with a painful injury) is by positioning the arm over the head.

Acton JD, McNally MA. Baumann's confusing legacy. Injury 2001;32(1):41–43

Baumann E. Beiträge zur Kenntnis der Frakturen am Ellenbogengelenk. Allgemeines und Fractura supracondylica. Beitr Klin Chir 1929;146:1–50

Williamson DM, Coates CJ, Miller RK, Cole WG. Normal characteristics of the Baumann (humerocapitellar) angle: an aid in assessment of supracondylar fractures. J Pediatr Orthop 1992;12(5):636–639

Reference Lines and Angles for the Diagnosis of Fractures and Deformities

Various reference lines have been described for the detection of joint deformity and fragment displacement on conventional radiographs. These lines are particularly helpful in evaluations of the pediatric elbow joint.

Anterior Humeral Line (Rogers Line)

The Rogers line is drawn tangent to the anterior border of the humeral shaft on a lateral radiograph of the elbow joint (**Fig. 6.4**). Normally this line passes through the middle third of the humeral capitulum. If the capitulum is displaced posteriorly (extension fracture), the Rogers line will pass through its anterior third. If the capitulum is displaced anteriorly (flexion fracture), the line will transect its posterior third.

Rogers LF, Malave S Jr, White H, Tachdjian MO. Plastic bowing, torus and greenstick supracondylar fractures of the humerus: radiographic clues to obscure fractures of the elbow in children. Radiology 1978;128(1):145–150

Radius–Capitulum Axis

An extension of the longitudinal axis of the proximal radius should pass through the center of the humeral capitulum in the AP and lateral radiographs in all joint positions (**Fig. 6.5**). Dislocations of the radial head can be diagnosed based on deviations of this axis.

> **!**
> With congenital dislocation, the angular deformity is typically accompanied by dysplasia of the radial head (bulbous shape).

Storen G. Traumatic dislocation of the radial head as an isolated lesion in children; report of one case with special regard to roentgen diagnosis. Acta Chir Scand 1959;116(2):144–147

Elbow Joint

6

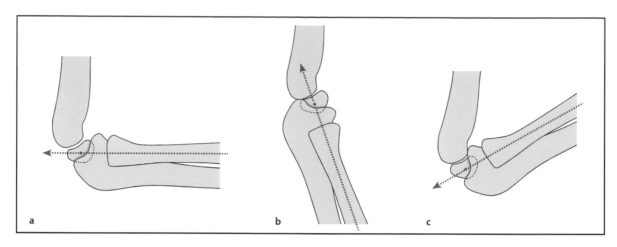

Fig. 6.5a–c Radius–capitulum axis. An extension of the radial axis on lateral radiographs will normally pass through the center of the humeral capitulum in any joint position.

O'Driscoll Classification of Posterolateral Rotatory Instability

Posterolateral instability is by far the most common form of instability in the elbow joint. Cadaveric studies have shown that the underlying injury starts with a tear of the lateral collateral ligament and progresses medially in response to additional forces. O'Driscoll described the progression of this injury as a circle of disruption called the Horii circle (**Fig. 6.6**). According to O'Driscoll, the development of posterolateral rotatory instability proceeds in three stages as shown in **Fig. 6.7**.

O'Driscoll SW, Jupiter JB, King GJ, Hotchkiss RN, Morrey BF. The unstable elbow. J Bone Joint Surg Am 2000;82(5):724–738

O'Driscoll SW, Jupiter JB, King GJ, Hotchkiss RN, Morrey BF. The unstable elbow. Instr Course Lect 2001;50:89–102

O'Driscoll SW, Morrey BF, Korinek S, An KN. Elbow subluxation and dislocation. A spectrum of instability. Clin Orthop Relat Res 1992;280(280):186–197

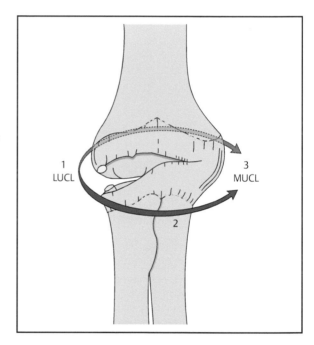

Fig. 6.6 "Horii circle" described by O'Driscoll. Schematic representation of the pathogenic mechanism of posterolateral instability.
LUCL = Lateral ulnar collateral ligament
MUCL = Medial ulnar collateral ligament

Stage	Description	
Normal		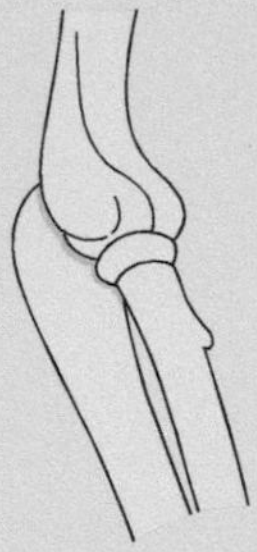
1	Tear of the lateral ulnar collateral ligament (LUCL). Posterolateral subluxation occurs and reduces spontaneously, regardless of whether the rest of the radial collateral ligament is intact or not	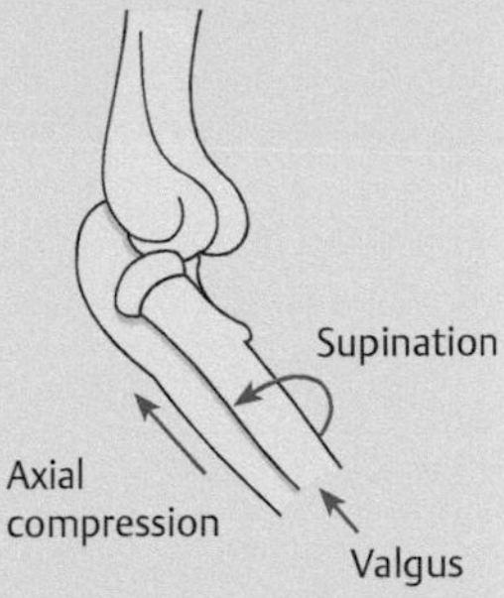
2	Additional lesions of the anterior and posterior capsular structures. There is incomplete posterolateral dislocation with displacement of the coronoid process onto the trochlea, creating a "perched dislocation"	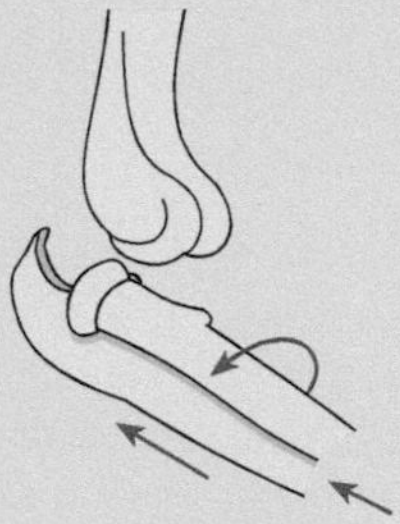
3A	Soft-tissue disruption extends to the medial-sided ligamentous structures, tearing all but the anterior portion of the medial collateral ligament. The elbow dislocates posteriorly, rotating about the intact anterior band	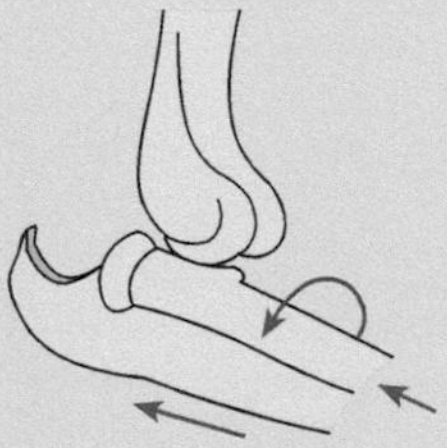
3B	All portions of the medial collateral ligament are disrupted. Reduction is followed by varus, valgus and rotatory instability because all ligaments and capsular structures are destroyed	

Fig. 6.7 O'Driscoll classification of posterolateral rotatory instability.

Elbow Joint

6

107

7 Wrist and Hand[1]

Joint Angles of the Distal Radius

Radial Inclination

Radial inclination (synonyms: radial deviation, radial tilt, ulnar inclination, radial angle; **Fig. 7.1**) is measured on a dorsopalmar radiograph of the wrist in the neutral position. First the longitudinal axis of the radius is drawn as a reference line. The second reference line is drawn from the tip of the radial styloid process to the ulnar margin of the distal radius, passing through the midpoint between the dorsal and palmar radial cortical margins. Radial inclination is measured as the angle between the second reference line and a line perpendicular to the longitudinal axis of the radius.

Radial inclination
Normal value: 23° (15–35°)

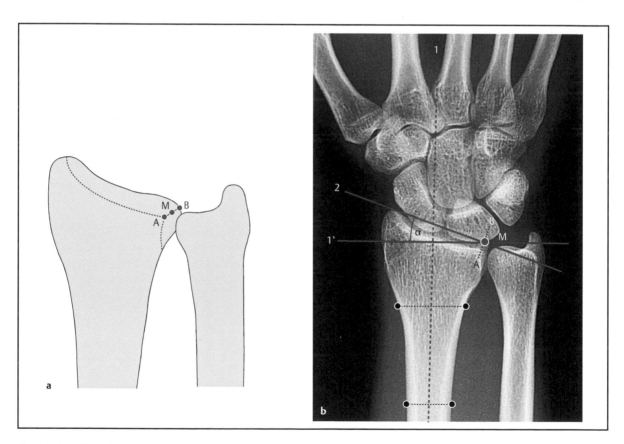

Fig. 7.1a,b Radial inclination.

A = Anterior margin of the ulnar radius
B = Posterior margin of the ulnar radius
M = Midpoint of line A–B
1 = Longitudinal axis of the distal radius
1' = Line perpendicular to 1

2 = Connecting line from M to the radial styloid process
α = Angle between 1' and 2
a Diagram for determining M.
b Dorsopalmar radiograph.

[1] Based on Schmitt R and Lanz U. Diagnostic Imaging of the Hand. Stuttgart: Thieme, 2007.

DiBenedetto MR, Lubbers LM, Ruff ME, Nappi JF, Coleman CR. Quantification of error in measurement of radial inclination angle and radiocarpal distance. J Hand Surg [Br] 1991;16A:399–400

Schmitt R, Prommersberger KJ. Karpale Morphometrie und Funktion. In: Bildgebende Diagnostik der Hand. 2nd ed. Stuttgart: Thieme; 2004: 122–130

Palmar Tilt of the Distal Radius

The palmar tilt of the distal radius (synonyms: volar tilt, volar angle, dorsal tilt, dorsal angle, palmar slope, palmar inclination; **Fig. 7.2**) is evaluated on a lateral radiograph of the hand in the neutral position. The angle is measured between a reference line tangent to the dorsal and palmar margins of the distal radius and a line perpendicular to the longitudinal axis of the radius.

Palmar tilt
Normal value: 11° (0–20°)

Baratz ME, Larsen CF. Wrist and hand measurements and classification schemes. In: Gilula LA, Yuming Y. Imaging of the Hand and Wrist. Philadelphia: Saunders; 1996: 225–259

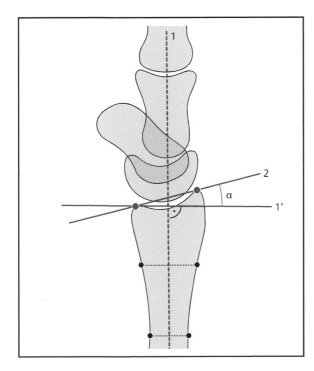

Fig. 7.2 Palmar tilt of the distal radius.
1 = Longitudinal axis of the distal radius
1' = Line perpendicular to 1
2 = Line tangent to the anterior and posterior radial margins
α = Palmar tilt of the distal radius

Schmitt R, Prommersberger KJ. Karpale Morphometrie und Funktion. In: Bildgebende Diagnostik der Hand. 2nd ed. Stuttgart: Thieme; 2004: 122–130

Ulnar Variance according to Gelberman

Ulnar variance, also called the radioulnar index, is a measurement of the relative lengths of the radius and ulna determined on a dorsopalmar radiograph of the wrist. A neutral rotation view is necessary because pronation and supination movements of the forearm alter the relative length of the ulna, causing erroneous measurements in other joint positions.

> An abnormal length of the ulna is associated with different pathologies of the wrist (Kienböck disease, negative ulnar variance; ulnolunate impaction syndrome and triangular fibrocartilage tears, positive ulnar variance). Furthermore, considering the ulnar variance is helpful in assessing the degree of posttraumatic instability of the distal radioulnar joint following distal radius fractures.

Various methods for determining ulnar variance have been described and evaluated. The Gelberman method described below is easy to perform. Steyers and Blair compared various techniques and found that, like the other methods evaluated, the Gelberman method yielded reliable results.

Gelberman defines ulnar variance as the distance between two lines perpendicular to the long axis of the radius (**Fig. 7.3**). On the radial side, a line perpendicular to the radial axis is drawn through the ulnar margin of the radius. It should pass through the midpoint between the dorsal and palmar edges of the ulnar radial margin (see p. 108). On the ulnar side, a line perpendicular to the radial long axis is drawn tangent to the distal articular surface of the ulna.

Ulnar variance	
● *Normal value:*	Length discrepancy ≤ 2 mm
● *Positive ulnar variance:*	Ulna longer than the radius > 2 mm
● *Negative ulnar variance:*	Ulna shorter than the radius > 2 mm

Baratz ME, Larsen CF. Wrist and hand measurements and classification schemes. In: Gilula LA, Yuming Y. Imaging of the Hand and Wrist. Philadelphia: Saunders; 1996: 225–259

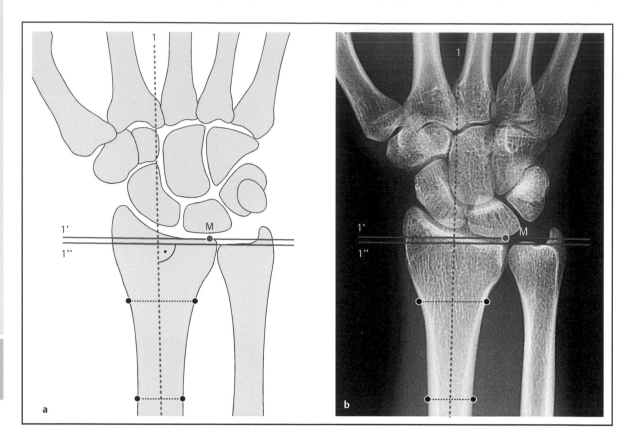

Fig. 7.3a,b Ulnar variance (Gelberman method).

1 = Longitudinal axis of the radius
1' = Line perpendicular to 1 through M
1" = Line perpendicular to 1 and tangent to the distal articular
surface of the ulna

M = Midpoint between the anterior and posterior margins of the
ulnar radius
a Diagram.
b Dorsopalmar radiograph.

Gelberman RH, Salamon PB, Jurist JM, Posch JL. Ulnar variance in Kienböck's disease. J Bone Joint Surg Am 1975;57(5):674–676
Schmitt R, Prommersberger KJ. Karpale Morphometrie und Funktion. In: Bildgebende Diagnostik der Hand. 2nd ed. Stuttgart: Thieme; 2004: 122–130
Steyers CM, Blair WF. Measuring ulnar variance: a comparison of techniques. J Hand Surg Am 1989;14(4):607–612

!

Any break in the contour of a carpal arc is suggestive
of carpal instability.

Gilula LA. Carpal injuries: analytic approach and case exercises. AJR Am J Roentgenol 1979;133(3):503–517

Carpal Arcs of Gilula

With a normal arrangement of the carpal bones, three smooth, parallel arcs can be traced along the proximal and distal rows of carpal bones depicted on a dorsopalmar radiograph of the wrist (**Fig. 7.4**). The first arc follows the proximal contours of the proximal row of carpal bones. The second arc follows the distal contours of the same bones, and the third arc traces the proximal contours of the distal carpal bones (capitate and hamate).

Carpal Angles

The wrist is evaluated for derangement of the carpal joints by determining the carpal angles on a lateral radiograph of the wrist. The carpal angles are formed by the longitudinal axes of the radius, lunate, scaphoid and capitate (**Fig. 7.5**).

Two methods can be used to determine the longitudinal axes of the carpal bones: tangential and axial. In the tangential method, the longitudinal axes of the carpal bones are defined as follows (**Fig. 7.6a**). The scaphoid axis is found by drawing a line tangent to the palmar contour

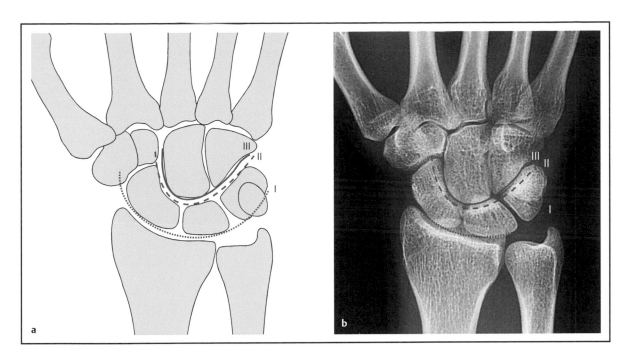

Fig. 7.4a,b Carpal arcs of Gilula.

a Diagram.

b Dorsopalmar radiograph.

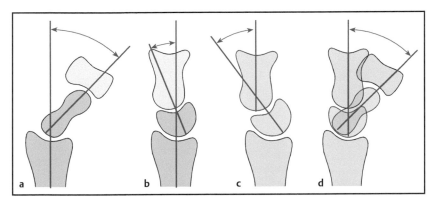

Fig. 7.5a–d Carpal angles.
Schematic representation.
a Radioscaphoid angle.
b Radiolunate angle.
c Capitolunate angle.
d Scapholunate angle.

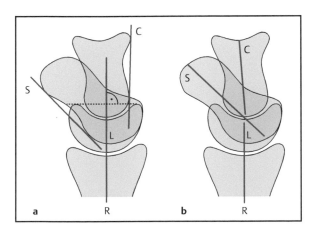

Fig. 7.6a,b Determining the longitudinal axes of the radius (R), lunate (L), scaphoid (S), and capitate (C).
a Tangential method.
b Axial method.

Table 7.1 Normal values of the carpal angles

Angle	Normal value (°)	Normal range (°)
Radiolunate	0	– 15 to + 15
Radioscaphoid	45	30–60
Scapholunate	47	30–60
Capitolunate	0	– 15 to + 15

Larsen CF, Mathiesen FK, Lindequist S. Measurements of carpal bone angles on lateral wrist radiographs. J Hand Surg Am 1991;16(5):888–893

Linscheid RL, Dobyns JH, Beabout JW, Bryan RS. Traumatic instability of the wrist. Diagnosis, classification, and pathomechanics. J Bone Joint Surg Am 1972;54(8):1612–1632

Schmitt R, Prommersberger KJ. Karpale Morphometrie und Funktion. In: Bildgebende Diagnostik der Hand. 2nd ed. Stuttgart: Thieme; 2004: 122–130

of the scaphoid, the capitate axis by drawing a line tangent to its dorsal contour. The lunate axis is found by drawing a line perpendicular to the line connecting the anterior and posterior horns of the lunate bone. In the axial method, the longitudinal axes of the carpal bones are defined as lines connecting the midpoints of the proximal and distal articular surfaces (**Fig. 7.6b**). The longitudinal axis of the distal radius is used in both methods. The angles listed in **Table 7.1** are then evaluated to check for malalignment of the carpal bones.

Baratz ME, Larsen CF. Wrist and hand measurement and classification schemes. In: Gilula LA, Yuming Y. Imaging of the Hand and Wrist. Philadelphia: Saunders; 1996: 225–259

Carpal Height

Some types of wrist pathology are associated with decreased height of the proximal row of carpal bones. The following indices can be used to quantify this change:

Carpal Height Ratio of Youm

The carpal height ratio of Youm is found by dividing carpal height measured in line with the third metacarpal axis by the length of the third metacarpal (**Fig. 7.7**).

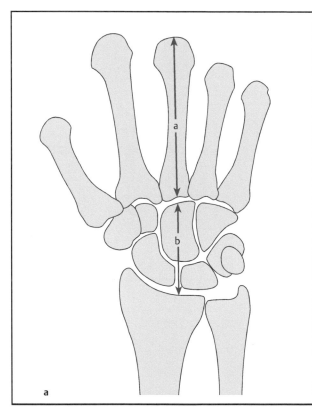
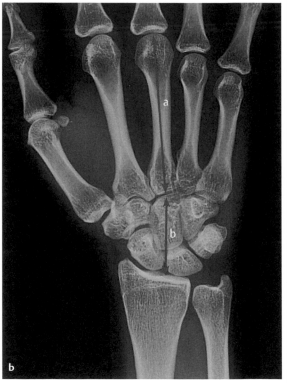

Fig. 7.7a,b Carpal height ratio of Youm.

a = Length of the third metacarpal
b = Total carpal height
b/a = Carpal height ratio of Youm

a Diagram.
b Dorsopalmar radiograph.

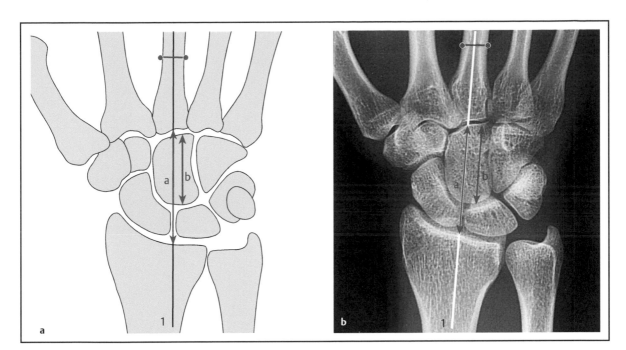

Fig. 7.8a,b Carpal height ratio of Natrass.

1 = Axis of the third metacarpal shaft
a = Carpal height (measured in line with the shaft axis)
b = Capitate length

a/b = Carpal height ratio of Natrass
a Diagram.
b Dorsopalmar radiograph.

Carpal height ratio of Youm
Normal value: 0.54 ± 0.03

Youm Y, McMurthy RY, Flatt AE, Gillespie TE. Kinematics of the wrist. I. An experimental study of radial-ulnar deviation and flexion-extension. J Bone Joint Surg Am 1978;60(4):423–431

Carpal Height Ratio of Natrass

To calculate this ratio, the carpal height (a) is divided by the capitate length (b) (**Fig. 7.8**). The axis of the third metacarpal shaft is defined first, and the carpal height is measured in line with that axis as the distance from the base of the third metacarpal to the distal radial articular surface. Capitate length is defined as the greatest distance between its distal and proximal articular surfaces.

Carpal height ratio of Natrass
Normal value: a/b = 1.57 ± 0.05

Natrass GR, King GJ, McMurtry RY, Brant RF. An alternative method for determination of the carpal height ratio. J Bone Joint Surg Am 1994;76(1):88–94

Ulnar Translation Index of Chamay

Ulnar translation of the carpus may occur in the setting of degenerative, posttraumatic, or destructive inflammatory disorders. Chamay developed an index for quantifying the degree of ulnar translation (**Fig. 7.9**). First the center of the capitate head (M) is located, and the distance (a) is measured from that point to a line parallel to the long axis of the radius, through the radial styloid process. That distance (a) is divided by the length of the third metacarpal (b) to obtain the ulnar translation index.

Ulnar translation index of Chamay	
• *Normal value:*	a/b = 0.28 ± 0.03
• *Abnormal values:*	a/b > 0.31

Chamay A, Della Santa D, Vilaseca A. Radiolunate arthrodesis. Factor of stability for the rheumatoid wrist. Ann Chir Main 1983;2(1):5–17

Wrist and Hand

7

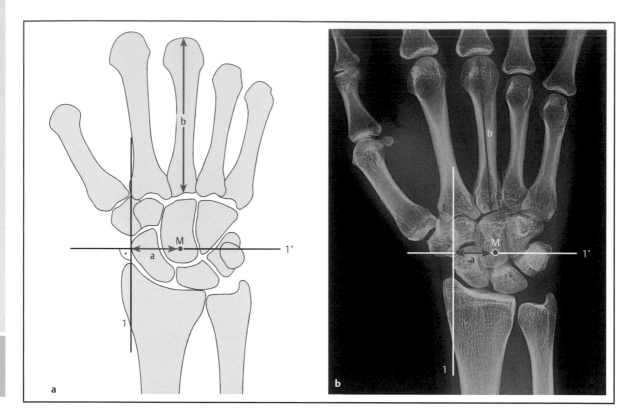

Fig. 7.9a,b Ulnar translation index of Chamay.

M = Center of the capitate head
1 = Line parallel to the long axis of the radius through the radial styloid process
1' = Line perpendicular to 1 through M

a = Distance from M to 1
b = Length of the third metacarpal
a/b = Ulnar translation index of Chamay
a Diagram.
b Dorsopalmar radiograph.

Carpal Instability

Carpal instability is defined as a derangement of the carpus with malalignment of the carpal elements during normal use of the wrist, i.e., throughout the arc of physiologic motions and subjected to physiologic stresses. Because carpal instabilities are based on complex pathogenic mechanisms that are not fully understood, they may be classified according to various criteria. The Amadio classification of carpal instability (see below) is an established system based on the integrity of the proximal carpal row.

Static and *dynamic* forms of instability are distinguished according to degree of severity. Whereas the malalignment is present at rest in the static form, it occurs only during certain movements in the dynamic form.

Amadio Classification of Carpal Instability (Supplemented by Schmitt)

This established classification of carpal instability has as its central criterion the integrity of the proximal carpal row. Accordingly, the carpal instability may be described as dissociative (CID) or nondissociative (CIND). Both types of derangement, which are usually chronic, are contrasted with complex (CIC) and axial instabilities that involve acute (traumatic) dislocations and fracture–dislocations (**Table 7.2**):

- *CID:* In dissociative instabilities, the continuity of the proximal carpal row is disrupted. This may be because of ligament ruptures (scapholunate and lunotriquetral ligaments) or scaphoid fractures or nonunions.
- *CIND:* In nondissociative instabilities, the proximal carpal row is intact but is rotated or subluxated as a whole relative to the distal carpal row or forearm. The acronym CIND-DISI means that the entire proximal carpal row rotates dorsally (into extension), while CIND-PISI means that the entire row rotates toward the palmar side (into flexion). The underlying lesions

Table 7.2 Amadio classification of carpal instabilities (supplemented by Schmitt)

Type of instability	Acronym	Location	Acronym
Dissociative	CID	Scapholunate (SLD)	CID-DISI
		Lunotriquetral (LTD)	CID-PISI
Nondissociative	CIND	Radiocarpal (RCI)	CIND-DISI, CIND-PISI
		Midcarpal (MCI)	CIND-DISI, CIND-PISI
		Capitolunate (CLIP)	CIND-CLIP
		Ulnar (UTL)	CIND-trans
Complex	CIC	Perilunar	CIC-DISI, CIC-PISI
Axial	Ulnar		–
	Radial		–
	Combined ulnar–radial		–

CIC = Carpal instability complex
CID = Carpal instability dissociative
CIND = Carpal instability nondissociative
CLIP = Capitolunate instability pattern

DISI = Dorsiflexed intercalated segment instability
PISI = Palmar-flexed intercalated segment instability
UTL = Ulnar translation

may be injuries of the extrinsic ligaments or dysplasias or displacements of the radial articular surface.
- *CIC:* Complex instabilities.
- *Axial malalignment.*

Amadio PC. Carpal kinematics and instability: a clinical and anatomic primer. Clin Anat 1991;4(1):1–12
Schmitt R, Stäbler A, Krimmer H. Carpal instability. In: Schmitt R and Lanz U. Diagnostic Imaging of the Hand. Stuttgart: Thieme; 2007: 274–291

Mayfield Stages of Progressive Perilunar Instability

Progressive perilunar instability refers to a dislocation involving the capitate and lunate bones. Because the wrist is stabilized by a complex system of ligaments, complete dislocation of the lunate can occur only in the presence of an extensive ligament injury. Mayfield described four stages of progressive perilunar instability characterized by specific, successive patterns of ligamentous and associated injuries. Progressive perilunar instability begins on the radial side with tearing of the scapholunate ligament (**Figs. 7.10 and 7.11**).

Mayfield JK, Johnson RP, Kilcoyne RK. Carpal dislocations: pathomechanics and progressive perilunar instability. J Hand Surg Am 1980;5(3):226–241
Schmitt R, Stäbler A, Krimmer H. Carpal instability. In: Schmitt R and Lanz U. Diagnostic Imaging of the Hand. Stuttgart: Thieme; 2007: 274–291

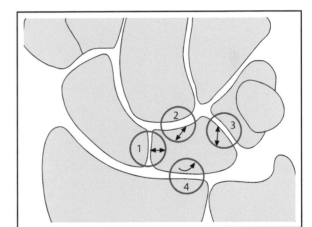

Fig. 7.10 Mayfield stages of progressive perilunar instability (full explanation given in Fig. 7.11). Schematic representation.

Instabilities of the Central Carpal Column

An abnormal position of the lunate in the central column of the carpus is designated by the acronym PISI (palmar-flexed intercalated segment instability) or DISI (dorsiflexed intercalated segment instability), depending on the direction of rotation (see above; **Fig. 7.12**). The wrist is evaluated for this abnormality on a lateral radiograph in the neutral position.
- *DISI configuration:* dorsal rotation of the lunate (into extension) with a radiolunate angle > 15°. This is a typical finding in scapholunate dissociation.
- *PISI configuration:* palmar rotation of the lunate (into flexion) with a radiolunate angle < – 15°. This is much rarer than the DISI pattern and occurs in the setting of midcarpal and ulnar-side instabilities.

Wrist and Hand

7

Stage	Type of instability	Ruptured ligament(s)	Radiographic findings	Schematic drawing
1	Scapholunate dissociation	Scapholunate ligament (SCL)	Scapholunate diastasis (DP view), rotary subluxation of the scaphoid, dorsal subluxation of the proximal scaphoid pole (lateral view)	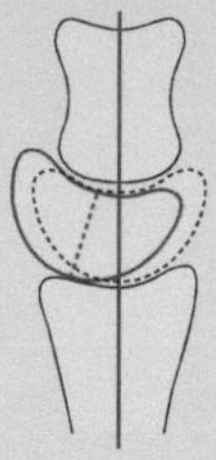
2	Scapholunate dissociation and midcarpal (sub)luxation	Scapholunate ligament (SCL) and radioscaphocapitate ligament (RSCL)	Same as stage 1 plus (sub)luxation of the capitate	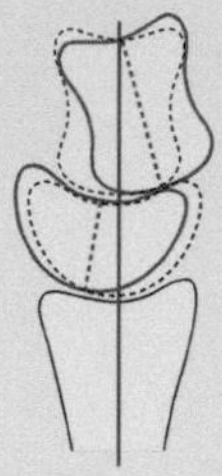
3	Scapholunate dissociation and midcarpal (sub)luxation plus lunotriquetral dissociation	Scapholunate ligament (SCL), radioscaphocapitate ligament (RSCL), lunotriquetral ligament (LTL), and radiolunotriquetral ligament (RLTL)	Same as stage 2 plus volar triquetral fracture or disruption of the radiotriquetral and lunotriquetral ligaments	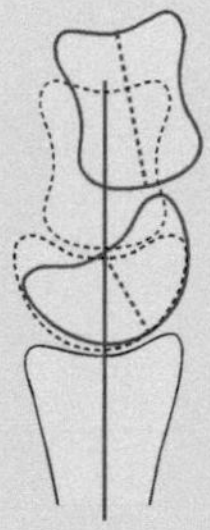
4	Complete dislocation of the lunate	Scapholunate ligament (SCL), radioscaphocapitate ligament (RSCL), lunotriquetral ligament (LTL), radiolunotriquetral ligament (RLTL), and dorsal radiotriquetral ligament (DRTL)	Volar dislocation of the lunate, capitate parallel to the radial axis	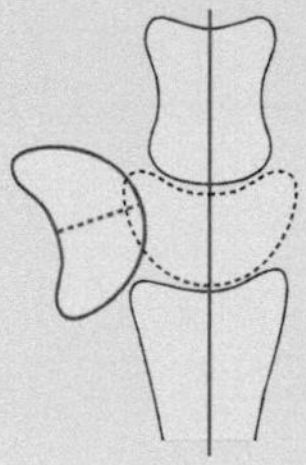

Fig. 7.11 Mayfield stages of progressive perilunar instability.

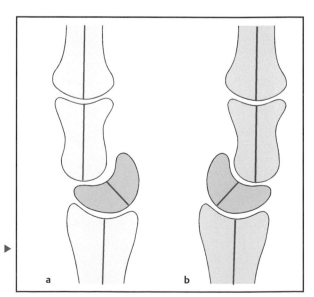

Fig. 7.12a,b Instabilities of the central carpal column.
a DISI malalignment (dorsiflexed intercalated segment instability).
b PISI malalignment (palmar-flexed intercalated segment instability).

Table 7.3 Watson and Black classification of scapholunate dissociation (expanded by Schmitt)

Stage	Basis for classification	Pathoanatomy	Imaging	Clinical manifestations
1	Partial tear	Tear of the palmar segment of the scapholunate segment	No radiographic changes. Diagnosed by arthroscopy or MR arthrography (limited)	Usually none
2	Complete tear, dynamic	Complete tear of the scapholunate ligament. Little or no involvement of extrinsic ligaments	No radiographic changes. Diagnosed by arthroscopy, kinematography or MR arthrography	Click or snap and weak grip during wrist movement

3	Complete tear, static without degenerative changes	Complete tear of the scapholunate ligament. Significant involvement of extrinsic ligaments	Conventional radiograph
			• DP view:
			  • Increased scapholunate distance (Terry Thomas sign)
			  • Scaphoid ring sign
			  • Scaphoid length shortened
			• Lateral view:
			  • Radioscaphoid angle > 60°
			  • DISI configuration
			  • Radiolunate angle > 15°
			  • Capitolunate angle > 60°
				Weak grip, swelling and pain even at rest, progressive course

4	Complete tear, static, with degenerative changes	Degenerative arthritis: radioscaphoid (IVa), midcarpal spread (IVb) Culminates in carpal collapse (SLAC wrist)	Same as stage 3 plus degenerative changes: • Radioscaphoid (IVa) • Midcarpal (IVb) • SLAC wrist • Decreased carpal height (abnormal Youm index)	Progressive swelling and limited motion. Chronic pain

MR = Magnetic resonance
DP = Dorsopalmar

DISI = Dorsiflexed intercalated segment instability
SLAC = Scapholunate advanced collapse

Classification of Scapholunate Dissociation

Scapholunate dissociation, caused by insufficiency of the scapholunate ligament, is the most common form of carpal instability. The severity of scapholunate insufficiency is graded by the Watson and Black classification, which Schmitt expanded by adding stage 4 degenerative changes (**Table 7.3**).

Stage 1

Stage 1, a partial tear of the scapholunate ligament, cannot be reliably diagnosed by imaging. The best method for detecting a partial tear of the scapholunate ligament is arthroscopy. MR arthrography can also detect these lesions, but with lower sensitivity.

Stage 2

Stage 2 is a complete tear of the scapholunate ligament without significant associated injuries. Plain radiographs are negative as in stage 1, but lesions can be demonstrated by MRI, stress radiography or kinematography. Stress radiographs can be reduced to a dorsopalmar projection of the wrist during forcible fist closure or a dorsopalmar projection while the patient grips a tennis ball. If scapholunate insufficiency is present, the scapholunate distance will be increased to > 3 mm on these views.

Kinematography can document the brief occurrence of carpal dissociation during various wrist movements, which is characteristic for a stage 2 scapholunate dissociation. A dorsopalmar kinematogram taken during radial and ulnar deviation of the hand will show widening of the scapholunate joint space to > 3 mm, whereas a lateral kinematogram will show transient dorsal rotary subluxation of the scaphoid and a DISI position of the lunate.

Stage 3

It is only in stage 3, marked by a complete disruption of the scapholunate ligament and extensive injuries to the extrinsic ligaments, that standard radiographs of the wrist (dorsopalmar and lateral views) will show characteristic findings. The main parameter at this stage of static instability is an increase in the scapholunate angle. Other features are an increased scapholunate distance ("Terry Thomas sign"), an increased radioscaphoid angle due to palmar flexion of the scaphoid, and a DISI configuration of the central carpal column caused by dorsal extension of the lunate:

Stage 3 scapholunate dissociation

- *Scapholunate angle:* > 60°; normal range: 30–60°
- *Terry Thomas sign:* widening of the scapholunate joint space > 3 mm; normal value < 2 mm; borderline: 2–3 mm
- *Radioscaphoid angle:* > 60°; normal range: 30–60°
- *DISI configuration of central carpal column:* radiolunate angle > 15°; normal range: – 15 to + 15°

! The Terry Thomas sign is an inconsistent finding. Stress radiographs or a Monheim projection are often necessary to detect widening of the scapholunate joint space.

Stage 4

Over time, secondary degenerative changes develop in joint areas subjected to unphysiologic loads. The radiographic detection of these changes signals the presence of stage 4 disease. Initial osteoarthritic changes develop between the radius and scaphoid (stage 4A), and descent of the capitate and hamate toward the widened scapholunate joint space leads to increasing involvement of the midcarpal compartment (stage 4B). Progressive loss of wrist height eventually leads to carpal collapse, known as the "SLAC wrist" (ScaphoLunate Advanced Collapse).

Schmitt R, Stäbler A, Krimmer H. Carpal instability. In: Schmitt R and Lanz U. Diagnostic Imaging of the Hand. Stuttgart: Thieme; 2007: 274–291

Watson HK, Black DM. Instabilities of the wrist. Hand Clin 1987;3(1):103–111

Lichtman and Ross Classification of Lunate Osteonecrosis (Kienböck Disease)

The Lichtman and Ross classification of lunate osteonecrosis has become well established in recent years (**Fig. 7.13**) and has largely replaced the traditional Decoulx classification.

The Lichtman classification is based on conventional radiographs of the wrist in two planes. But additional information provided by other imaging modalities (contrast-enhanced MRI and computed tomography) should be considered in this classification. Symptomatic patients with negative radiographs should undergo MRI to detect or exclude stage 1 lunate osteonecrosis. In stages 2 through 4B, radiographs should be supplemented by high-resolution computed tomography scans as these are more sensitive than conventional X-rays for detecting changes in bone structure, complete and incomplete fractures, and initial degenerative changes, permitting an earlier diagnosis of stages 2, 3A, and 4.

- *Stage 1:* characterized by localized or diffuse bone-marrow edema. The lunate still has a normal shape and trabecular structure. Only MRI is diagnostic at this stage.
- *Stage 2:* characterized by changes in bone structure (cystic changes and zones of osteosclerosis). The shape of the bone is essentially unchanged.
- *Stage 3:* infraction of the lunate (typically in the proximal circumference) determines the onset of stage 3. Later, this is followed by fragmentation and progressive collapse of the bone.
- *Stage 3A:* detectable fracture with possible initial decrease in lunate height; carpal integrity is maintained.
- *Stage 3B:* progressive collapse of the lunate, causing a decrease in carpal height and carpal instability. The scaphoid increasingly deviates toward the palmar side ("ring sign"), and the triquetrum toward the ulnar side.
- *Stage 4:* complete collapse of the lunate or complete fragmentation, accompanied by secondary osteoarthritic changes (osteophyte formation, joint-space narrowing, subchondral sclerosis).

Differentiation of stages 3A and 3B

- *Stahl height index:* ratio of longitudinal and sagittal diameters of the lunate; normal value: 0.53; abnormal: < 0.5
- Ulnar translation index of Chamay (see pp. 113–114)
- Carpal height ratio of Youm (see pp. 112–113)

These indices are abnormal in stage 3B.

Stage	Internal structure of lunate	External shape of lunate	Other carpal bones	Schematic drawing
1	Normal by radiograph and CT. MRI is diagnostic	Normal	Normal	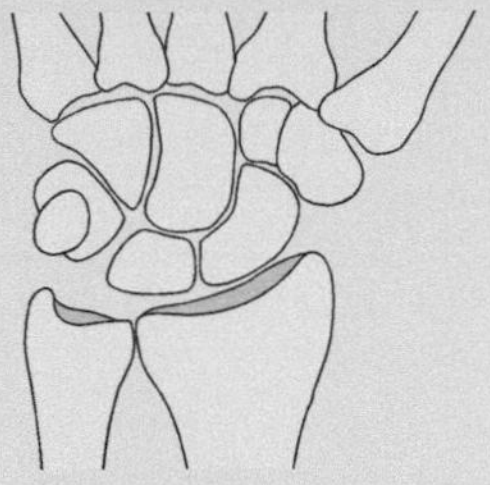
2	Density changes with diffuse osteosclerosis and cystic inclusions (possible early fracture line on lunate radial border)	Normal	Normal	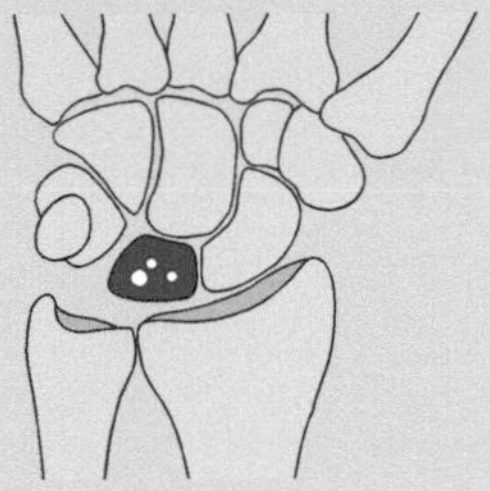
3A	Fracture line on the proximal circumference	Slightly deformed, incipient collapse	Without fixed scaphoid rotation, normal carpal alignment	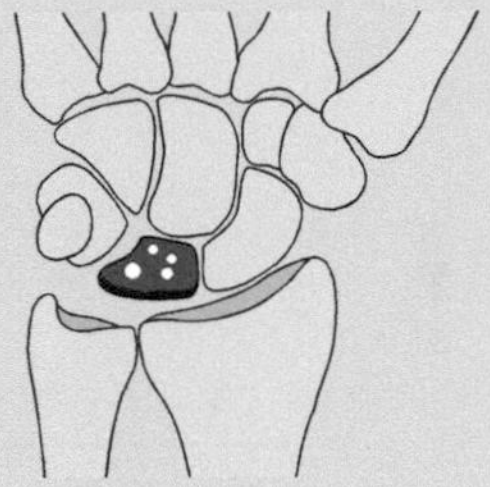
3B	Fractured, increased density	Increasingly deformed, progressive collapse	With fixed scaphoid rotation, carpal collapse	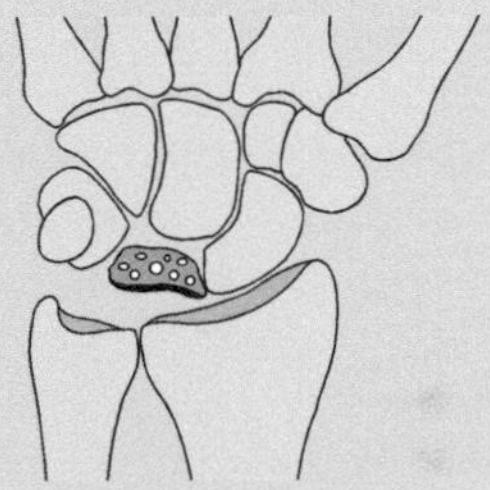
4	Extremely dense, severe lunate collapse	Osteophyte formation	Carpal collapse, osteoarthritis (osteophyte formation and sclerosis) in the remaining carpus	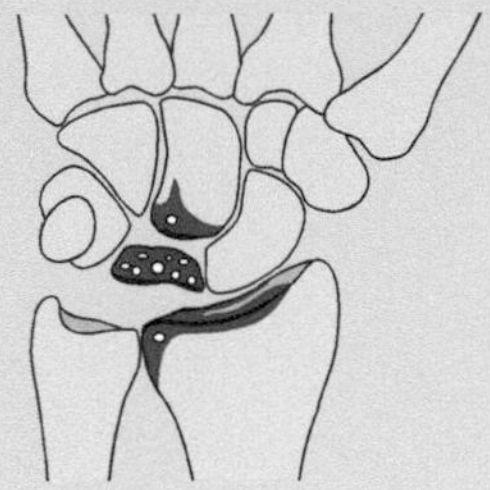

Fig. 7.13 Lichtman classification of lunate osteonecrosis (Kienböck disease).

Lichtman DM, Ross G. Revascularization of the lunate in Kienböck disease. In: Gelberman RH, ed. The Wrist. New York: Raven Press; 1994: 363–372

Schmitt R, Krimmer H. Osteonecrosis of the hand skeleton. In: Schmitt R and Lanz U. Diagnostic Imaging of the Hand. Stuttgart: Thieme; 2007: 351–365

Wrist and Hand

7

Palmer Classification of Triangular Fibrocartilage Complex Lesions

The triangular fibrocartilage complex (TFCC) is formed by the central, avascular triangular fibrocartilage and well-vascularized peripheral elements that include the stabilizing ligaments (ulnolunate ligament, ulnotriquetral ligament, palmar and dorsal radioulnar ligaments, ulnar collateral ligament), the meniscus homolog, and the extensor carpi ulnaris tendon sheath. Degenerative and traumatic lesions may affect any of the elements that comprise the TFCC.

The most widely used system for classifying TFCC abnormalities is the Palmer classification, which takes into account the etiology of TFCC lesions (traumatic versus degenerative) and the vascularity of the affected structures (avascular versus vascularized). Because lesions in the vascularized periphery of the complex tend to heal well whereas lesions of the avascular center heal poorly, vascularity is a key factor in directing the therapeutic approach (**Fig. 7.14**).

The best techniques for imaging the TFCC are MRI and MR arthrography. Whereas lesions of the (avascular) triangular fibrocartilage are best demonstrated by MR arthrography (two-compartment study with puncture of the radiocarpal joint and distal radioulnar joint), peripheral TFCC lesions are detected most sensitively on contrast-enhanced MR images based on the enhancement of fibrovascular repair tissue. Conventional MRI using fat-saturated proton-density sequences can detect lesions of the avascular triangular fibrocartilage as well but is less sensitive than MR arthrography.

Palmer AK. Triangular fibrocartilage complex lesions: a classification. J Hand Surg Am 1989;14(4):594–606

Metacarpal Sign

A (positive) metacarpal sign (**Fig. 7.15**) means that the fourth and fifth metacarpals are shortened relative to the third metacarpal, reflecting a disturbance of metacarpal growth.

The metacarpal sign is evaluated by drawing a line tangent to the heads of the fourth and fifth metacarpals on the dorsopalmar radiograph of the hand. In a normal hand, this metacarpal tangent will pass distal to the head of the third metacarpal (negative metacarpal sign). If the line just touches the head of the third metacarpal, the finding is considered borderline. If it passes through the head of the third metacarpal (positive metacarpal sign), relative shortening of the metacarpals is present.

! When the metacarpal sign was first described, a positive sign was considered typical of various endocrine disorders including pituitary dwarfism, gonadal dysgenesis and pseudohypoparathyroidism. Since then, however, it has been shown that this finding is common in other patient groups without endocrine abnormalities and even has a fairly high prevalence in the normal population. As a positive metacarpal sign is often found in diseases associated with growth delay, it is considered a nonspecific sign of a metacarpal growth disturbance.

Classification of Finger Pulley Injuries

The flexor tendon sheaths of the fingers are tethered to the bone by fibrous tissue bands (annular and cruciform pulleys) located on the volar side of the fingers (**Fig. 7.16**). Four or five annular pulleys (A1–A5) and three thinner cruciform pulleys (C1–C3) can be identified. The A2 annular pulley is considered the most important structure for transmitting forces to the bone, followed by the A3 and A4 pulleys. The A1 and A5 pulleys, like the cruciform pulleys, have only a minor role in stabilizing the flexor tendon sheaths on the volar side of the phalanges.

Two imaging techniques that can reliably detect finger pulley injuries are dynamic ultrasonography and MRI.

Dynamic Ultrasound Evaluation of Finger Pulley Injuries

Finger pulley injuries can be diagnosed with high sensitivity by performing a dynamic ultrasound examination of the finger at rest and during active forced flexion (**Fig. 7.17**). The examination is performed with a high-resolution transducer (12–14 MHz). The transducer is placed longitudinally on the volar side of the injured finger, and the distance between the flexor tendon and phalanx is measured at the level of the A2 (A3) and A4 annular pulleys. The measurement is performed in the resting position and then during active forced flexion, in which the patient presses the fingertip against the resistance of the examiner's finger. When a pulley injury is present, the tendon sheath will "bowstring" away from the bone during active flexion. A tendon–phalanx (TP) distance >1 mm in the resting position suggests a pulley lesion, and a specified increase in this distance with forced flexion is interpreted as a complete rupture of the annular ligament. Isolated ruptures of the A3 pulley are rare. If an abnormal TP distance is measured over the A2 pulley, the distance should also be measured at the A3 level to detect a possible combined rupture. If the TP distance is > 5 mm over the A2 or A3 pulley, it should be assumed that both

Wrist and Hand

7

Class	Type	Pathoanatomy	Schematic drawing	Vascularization of damaged zone	Treatment
Traumatic	1A	Vertical tear of the TFCC near its radial attachment	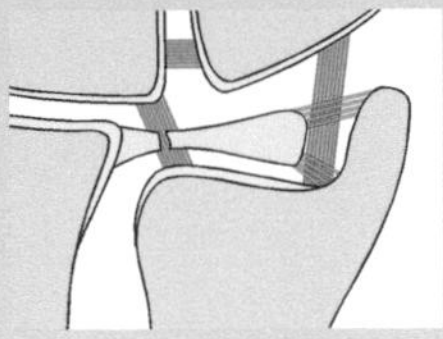	Avascular	Debridement
	1B	Avulsion of the TFCC from its ulnar insertion with or without fracture of the ulnar styloid at its base	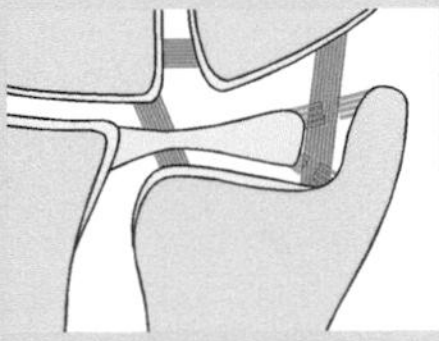	Vascularized	Surgical reattachment
	1C	Peripheral tears of the TFCC, i.e., tear of the ulnolunate and/or ulnotriquetral ligament	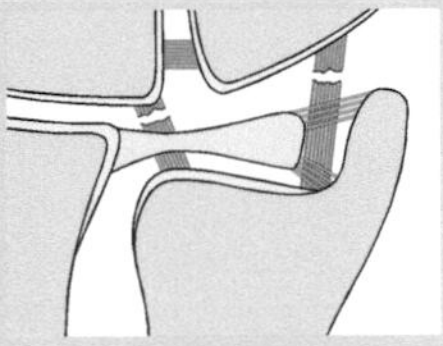	Vascularized	Acute: ligament repair; Chronic: ulnar shortening
	1D	Avulsion of the TFCC from the sigmoid notch of the radius (often with fracture of the distal radius)	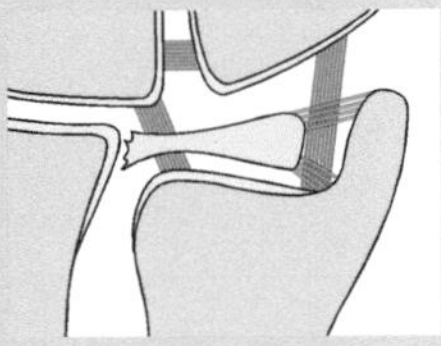	Avascular	Debridement
Degenerative	2A	Wear of the horizontal portion of the TFCC	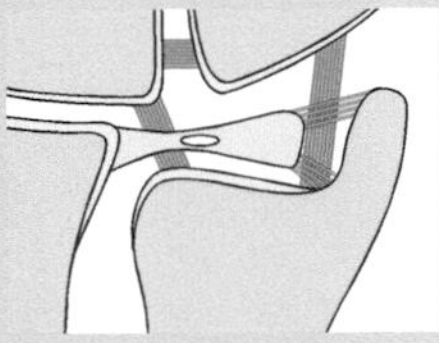	Avascular	(Debridement)
	2B	TFCC wear and lunate and/or ulnar chondromalacia	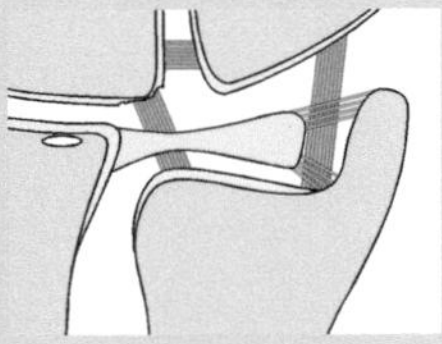	Avascular	Debridement, ulnar shortening if required
	2C	Perforation of the horizontal portion of the TFCC and lunate and/or ulnar chondromalacia	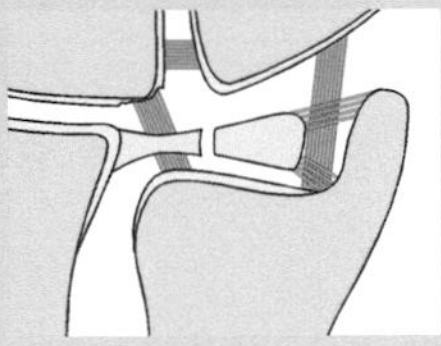	Avascular	Debridement, ulnar shortening if required
	2D	Perforation of the horizontal portion of the TFCC, disruption of the lunotriquetral ligament, and lunate and/or ulnar chondromalacia	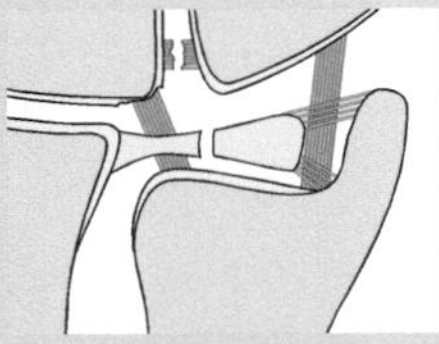	TFC avascular, ligament vascularized	Debridement, lunotriquetral partial arthrodesis
	2E	Perforation of the horizontal portion of the TFCC, disruption of the lunotriquetral ligament, lunate and/or ulnar chondromalacia, and ulnocarpal arthritis	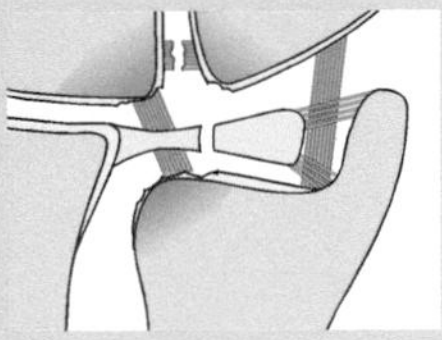	TFC avascular, ligament vascularized	Debridement, lunotriquetral partial arthrodesis

Fig. 7.14 Palmer classification of triangular fibrocartilage complex lesions.

Wrist and Hand

7

Wrist and Hand

7

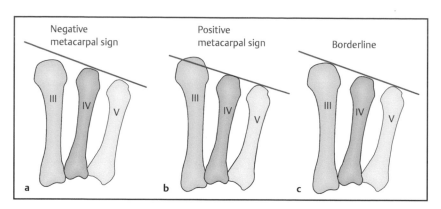

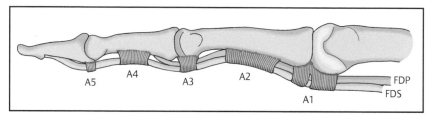

Fig. 7.15a–c Metacarpal sign. Schematic representation.
a Negative metacarpal sign (normal).
b Positive metacarpal sign (abnormal). The positive metacarpal sign is suggestive of abnormal metacarpal growth.
c Borderline finding (normal or abnormal?).

Fig. 7.16 Annular pulleys A1–A5. Schematic representation.
FDP = Flexor digitorum profundus tendon
FDS = Flexor digitorum superficialis tendon

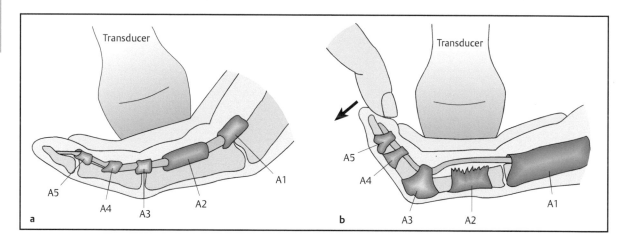

Fig. 7.17a,b Dynamic ultrasound examination of the annular pulley system.

a Resting position.

b Active forced flexion.

pulleys are ruptured. The corresponding cutoff values are shown in **Table 7.4**.

Klauser A, Frauscher F, Bodner G, et al. Finger pulley injuries in extreme rock climbers: depiction with dynamic US. Radiology 2002;222(3):755–761

MRI of Finger Pulley Injuries

> **!** Even high-resolution MRI cannot consistently define the finger pulleys because of their small dimensions and the difficulty of distinguishing them from flexor tendons, which have similar low signal intensity.

As in ultrasonography, an increased tendon phalanx (TP) distance on MRI provides an important indirect sign of a pulley rupture, and differentiation is aided by imaging the finger in the flexed position. A TP distance ≥ 1 mm

Table 7.4 Ultrasound evaluation of finger pulley injuries

Pulley level	Tendon–phalanx distance in the resting position		Tendon–phalanx distance during active forced flexion	
A2	≥ 1 mm	Suspicious for rupture	< 3 mm	Incomplete rupture
			> 3 mm	Complete rupture
A2 and A3	≥ 1 mm	Suspicious for rupture	< 5 mm	Incomplete rupture
			> 5 mm	Complete rupture
A4	≥ 1 mm	Suspicious for rupture	< 2.5 mm	Incomplete rupture
			> 2.5 mm	Complete rupture

measured over an annular pulley in the resting position is suggestive of a pulley injury. The lesions can be further differentiated by MRI based on the longitudinal extent of the bowstring effect during finger flexion. The area of increased TP distance does not reach the base of the proximal phalanx with an incomplete rupture of the A2 pulley, but it does with a complete rupture. With a combined rupture of the A2 and A3 pulleys, the TP distance is also increased at the level of the proximal interphalangeal joint. An A4 pulley rupture is present when the area of increased TP distance involves the pulley area at the level of the middle phalanx.

Another way to make or support the diagnosis is by using the cutoff values (TP distance during forced flexion) described above for the ultrasound technique.

Gabl M, Rangger C, Lutz M, Fink C, Rudisch A, Pechlaner S. Disruption of the finger flexor pulley system in elite rock climbers. Am J Sports Med 1998;26(5):651–655

Klauser A, Frauscher F, Hochholzer T, Helweg G, Kramer J, Zur Nedden D. Diagnosis of climbing related overuse injuries. [Article in German] Radiologe 2002;42(10):788–798

Wrist and Hand

7

8 Spine

Physiologic Curves of the Spine in the Sagittal Plane

Cervical Lordosis

The degree of cervical lordosis can be measured on a lateral radiograph of the cervical spine or full spine. The most common technique is to measure the angle between a reference line through the atlas and a reference line parallel to the lower endplate of the C7 vertebra (**Fig. 8.1**).

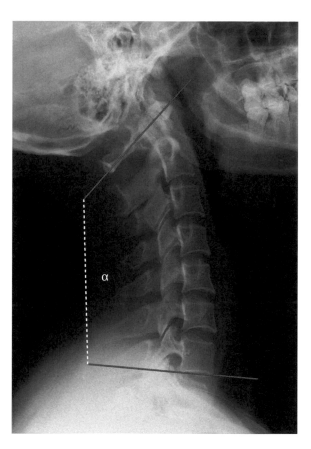

Fig. 8.1 Measurement of the cervical lordosis angle. The angle is formed by a reference line through the center of the atlas and a line along the lower endplate of the C7 vertebra.

Cervical lordosis	
• Mean value:	40°
• Normal range:	35–45°

! Positioning the patient for a lateral radiograph of the cervical spine, with the arms and shoulders drawn downward, often alters the posture in a way that straightens the physiologic lordosis of the cervical spine. As a consequence, decreased cervical lordosis on a lateral radiograph should be considered abnormal only when interpreted within the context of other findings.

Thoracic Kyphosis

Thoracic kyphosis is evaluated on a lateral radiograph by measuring the angle between the upper endplate of the T4 vertebra and the lower endplate of the T12 vertebra (**Fig. 8.2**). This angle is highly variable. Stagnara et al reported the following normal values:

Thoracic kyphosis	
• Mean value:	37°
• Normal range:	30–50°

Stagnara P, De Mauroy JC, Dran G, et al. Reciprocal angulation of vertebral bodies in a sagittal plane: approach to references for the evaluation of kyphosis and lordosis. Spine 1982;7(4):335–342

Vialle R, Levassor N, Rillardon L, Templier A, Skalli W, Guigui P. Radiographic analysis of the sagittal alignment and balance of the spine in asymptomatic subjects. J Bone Joint Surg Am 2005;87(2):260–267

Lumbar Lordosis

Lordosis of the lumbar spine can be quantified on lateral radiographs. A common technique is to measure the angle formed by the upper endplate of L1 and the upper endplate of S1 or the lower endplate of L5 (**Fig. 8.3**).

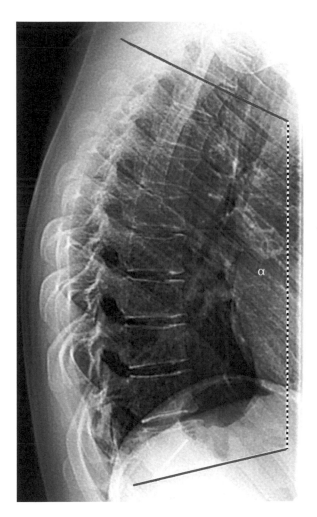

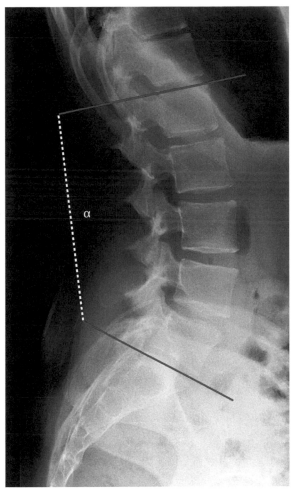

Fig. 8.2 Thoracic kyphosis angle. The angle is measured between the upper endplate of T4 and the lower endplate of T12.

Fig. 8.3 Measurement of the lumbar lordosis angle. The angle is measured on a lateral radiograph of the lumbar spine between the upper endplate of L1 and the superior margin of the S1 sacral segment.

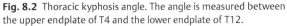

Lumbar lordosis (measured between L1 and L5)	
• *Mean value:*	43°
• *Normal range:*	14–69°

Vialle R, Levassor N, Rillardon L, Templier A, Skalli W, Guigui P. Radiographic analysis of the sagittal alignment and balance of the spine in asymptomatic subjects. J Bone Joint Surg Am 2005;87(2):260–267

Scoliosis

Cobb Angle

The American Scoliosis Research Society (ASRS) recommends the Cobb method as the standard measuring technique for quantifying spinal curvature in the frontal plane to obtain uniform and comparable values.

The measurement is performed on a standing anteroposterior (AP) radiograph of the full spine. The Cobb angle is measured between the vertebral bodies that are most tilted toward the concavity of the curve, or between the upper and lower endplates of these "end vertebrae" (**Fig. 8.4**). By definition, the reference lines are drawn along the superior endplate of the upper end vertebra and the inferior endplate of the lower end vertebra. The angle formed by lines drawn perpendicular to the reference lines is the Cobb angle.

Spine

8

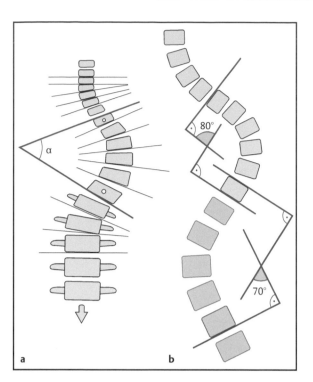

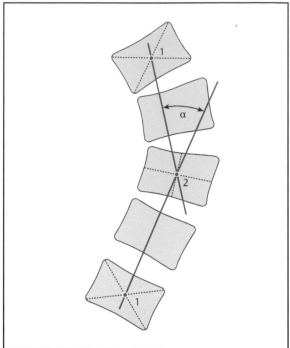

a　　　　　　b

Fig. 8.4a,b Measurement of the Cobb angle in scoliosis.
a The Cobb angle is measured between the most tilted vertebrae (= end vertebrae) above and below the apex of the curve.
b Sample measurement of scoliosis with an s-shaped curve. By definition, the angles are measured between the superior endplate of the upper end vertebra and the inferior endplate of the lower end vertebra.

Fig. 8.5 Measurement of the Ferguson angle.
1 = Center of the end vertebra (found by drawing diagonals across the vertebral body)
2 = Center of the apical vertebra (found by bisecting the sides and endplates of the vertebra)

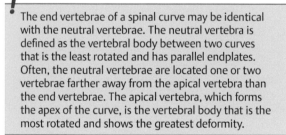

The end vertebrae of a spinal curve may be identical with the neutral vertebrae. The neutral vertebra is defined as the vertebral body between two curves that is the least rotated and has parallel endplates. Often, the neutral vertebrae are located one or two vertebrae farther away from the apical vertebra than the end vertebrae. The apical vertebra, which forms the apex of the curve, is the vertebral body that is the most rotated and shows the greatest deformity.

Cobb JR. Outline for the study of scoliosis. In: American Academy of Orthopedic Surgeons. Instructional Course Lectures. Vol. 5. Ann Arbor, MI: Edwards; 1948

Ferguson Angle

The Ferguson angle can be determined as an alternative to the Cobb angle. This measurement starts by identifying the end vertebrae and apical vertebra of the spinal curve. The end vertebrae are the vertebral bodies in the upper and lower parts of the curve that appear the most tilted in the frontal plane. The apical vertebra lies at the apex of

the curve and shows the greatest degree of rotation and deformity but the least amount of tilt. The centers of the end vertebrae and neutral vertebra are found as shown in **Fig. 8.5**. The centers of the end vertebrae, which have near-parallel upper and lower endplates, are located by finding the intersection of diagonal lines through the vertebral body. Because the apical vertebra is more deformed, its center is defined by the intersection of lines bisecting the sides and endplates of the vertebral body. Two lines are then drawn connecting the centers of the end vertebrae and apical vertebra. These lines intersect at an angle, the complement of which equals the Ferguson angle (**Fig. 8.5**).

Ferguson AB. The study and treatment of scoliosis. South Med J 1930;23:116–120

Risser Sign

The Risser sign can be used to assess skeletal maturity on a full-spine radiograph without the need for additional views. Risser observed in 1958 that ossification of the iliac apophysis begins as a bony "cap" on the anterolateral aspect of the iliac crest and progresses posteromedially toward the spine. Fusion of the apophysis to the ilium then progresses in a reverse direction.

Risser did not divide this process into grades or stages in his original publication. As a result, the classifications that appeared in later publications and textbooks show considerable variation. The classification shown in **Fig. 8.6** is widely used and divides the iliac apophysis into fourths.

Risser recognized that ossification of the vertebral apophyses roughly paralleled the ossification of the iliac apophyses, so that the Risser sign could be used to assess the remaining growth potential of the spine. Because scoliosis tends to progress during the adolescent growth spurt, a higher Risser stage correlates with a more favorable prognosis.

!
The apophyses on the iliac crest appear ~ 4 months after the peak of the adolescent growth spurt (age 12–15 years), which roughly coincides with menarche in females. By the time the apophysis starts to fuse with the iliac crest, marking the transition to stage 5, the adolescent growth spurt is completed. Very little additional growth occurs after that time (no more than 1–2 cm of longitudinal spine growth). Definitive fusion of the iliac apophysis to the ilium takes ~ 2 years on average and is generally complete by 21–25 years of age.

Risser JC. The iliac apophysis: an invaluable sign in the management of scoliosis. Clin Orthop Relat Res 1958;11:111–119

Fig. 8.6 Staging skeletal maturity with the Risser sign.

Stage	Description
0	Bony iliac apophysis not yet visible on radiographs 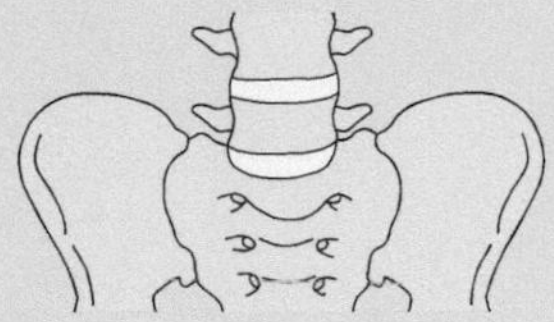
1	Initial (< 25%) ossification of the iliac apophysis
2	From 25% to 50% ossification of the iliac apophysis 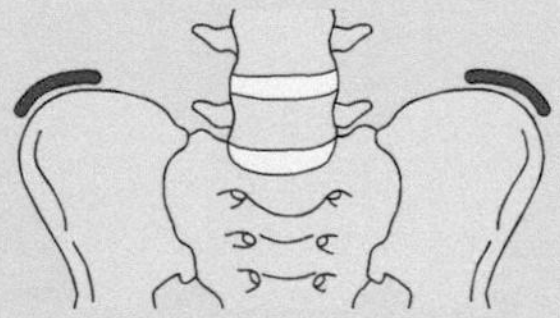
3	From 50% to 75% ossification of the iliac apophysis 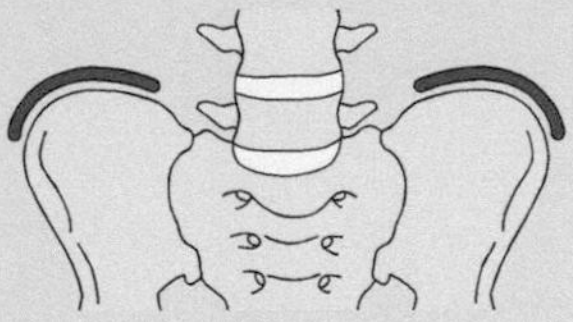
4	More than 75% ossification of the iliac apophysis 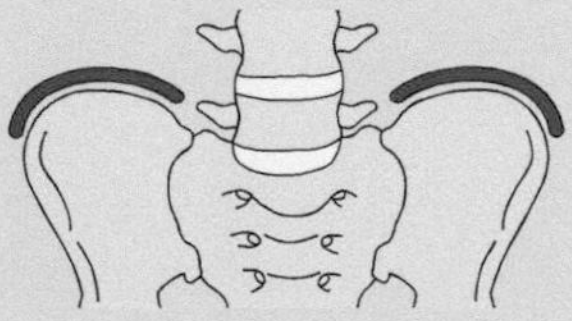
5	Iliac apophysis fuses to the iliac crest 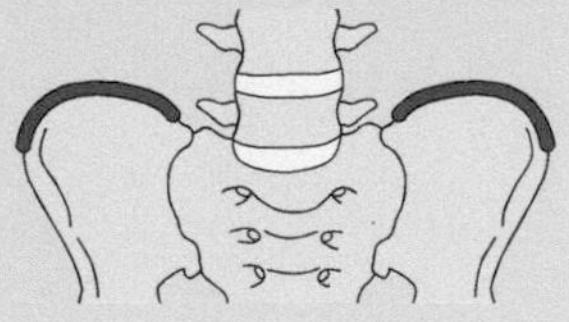

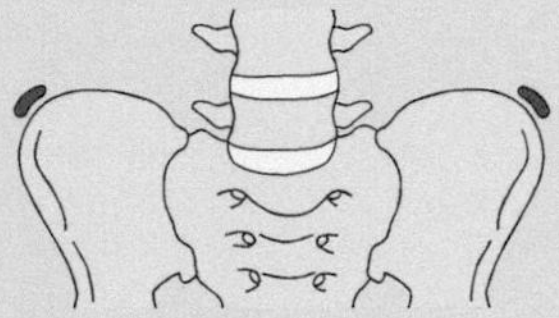

Spine

8

Nash–Moe Method of Measuring Vertebral Rotation

The Nash–Moe method is used to assess the rotation of the apical vertebra of a scoliotic curve. Located at the apex of the curve, the apical vertebra undergoes the greatest degree of rotation and deformity and the least amount of tilt.

Rotation is assessed by dividing the vertebral body into six sections on the AP radiograph. The relative displacement of the pedicles is evaluated. The pedicle on the convex side of the scoliosis is displaced toward the center of the vertebral body. The pedicle on the concave side is displaced toward that side and is no longer projected onto the vertebral body as an elliptical outline. The rotation is graded on a five-point scale (**Fig. 8.7**), and the degree of rotation can be directly determined as a percentage displacement (**Fig. 8.8**).

Nash CL Jr, Moe JH. A study of vertebral rotation. J Bone Joint Surg Am 1969;51(2):223–229

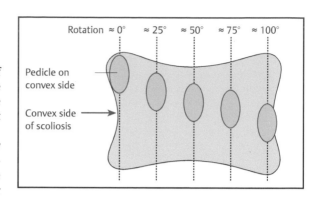

Fig. 8.8 Quantitative assessment of vertebral rotation (in %) by the Nash–Moe method. Schematic drawing.

Perdriolle Method of Measuring Vertebral Rotation

The rotation of a vertebral body can be read directly from the Perdriolle torsion meter on an AP radiograph of the spine (**Fig. 8.9**). First the midline of the pedicle on the convex side of the scoliosis is determined. The edges of the torsion meter are then aligned with the innermost points on the lateral vertebral margins, designated A and A'. The reference line that passes through the midline of the convex pedicle indicates the degree of vertebral body rotation.

Richards BS. Measurement error in assessment of vertebral rotation using the Perdriolle torsionmeter. Spine 1992;17(5): 513–517

Coronal Trunk Balance

The lateral deviation of the trunk relative to the lower body half can be quantified on an AP full-spine radiograph by assessing the coronal trunk balance (plumb line). A vertical line is dropped from the center of the T1 vertebra, and the distance from that line to the center of the S1 segment is measured in centimeters. Normally the coronal trunk balance should equal zero. Although normal values have not yet been published in the literature, a value > 1 cm is considered definitely abnormal.

Scoliosis Classifications

■ Topographic Classification

A simple classification of scoliosis is based on the level of the apical vertebra. The Scoliosis Research Society (SRS) uses the classification outlined in **Table 8.1** and illustrated in **Fig. 8.10**.

Grade	Description
0	Symmetrical appearance of the pedicles
1	Slight asymmetry of the pedicles; the pedicle (convex side) is displaced slightly toward the concave side
2	The pedicle on the convex side is in the middle third of the corresponding half of the vertebral body; the concave pedicle is barely visible
3	The pedicle on the convex side is at the center of the vertebral body; the concave pedicle is no longer visualized
4	The pedicle on the convex side has crossed the vertebral body midline

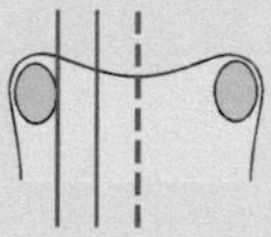

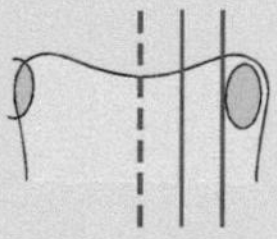

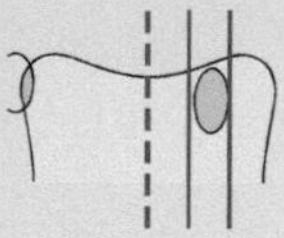

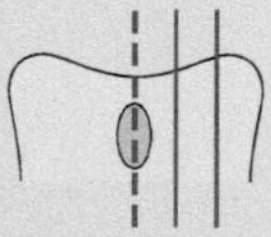

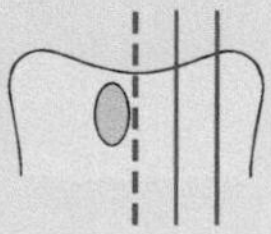

Fig. 8.7 Grading vertebral rotation by the Nash–Moe method.

Spine

8

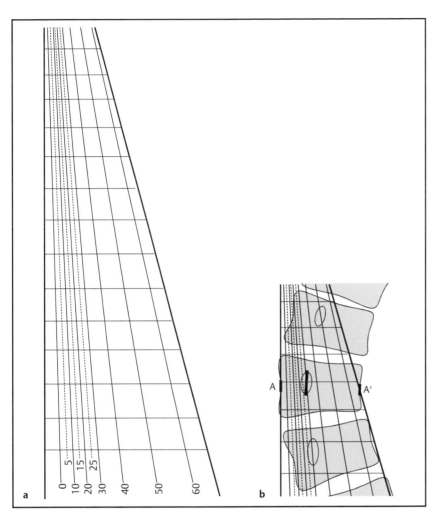

Fig. 8.9a,b Vertebral rotation measurement with the Perdriolle torsion meter.

a Torsion meter marked in degrees.

b With the edges of the torsion meter placed at A and A′ (the innermost points on the lateral vertebral margins), the degree of scoliosis is indicated by the scale line passing through the center of the pedicle on the convex side.

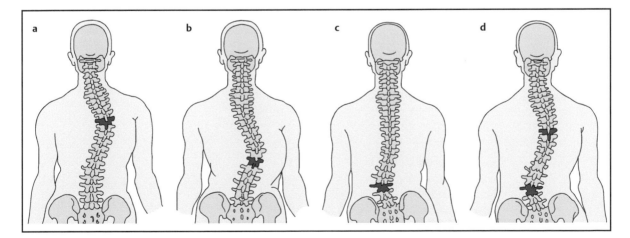

Fig. 8.10a–d Topographic classification of scoliosis.

a Thoracic scoliosis.

b Thoracolumbar scoliosis.

c Lumbar scoliosis.

d Double curve with a lumbar and thoracic component.

Table 8.1 Topographic classification of scoliosis

Level of apical vertebra	Type of scoliosis
T2–T11/12 disc	Thoracic scoliosis
T12–L1	Thoracolumbar scoliosis
L1/L2 disc–L4	Lumbar scoliosis

■ King Classification

The King classification of idiopathic scoliosis is based on radiographs of the full spine and side-bending radiographs (**Fig. 8.11**). Five types of scoliosis are distinguished in this classification, which takes into account the Cobb angle and the flexibility index determined on side-bending radiographs.

Fig. 8.11 King classification of idiopathic scoliosis.

Type	Description
1	• S-shaped curve in which the lumbar curve (Cobb angle) is larger than the thoracic curve • Both curves cross the midline • The thoracic curve is more flexible than the lumbar curve on side bending (flexibility index < 0)
2	• S-shaped curve in which the thoracic curve (Cobb angle) is larger than the lumbar curve • Both curves cross the midline • The lumbar curve is more flexible than the thoracic curve on side bending (flexibility index ≥ 0) 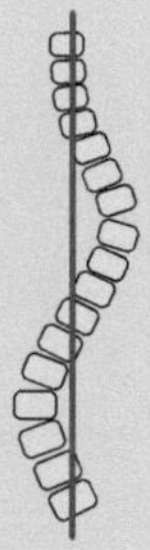
3	• Thoracic curve in which the compensatory lumbar curve does not cross the midline ("overhang") 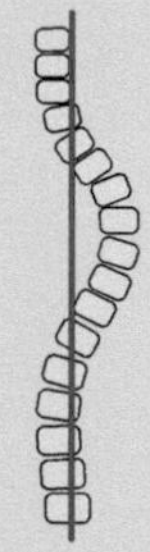
4	• Long thoracic curve in which L4 tilts into the thoracic curve • L5 is centered over the sacrum 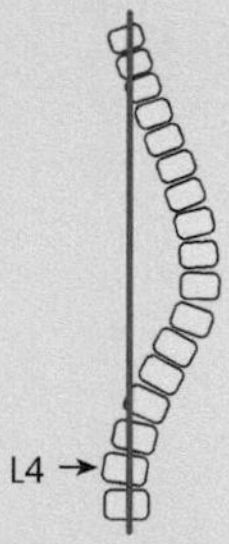
5	• Double thoracic curve in which T1 is tilted into the convexity of the upper curve • The upper curve is structural on side bending 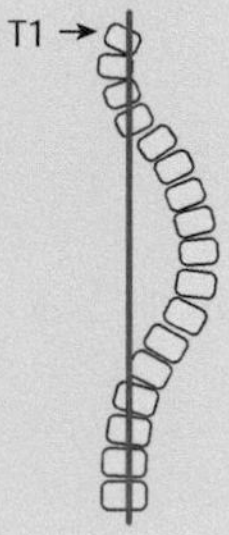

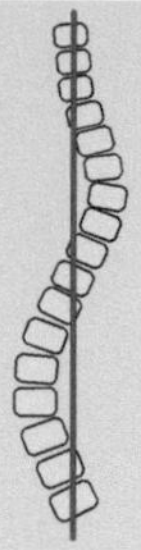

!
The classification of King et al, developed for the standardization of operative treatments, is widely used in describing curve types even though the surgical options recommended in the original work have become obsolete. The limitations of the King classification are well known. For example, it disregards important subtypes such as s-shaped scoliosis with thoracic and lumbar major curves. The classification has also been found to have low interobserver reliability, prompting the development of various modifications and even new classifications (Lenke classification, see below).

King HA, Moe JH, Bradford DS, Winter RB. The selection of fusion levels in thoracic idiopathic scoliosis. J Bone Joint Surg Am 1983;65(9):1302–1313

■ Lenke Classification of Adolescent Idiopathic Scoliosis

Given the limitations of the King classification, Lenke et al introduced a new scoliosis classification in 2001. It is based on full-spine radiographs in two planes and on right and left side-bending radiographs. The Lenke classification is much more complex than the King system. It describes a total of 42 subtypes, which are identified in three steps:
1. Determining the curve type (1–6)
2. Evaluating the lumbar changes ("lumbar spine modifier")
3. Evaluating the lateral profile ("sagittal thoracic modifier")

The components are assessed separately and then combined to form a classification triad, such as 2A+ or 2B–.

Step 1: Determining the Curve Type (1–6)

The curve type is determined by the location of the curve (level of the apical vertebra) and the flexibility of the curve. The level of the apical vertebra is first localized to a specific region:
- *Proximal thoracic curve:* apical vertebra is between T2 and T6

- *Main thoracic curve:* apical vertebra is between T6 and the T11/12 disc
- *Thoracolumbar curve:* apical vertebra is between T12 and L1
- *Lumbar curve:* apical vertebra is between the L1/2 disc and L4

To determine the curve type, the Cobb angle is measured for each curve and the greatest curve is defined as the major curve. Associated minor curves are then classified as structural or nonstructural by assessing their flexibility. A structural minor curve is present if the residual curve on the side-bending radiographs is > 25° or if the kyphosis angle of the curve on the lateral radiograph is > 20°. Six curve types can be assigned based on the above parameters (**Fig. 8.12**).

Step 2: Assessing the Lumbar Spine Modifier

The lumbar spine modifier is added to assess the lumbar deviation of the spine in the coronal plane. The central sacral vertical line (CSVL) is drawn up from the center of the S1 sacral segment on an AP spinal radiograph. The vertebral body divided most evenly by the CSVL is considered a stable vertebra. If the CSVL passes through an intervertebral disc, it is assumed that the vertebra just below that disc is a stable vertebra. The vertebra or disc located most lateral to the CSVL is then defined as the apex of the curve. The relationship between the CSVL and the apex of the lumbar curve defines the lumbar spine modifier. The three subtypes described in **Table 8.2** are distinguished by the position of the CSVL (see also **Fig. 8.12**).

Step 3: Assessing the Sagittal Thoracic Modifier

In the third step, the degree of kyphosis is evaluated on a lateral radiograph by assigning a minus sign (–), N (normal), or a plus sign (+). The kyphosis angle is measured between the T5 and T12 vertebrae.

Kyphosis angle	
• *Minus (–) sign:*	Kyphosis angle < 10°
• *N (normal):*	Kyphosis angle 10–40°
• *Plus (+) sign:*	Kyphosis angle > 40°

Table 8.2 Subtypes of the Lenke lumbar spine modifier

Subtype	Vertical line (CSVL)	Lumbar curve
A	Runs between the lumbar pedicles to the stable vertebra	No to minimal curve
B	Falls between medial border of lumbar concave pedicle and lateral margin of apical vertebral body or bodies (if apex is a disc)	Moderate curve
C	Runs completely medial to the concave aspect of the apical vertebral body or bodies (if apex is a disc)	Large curve

Spine

8

Type	Curve type	Description	Lumbar spine modifier		
			A (little or no curve)	B (moderate curve)	C (large curve)
1	Main thoracic	The main thoracic curve is the major curve and is structural. Proximal thoracic and thoracolumbar/lumbar curves are minor and nonstructural			
2	Double thoracic	The main thoracic curve is the major curve, the proximal thoracic curve is minor and structural, and the thoracolumbar/lumbar is minor and nonstructural			
3	Double major	The main thoracic and thoracolumbar/lumbar curves are structural, and the proximal thoracic curve is nonstructural. The main thoracic is the major curve and is greater than, equal to, or no more than 5° less than the thoracolumbar/lumbar curve			
4	Triple major (triple curve)	All three curves (proximal thoracic, main thoracic, and thoracolumbar/lumbar) are structural. The main thoracic or the thoracolumbar/lumbar curve may be the major curve			
5	Thoracolumbar/lumbar (TL/L)	The thoracolumbar/lumbar curve is the major curve and is structural. The proximal thoracic and main thoracic curves are minor nonstructural curves			
6	Thoracolumbar/lumbar–main thoracic (TL/L–MT)	The thoracolumbar/lumbar and the main thoracic curves are structural. The thoracolumbar/lumbar curve is the major curve and measures at least 5° more than the main thoracic curve. The proximal thoracic curve is nonstructural			

Curve type	Proximal thoracic	Main thoracic	Thoracolumbar/ lumbar	Description
1	Nonstructural	Structural (major)	Nonstructural	Main thoracic (MT)
2	Structural	Structural (major)	Nonstructural	Double thoracic (DT)
3	Nonstructural	Structural (major)	Structural	Double major (DM)
4	Structural	Structural (major)	Structural	Triple major (TM)
5	Nonstructural	Nonstructural	Structural (major)	Thoracolumbar/lumbar (TL/L)
6	Nonstructural	Structural	Structural (major)	Thoracolumbar/lumbar–main thoracic (TL/L–MT)

Structural criteria (minor curves)

Proximal thoracic:	– Side-bending Cobb ≥ 25° – T2–T5 kyphosis ≥ +20°
Main thoracic:	– Side-bending Cobb ≥ 25° – T10–L2 kyphosis ≥ +20°
Thoracolumbar/ lumbar:	– Side-bending Cobb ≥ 25° – T10–L2 kyphosis ≥ +20°

Modifiers

Lumbar spine modifier	CSVL = central sacral vertical line		Sagittal thoracic modifier (kyphosis angle T5/T12)	
A	CSVL between pedicles			
B	CSVL touches apical body(ies)		– (Hypo)	< 10°
C	CSVL completely medial to apical vertebra		N (Normal)	10°– 40°
			+ (Hyper)	> 40°

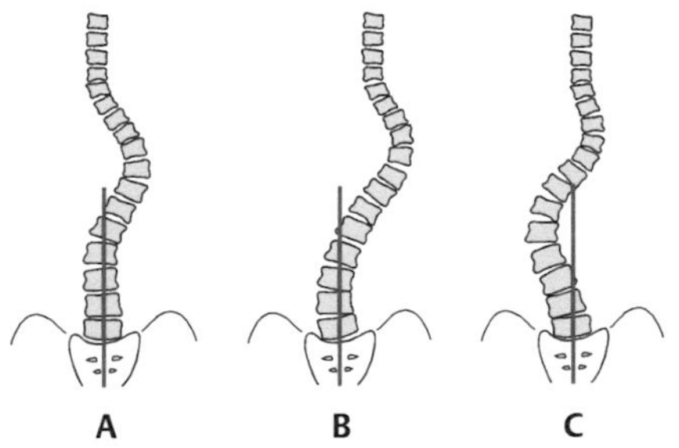

◀ **Fig. 8.12** Lenke classification of scoliosis.

Opposite: Curve types in the Lenke classification. Subtypes depend on the lumbar spine modifier, or the degree of lumbar deviation in the coronal plane (subtypes A–C).

Above: Synopsis of the Lenke classification. The major curve is determined by the largest Cobb angle and is always structural. Classification triad = curve type (1–6) + lumbar spine modifier (A, B or C) + sagittal thoracic modifier (–, + or N). Example: 1B+.

Spine

8

! On the whole, the Lenke classification is more reliable than the King classification and is helpful in the selection of modern corrective surgical techniques.

Lenke LG, Betz RR, Harms J, et al. Adolescent idiopathic scoliosis: a new classification to determine extent of spinal arthrodesis. J Bone Joint Surg Am 2001;83-A(8):1169–1181

Intervertebral Disc Heights

Dihlmann and Bandick (1995) investigated the normal progression of intervertebral disc heights in the motion segments of the cervical and lumbar spine. As indicated by the box below and **Fig. 8.13**, both regions generally show a harmonious increase of disc heights in the craniocaudal direction. It is only in the terminal segment of each region (C7/T1 and L5/S1) that the normal disc height may at most equal that of the next highest segment.

Normal progression of disc heights described by Dihlmann and Bandick

- *Cervical spine:*
  C2/C3 < C3/C4 < C4/C5 < C5/C6 < C6/C7 ≥ C7/T1
- *Lumbar spine:*
  L1/L2 < L2/L3 < L3/L4 < L4/L5 ≥ L5/S1

Based on this pattern, an abnormal loss of substance can be diagnosed by noting a change in the intervertebral disc height relative to the adjacent disc. An abrupt,

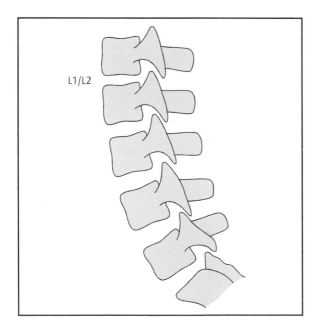

L1/L2

Fig. 8.13 Normal craniocaudal progression of lumbar disc heights (source: Dihlmann 2002).

discontinuous decrease or increase in the relative height of a disc space may be the earliest radiographic sign of an inflammatory or degenerative process or other pathology affecting the disc or vertebral body. An increase in disc height may signal an early stage of spondylodiscitis. A decrease in disc height may be caused by (bacterial) spondylitis or degenerative disc changes. Traumatic spinal injuries may also be associated with changes in disc height.

It is not possible to make accurate quantitative measurements of all the disc heights on lateral radiographs of the lumbar spine. Only the height of the disc within the central ray can be accurately measured while objects outside the central ray appear distorted because of projection effects.

In a larger study conducted by Biggemann et al (1997), the progression of disc heights that Dihlmann and Bandick described as normal in 1995 could be found in only 35% of men and 55% of women. This is mainly because the height of healthy intervertebral discs is subject to a relatively large range of biological variation. On analyzing the height differences between adjacent discs, Biggemann et al found that disc heights increased from above downward at the L1/L2 and L4/L5 levels, in agreement with Dihlmann and Bandick. But this rule does not apply at the L5/S1 level. To avoid false-positive results, the authors suggest that an equal, decreased, or increased disc height at L5/S1 relative to L4/L5 should be accepted as physiologic. Approximately 71% of men and 86% of healthy women would be classified as radiographically normal by this criterion.

Besides the relative comparison of disc heights with adjacent segments, absolute heights can also be measured. It should be noted, however, that high accuracy cannot be achieved because of projection errors. To correct for the wedge shape dimensions can be approximated by measuring the anterior and posterior disc heights and taking the average of the two measurements. For discs located farther from the central ray, the posterior end-plate margins of adjacent vertebrae appear to move closer together and may even overlap, resulting in negative measurements. Moreover, rotation or tilting of vertebrae or the spine will cause deviation from a true lateral projection, giving rise to additional errors. Frobin et al (1997) described a method for accurately measuring disc heights in the lumbar spine. This method is relatively complex, however, and adds little information to the relative comparison of disc heights.

! The pattern described by Dihlmann and Bandick (see above) can be evaluated on lateral radiographs of the spine and describes the physiologic progression of disc heights in the lumbar spine. Deviations from this pattern are suggestive of disc pathology. More recent studies have shown, however, that an increase of disc height may be a normal finding at the L5/S1 level. On the other hand, the increasing use of sectional imaging modalities in the spine has diminished the importance of indirect signs.

Biggemann M, Frobin W, Brinckmann P. The physiological pattern of lumbar intervertebral disk height. [Article in German] Rofo 1997;167(1):11–15

Dihlmann W, Bandick J. Die Gelenksilhouette: das Informationspotential der Röntgenstrahlen. Berlin: Springer; 1995

Frobin W, Brinckmann P, Biggemann M. Objective measurement of the height of lumbar intervertebral disks from lateral roentgen views of the spine. [Article in German] Z Orthop Ihre Grenzgeb 1997;135(5):394–402

Spondylolisthesis

Spondylolisthesis is the anterior displacement of a vertebra relative to the vertebrae below, generally caused by a morphologic abnormality in the pars interarticularis of the vertebral arch. Usually this consists of a defect in the isthmus of the vertebral arch between the superior and inferior articular processes (interarticular spondylolysis). Another possible cause is dysplasia characterized by elongation or shortening of the pars interarticularis. The prevalence of these two classic factors, with or without spondylolisthesis, is ~ 4–5%. The L4 or L5 vertebra is affected in ~ 90% of cases, with less frequent involvement of other lumbar or cervical vertebrae. An increased incidence of spondylolisthesis is found in gymnasts, ballet dancers, javelin throwers, weight lifters, and swimmers. Other causes of spondylolisthesis are listed in **Table 8.3**.

Because the different forms are on a continuum and may coexist with one another, the classification in **Table 8.3** is of limited clinical value. Spondylolisthesis with a degenerative cause is currently known as pseudospondylolisthesis and is considered a separate entity because of the absence of a vertebral arch defect.

The spondylolisthesis itself generally stops progressing after the cessation of skeletal growth. On the other hand, spondylolisthesis may lead to disc degeneration, which may in turn cause a slight progression of anterior slippage. It should also be noted that spondylolysis or isthmic dysplasia does not always lead to spondylolisthesis.

The diagnosis and follow-up of spondylolisthesis rely on lateral radiographs of the affected region. A standing radiograph (rather than supine) is recommended to detect any static changes caused by the process. It has been claimed that oblique radiographs of the lumbar spine in 45° rotation permit better evaluation of the pars interarticularis, but they rarely add information in patients with definite defects and high-grade spondylolisthesis and have been largely replaced by cross-sectional imaging studies.

At the cervical level, spondylolisthesis and spondylolysis most commonly affect the C6 vertebrae and are often accompanied by a median cleft in the neural arch and spinous process (spina bifida occulta). The slipped vertebra often shows a distorted shape with hypoplastic or aplastic pedicles, laminae, or articular processes.

As for the radiographic geometry of spondylolisthesis, methods have been devised for describing the anterior displacement of the vertebral body and for analyzing secondary static changes that may develop. As a rule, the latter methods can be applied and interpreted only for spondylolisthesis at the L5/S1 level.

Wiltse LL, Winter RB. Terminology and measurement of spondylolisthesis. J Bone Joint Surg Am 1983;65(6):768–772

Wiltse LL, Rothman SG. Lumbar and lumbosacral spondylolisthesis; classification, diagnosis and natural history. In: Wisel SW, Weinstein JN, Herkowitz HN et al, eds. Lumbar Spine. Vol. 2, 2nd ed. Philadelphia: W.B. Saunders; 1996: 621–651

Table 8.3 Causes of lumbar spondylolisthesis (after Wiltse)

Type	Description	Cause
1	Dysplastic	Congenital dysplasia of the articular process
2	Isthmic, lytic	Defect in the pars interarticularis, usually caused by repetitive loads or stress fractures, less commonly by acute trauma
3	Degenerative ("pseudospondylolisthesis")	Degenerative changes in the discs and facet joints
4	Traumatic	Vertebral arch fracture
5	Pathologic	General weakness of bone structure (Paget disease, osteoporosis, osteogenesis imperfecta) or focal defects (e.g., metastases)
6	Iatrogenic	Extensive resection for surgical decompression

Spine

Evaluating the Degree of Spondylolisthesis

■ Meyerding Classification

The anterior displacement of a vertebral body may be referred to as (o)listhesis, slip, or anterior translation. The Meyerding classification is the best-known system for grading the degree of anterior slip (**Fig. 8.14**). In this system the endplate of the vertebral body below the slipped vertebra is divided into four equal segments. The relationship of the posteroinferior corner of the slipped vertebra to the quadrants of the adjacent endplate determines the degree of spondylolisthesis. Complete forward and downward slippage of the L5 vertebra (spondyloptosis) produces a classic "inverted Napoleon's hat" sign in the AP radiograph (**Fig. 8.15**).

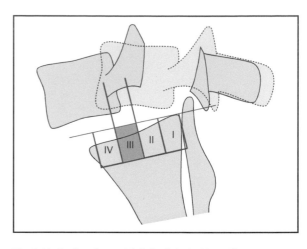

Fig. 8.14 Grades of spondylolisthesis in the Meyerding classification. Schematic representation of grades I–IV.

Meyerding HW. Spondylolisthesis: surgical treatment and results. Surg Gynecol Obstet 1932;54:371–377

■ Anterior Displacement

"Anterior displacement" as described by Taillard and later by Laurent expresses the percentage of vertebral slip relative to the underlying vertebral body (**Fig. 8.16a**). The distance of the posterior margin of the slipped vertebra from the posterior margin of the underlying vertebra (A) is divided by the length of the underlying vertebral body (B), and the result is multiplied by 100%.

Measurements may be distorted by the presence of a posterior spondylophyte or by posteroinferior dysplasia of the affected vertebra. Wiltse et al recommended the following technique for defining the posterior margin of the vertebral body in cases of this kind (**Fig. 8.16b**): First draw a line parallel to the anterior margin of the slipped vertebral body (a), then draw another line (b) along the upper endplate perpendicular to line a. The posterior margin is now defined by drawing a line c along the lower endplate that is parallel to line b and equal to it in length.

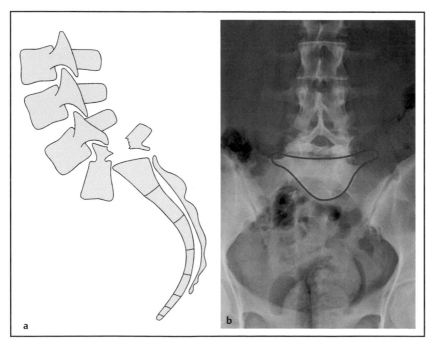

Fig. 8.15a,b Spondyloptosis.
a Diagram.
b "Inverted Napoleon's hat" sign on the anteroposterior radiograph.

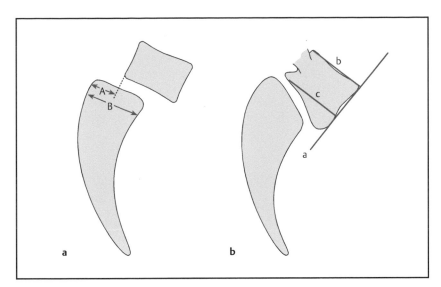

Fig. 8.16a,b Anterior displacement in spondylolisthesis.

a Schematic representation of anterior displacement described by Taillard. Anterior displacement measures ~ 40% in the example shown.
   A = Distance from the posterior sacral margin to the posterior margin of L5
   B = Diameter of sacrum
b Wiltse method for defining the posterior corner of the affected vertebra.
   a = Line parallel to anterior margin of vertebral body
   b = Line along the upper endplate, perpendicular to a
   c = Line along the lower endplate, parallel and of equal length to b

! Most authors prefer Taillard's "anterior displacement" method over the Meyerding classification owing to its greater accuracy. Measurements should be interpreted with caution, however, especially when evaluating small changes over time, as studies have shown up to 15% rates of interobserver and intraobserver variability (Danielson et al 1988, 1989).

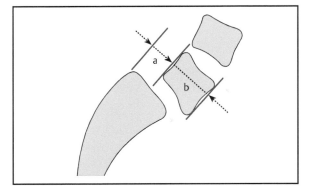

Fig. 8.17 Percentage slip (a/b ratio) described by Laurent and Einola. Schematic representation.
a = Distance between the posterior sacral margin and the posterior margin of L5
b = Sagittal diameter of the vertebral body

Danielson B, Frennered K, Irstam L. Roentgenologic assessment of spondylolisthesis. I. A study of measurement variations. Acta Radiol 1988;29(3):345–351

Danielson B, Frennered K, Selvik G, Irstam L. Roentgenologic assessment of spondylolisthesis. II. An evaluation of progression. Acta Radiol 1989;30(1):65–68

Laurent LE, Osterman K. Operative treatment of spondylolisthesis in young patients. Clin Orthop Relat Res 1976;117:85–91

Taillard W. Spondylolisthesis in children and adolescents. [Article in French] Acta Orthop Scand 1954;24(2):115–144

Wiltse LL, Winter RB. Terminology and measurement of spondylolisthesis. J Bone Joint Surg Am 1983;65(6):768–772

Wiltse LL, Rothman SG. Lumbar and lumbosacral spondylolisthesis; classification, diagnosis and natural history. In: Wisel SW, Weinstein JN, Herkowitz HN et al, eds. Lumbar Spine. Vol. 2, 2nd ed. Philadelphia: W.B. Saunders; 1996: 621–651

■ Method of Laurent and Einola

The Laurent–Einola method measures vertebral slip as a percentage (**Fig. 8.17**). The degree of spondylolisthesis is defined as the ratio of the anterior displacement of the affected vertebra to its sagittal diameter, multiplied by 100%. This method has not become established in clinical practice, however.

Laurent LE, Osterman K. Operative treatment of spondylolisthesis in young patients. Clin Orthop Relat Res 1976;117:85–91

Evaluating Secondary Static Changes

The static changes that develop in the setting of spondylolisthesis can be evaluated by various angles that are useful for follow-up and selecting patients for operative treatment.

■ Lumbosacral Kyphosis Angle

The lumbosacral kyphosis angle of Dick (**Fig. 8.18a**; Dick and Schnebel 1988, Dick and Elke 1997) is found by measuring the angle between the superior margin of the affected vertebra and the posterior surface of the sacrum. For spondylolisthesis at L5/S1, a kyphosis angle < 85° indicates a significant forward shift of the center of gravity. The patient tries to compensate for this by straightening the pelvis and lordosing the rest of the spine to return the center of gravity to a more posterior position (**Fig. 8.18b**).

This results in painful contracture of the lumbar paravertebral muscles and static problems that may require corrective surgery in severe cases.

Dick WT, Schnebel B. Severe spondylolisthesis. Reduction and internal fixation. Clin Orthop Relat Res 1988;232:70–79
Dick W, Elke R. Significance of the sagittal profile and reposition of grade III–V spondylolisthesis. [Article in German] Orthopade 1997;26(9):774–780

■ Ferguson Angle

Measurement of the Ferguson angle (also called the "sacrohorizontal angle") might depict increased angulation between the lumbar spine and sacrum (**Fig. 8.19**). The angle is measured between the upper endplate of S1 and a horizontal line. A value of ~ 34° is considered normal. Acute sacrum (sacrum acutum) describes a condition in which the static changes in advanced spondylolisthesis have led to increased lordosis and a decreased Ferguson angle. With an arched sacrum (sacrum arcuatum), the lumbosacral junction assumes a more curved shape due to an increase in the Ferguson angle. Besides spondylolisthesis, morphologic and postural changes are the most frequent causes of an acute or arched sacrum.

Wiltse LL, Winter RB. Terminology and measurement of spondylolisthesis. J Bone Joint Surg Am 1983;65(6):768–772

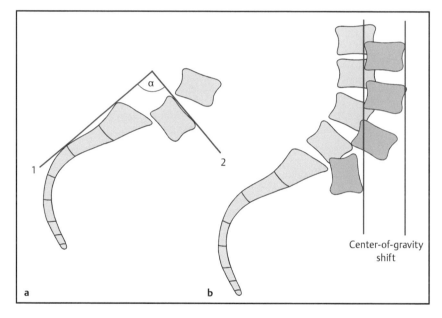

Fig. 8.18a,b Lumbosacral kyphosis angle.
a Determined by the Dick method.
  1 = Line tangent to the posterior surface of the sacrum
  2 = Line parallel to the upper endplate of L5
b Center of gravity in severe spondylolisthesis (dark) compared with the normal spine (light).

Center-of-gravity shift

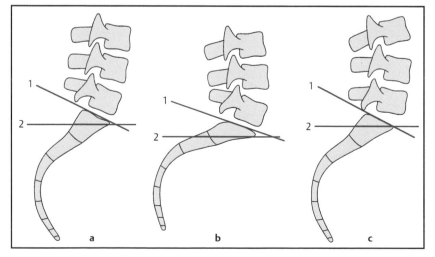

Fig. 8.19a–c Determination of the Ferguson angle.
1 = Upper endplate of S1
2 = Horizontal line
a Normal (~ 34°).
b Sacrum acutum.
c Sacrum arcuatum.

■ Sacral Inclination

Sacral inclination, or sacral tilt, describes the relationship of the sacrum to a vertical line in the sagittal plane (**Fig. 8.20**). It is used to measure the statically induced angulation of the lumbosacral junction that occurs in L5/S1 spondylolisthesis. Sacral inclination is evaluated on a lateral radiograph of the lumbar spine by drawing a straight line along the posterior margin of S1 and measuring the angle between that line and a vertical plumb line. The posterior margin of S1 may be difficult to discern on poorly exposed films. In this case an alternative reference line can be drawn through the midpoints of the upper and lower endplates of S1. As the anterior slip progresses, sacral inclination will decrease because of compensatory straightening of the pelvis. When the angle falls below 35°, surgical correction of the kyphosis should be considered based on recommendations in the orthopedic literature.

Wiltse LL, Winter RB. Terminology and measurement of spondylolisthesis. J Bone Joint Surg Am 1983;65(6):768–772

■ Sagittal Rotation

Sagittal rotation (also called roll, sagittal roll, or slip angle) can be determined by measuring the angle formed by the posterior margin of S1 and the anterior margin of L5 (**Fig. 8.21**). An angle of ~ 30° is considered normal in children and adolescents. The former method of measuring the angle between the upper endplate of S1 and the lower endplate of L5 is no longer recommended because of its poor reliability when L5 is hypoplastic.

Wiltse LL, Winter RB. Terminology and measurement of spondylolisthesis. J Bone Joint Surg Am 1983;65(6):768–772

■ Lumbar Lordosis

As spondylolisthesis increases, there is a marked increase in the degree of associated lordosis, especially in patients with a grade 3 or 4 slip. In the case of an L5/S1 spondylolisthesis, the angle describing the lumbar lordosis is measured between the upper endplate of L1 and the upper endplate of L5 (**Fig. 8.22**). With spondylolisthesis at the L4/L5 level, the upper endplate of L4 provides the lower reference line. The normal value (measured in a population without spondylolisthesis) is ~ 35°. It should be noted, however, that in patients with pronounced sagittal rotation of L5, the lordosis may extend up into the thoracic spine, making it necessary to distinguish "total" lordosis from lumbar lordosis.

Slim GP. Vertebral contour in spondylolisthesis. Br J Radiol 1973;46(544):250–254
Wiltse LL, Winter RB. Terminology and measurement of spondylolisthesis. J Bone Joint Surg Am 1983;65(6):768–772

■ Lumbar Index

Spondylolisthesis may be associated with a vertebral wedging deformity ("posterior hypoplasia") in which the height of the affected vertebral body is greater anteriorly than posteriorly. The lumbar index is measured by dividing the posterior height by the anterior height and multiplying the quotient by 100% (**Fig. 8.23**). Taillard and

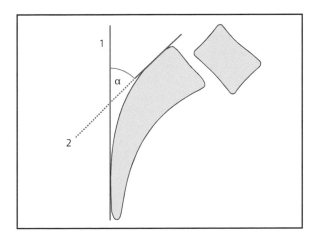

Fig. 8.20 Determination of sacral inclination.
1 = Vertical line
2 = Line tangent to the posterior margin of S1
α = Sacral inclination

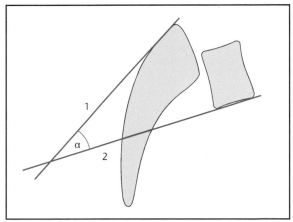

Fig. 8.21 Sagittal rotation.
1 = Line tangent to the posterior margin of S1
2 = Line tangent to the anterior margin of L5
α = Sagittal rotation

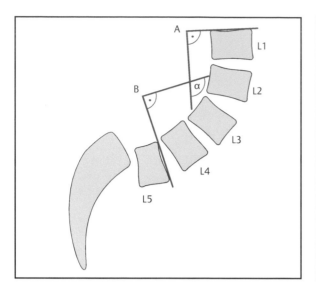

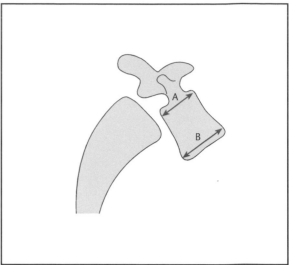

Fig. 8.22 Measurement of the lumbar lordosis angle between the upper endplate of L1 and the upper endplate of L5 in a patient with L5/S1 spondylolisthesis.
A = Line parallel to the upper endplate of L1
B = Line parallel to the upper endplate of L5
α = Lumbar lordosis angle

Fig. 8.23 Calculation of the lumbar index (LI).
LI = A/B × 100
A = Posterior height of the vertebral body
B = Anterior height of the vertebral body

Laurent and Osterman determined an average lumbar index of ~ 89.5% for the normal population. The average index in patients with spondylolisthesis was 72%. The lumbar index was < 70% only if the slip showed more than 30% of anterior displacement. This led the authors to conclude that increasing anterior displacement (especially > 30%) leads to secondary compression of the posterior elements of the affected vertebral body. The morphologic change may also involve a rounding of the anterior vertebral body contour.

Laurent LE, Osterman K. Operative treatment of spondylolisthesis in young patients. Clin Orthop Relat Res 1976;117:85–91
Taillard W. Spondylolisthesis in children and adolescents. [Article in French] Acta Orthop Scand 1954;24(2):115–144

■ **Summary**

The normal values for the various angles cited above, measured in a population 3–18 years of age, are outlined below. The lumbar index and lumbar lordosis increase with age.

Various angles and values used for evaluating spondylolisthesis
Mean values with 95% confidence interval, measured in 112 children (Wright and Bell 1991).
• *Sagittal rotation:* 32° (± 1.6°); range of 23–41°
• *Sacral inclination:* 52° (± 1.5°); range of 44–60°
• *Lumbar index:* 0.85% (± 0.01%); range of 0.78–0.92%
• *Lumbar lordosis:* 35° (± 1.8°); range of 25–45°
Lumbar index and lumbar lordosis are influenced by the age of the child.

Spine

8

! *Anterior slip*: Assessing the anterior slip of the affected vertebral body is of prime importance in the radiologic evaluation of spondylolisthesis. The Taillard method has largely replaced the Meyerding classification because of its better accuracy. It should be noted that most of the methods described have been normalized only for the lumbar spine and are applicable only in that region. Only the Meyerding and Taillard methods can be recommended for evaluating the rare cases of cervical spondylolisthesis. The Meyerding classification should not be used for pseudospondylolisthesis. The offset may be stated in millimeters.

Secondary static changes: Numerous angles have been devised for evaluating secondary static changes in the spine, but they are applicable only to the lumbosacral junction (in patients with L5/S1 spondylolisthesis). We recommend using the lumbosacral kyphosis angle or sacral inclination, as both angles are well represented in the literature and reliable reference values have been published for their therapeutic implications.

Therapeutic implications: In the radiographic evaluation of spondylolisthesis, it should be kept in mind that grade 1 or 2 spondylolisthesis is generally managed conservatively (restricted sports activity, back exercises, trunk muscle training, bracing). Surgical fusion is often recommended if complaints persist (especially root symptoms) or if the patient has Meyerding grade 3 or 4 spondylolisthesis (corresponding to 50% or more anterior displacement) before skeletal maturity, especially with a sacral kyphosis angle < 85° and sacral inclination <35°.

Dihlmann W. Gelenke—Wirbelverbindungen: klinische Radiologie einschliesslich Computertomographie—Diagnose, Differentialdiagnose. 3rd ed. Stuttgart: Thieme; 2002

Elke R, Dick W. The internal fixator for reduction and stabilization of grade III–IV spondylolisthesis and the significance of the sagittal profile of the spine. Orthop International 1996;4:165–176

Fredrickson BE, Baker D, McHolick WJ, Yuan HA, Lubicky JP. The natural history of spondylolysis and spondylolisthesis. J Bone Joint Surg Am 1984;66(5):699–707

Thurn P, Bücheler E. Röntgendiagnostik der Knochen und Gelenke. In: Thurn P, Bücheler E, eds. Einführung in die radiologische Diagnostik. Stuttgart: Thieme; 1986: 147–161

Wiltse LL, Winter RB. Terminology and measurement of spondylolisthesis. J Bone Joint Surg Am 1983;65(6):768–772

Wiltse LL, Rothman SG. Lumbar and lumbosacral spondylolisthesis; classification, diagnosis and natural history. In: Wisel SW, Weinstein JN, Herkowitz HN et al, eds. Lumbar Spine. Vol. 2, 2nd ed. Philadelphia: W.B. Saunders; 1996: 621–651

Wright JG, Bell D. Lumbosacral joint angles in children. J Pediatr Orthop 1991;11(6):748–751

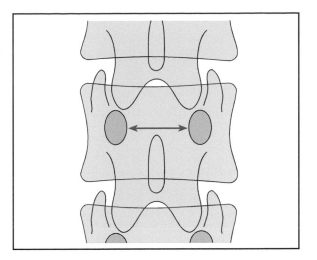

Fig. 8.24 Measurement of the interpedicular distance. Schematic representation.

Interpedicular Distance

Direct Measurement

The interpedicular distance is determined on an AP radiograph of the desired spinal region (cervical, thoracic, lumbar) by measuring the distance between the inner borders of both pedicles (**Fig. 8.24**). Elsberg and Dyke determined normal interpedicular distances for adults in 1934, and Simril and Thurston published normal values for children in 1955. The values vary with patient age and with the vertebral segment of interest. Slight sex-specific differences are also noted, with interpedicular distances averaging ~ 1 mm greater in males than in females. **Table 8.4** lists the normal values as 90th percentiles, which Hinck et al (1966) documented in 500 individuals. Values could not be determined for C1 or C2 because of their radiographic geometry. Normal values for interpedicular distances from C3 to L5 are shown graphically in **Fig. 8.25** for various age groups.

In theory, the interpedicular distances of thoracic vertebrae can be directly measured on a posterioranterior chest radiograph, but for technical reasons slightly higher values are measured than on an AP radiograph of the thoracic spine.

Spine

8

Table 8.4 Overview of the 90% tolerance limits for absolute interpedicular distances in males and females (source: Dihlmann 2002)

Vertebra	Age (years; males and females)							
	3–5	6–8	9–10	11–12	13–14	15–16	17–18	>18
C3	18–29	22–30	21–32	20–32	24–31	23–31	23–32	25–31
C4	19–30	23–31	21–32	21–33	25–32	24–32	24–33	26–32
C5	20–31	23–31	22–32	21–33	25–32	25–32	25–34	26–33
C6	20–31	24–31	22–32	21–33	25–32	24–33	25–34	26–33
C7	19–30	23–31	21–32	20–32	24–31	21–32	23–32	24–32
T1	17–26	19–26	20–27	20–27	19–28	18–29	20–26	20–28
T2	14–22	15–22	17–24	16–24	16–24	14–25	17–23	17–24
T3	13–21	14–21	15–21	14–22	15–23	15–22	15–21	16–22
T4	12–20	14–21	15–21	14–21	14–22	14–20	15–21	15–21
T5	12–20	13–20	14–20	13–21	14–22	14–21	15–21	14–21
T6	12–20	13–20	14–20	13–20	14–22	13–20	14–20	14–20
T7	12–20	13–21	14–20	13–20	14–22	13–21	15–21	14–20
T8	12–21	14–21	14–20	13–21	14–23	14–21	15–21	15–21
T9	12–21	14–21	13–21	14–21	15–23	14–22	15–21	15–21
T10	12–21	15–22	13–21	14–21	15–23	14–22	16–22	16–22
T11	13–22	16–23	14–23	15–22	16–25	16–23	17–23	17–24
T12	16–24	18–25	17–25	18–25	19–27	18–26	20–26	19–27
L1	17–24	17–27	19–28	19–27	20–27	20–28	20–29	21–29
L2	17–24	17–27	19–28	19–27	20–27	20–28	20–29	21–30
L3	17–24	17–27	19–28	20–27	21–28	21–29	20–29	21–31
L4	18–25	18–28	20–29	20–28	19–33	21–30	19–33	21–33
L5	21–28	22–32	24–33	24–34	22–36	23–35	23–37	23–37

Indirect Measurement

Besides the direct measurement of interpedicular distances, an alternative method is to determine the relative difference in interpedicular measurements between two adjacent vertebral bodies. The chart compiled by Lindgren in 1954 (**Table 8.5**) lists the normal relative differences from C4 to L5 in millimeters.

> **!** An abnormal increase in the interpedicular distance results from widening of the spinal canal and is found in numerous diseases. Besides neural tube defects such as diastematomyelia, syringomyelia, meningocele and myelomeningocele, dural ectasia may occur in Marfan syndrome, neurofibromatosis type 1, Ehlers–Danlos syndrome, ankylosing spondylitis, and osteogenesis imperfecta. Spinal trauma, such as a Chance fracture or compression fracture, may also cause an increased interpedicular distance. A narrowing of the normal interpedicular distance may occur in achondroplasia, thanatophoric dysplasia, and spinal stenosis.

In the relative method, the progression of measured values is compared with an age-dependent normal curve. An abrupt deviation of the actual curve (increased interpedicular distance) from the standard curve, or a progression of values opposite to the normal tendency, is strongly suggestive of an expansile interdural or intradural mass. One exception to this rule is that the pedicles at the apex of a kyphotic curve are often hypoplastic. Spinal torsion in scoliosis also causes interpedicular measurements to become less precise as the degree of torsion increases.

On the whole, methods based on the measurement of absolute values have not assumed greater importance than the relative method of Lindgren. Direct methods are influenced by various uncertainty factors such as film–focus distance, changes in object–film distance with body size, and the flattening of kyphotic and lordotic curves as the result of patient positioning. Additionally, measurement errors may occur in the determination of interpedicular distances.

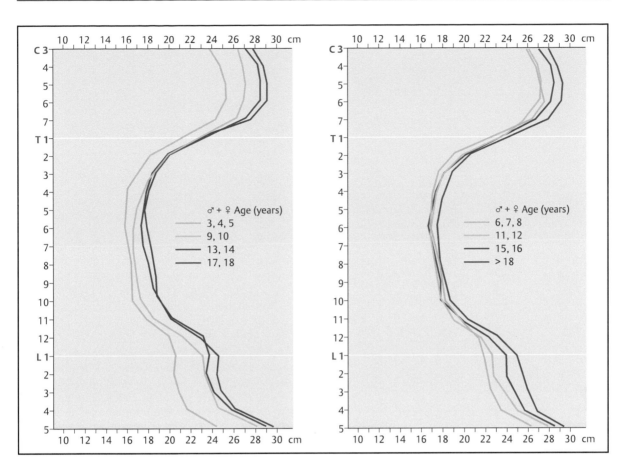

Fig. 8.25 Age-dependent curves for normal interpedicular distances from C3 to L5 (source: Dihlmann 2002).

Interpedicular Distance in Spondylolysis

There is evidence in the recent literature that patients with spondylolysis often have a small interpedicular distance. A predictive parameter is the relationship of the interfacet distance to interpedicular distance. An increase alters spinal statics and promotes the occurrence of spondylolysis in response to hyperextension trauma.

The interfacet distance is determined on an AP radiograph by measuring the transverse distance between the superior margins of the corresponding inferior articular processes (**Fig. 8.26**). Studies with relatively small case numbers have shown that an insufficient increase in interfacet distance between adjacent levels from L1/L2 to L5/S1, especially in relation to vertebral body width, is associated with a greater risk of developing spondylolysis.

Facet joint orientation or interfacet distance also has prospective importance in the possible development of degenerative changes such as osteochondrosis and facet joint osteoarthritis, which may be promoted by a constitutionally narrow spinal canal. A sagittal orientation of the facet joints and a small interfacet distance have a higher statistical association with pronounced degenerative changes.

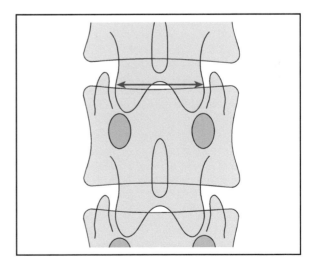

Fig. 8.26 Measurement of the distance between facet joints. Schematic representation.

Dihlmann W. Gelenke—Wirbelverbindungen: klinische Radiologie einschliesslich Computertomographie—Diagnose, Differentialdiagnose. 3rd ed. Stuttgart: Thieme; 2002

Spine

8

Table 8.5 Normal relations of the interpedicular distances of adjacent vertebrae (after Dihlmann)

Adjacent vertebral bodies	Interpedicular distance (mm)
C4/C5	~2
C5/C6	~2
C6/C7	~3
C7/T1	3–5
T1/T2	1–4
T2/T3	1–3
T3/T4	1–2
T4/T5	0–2
T5/T6	~1
T6/T7	~1
T7/T8	~1
T8/T9	0–2
T9/T10	0–3
T10/T11	0–3
T11/T12	2–5
T12/L1	1–4
L1/L2	0–3
L2/L3	0–3
L3/L4	0–3
L4/L5	0–5

Elsberg CA, Dyke CG. The diagnosis and localization of tumors of the spinal cord by means of measurements made on the x-ray films of the vertebrae and correlation of clinical and x-ray findings. Bull Neurol Inst NY 1934;3:359–394

Eubanks JD, Toy JO, Messerschmitt P, Cooperman DR, Ahn NU. Anatomic variance of interfacet distance and its relationship to facet arthrosis and disk degeneration in the lumbar spine. Orthopedics 2009;32(12):893–898

Fujiwara A, Tamai K, An HS, et al. Orientation and osteoarthritis of the lumbar facet joint. Clin Orthop Relat Res 2001;385(385):88–94

Hinck VC, Clark WM Jr, Hopkins CE. Normal interpediculate distances (minimum and maximum) in children and adults. Am J Roentgenol Radium Ther Nucl Med 1966;97(1):141–153

Kalichman L, Hunter DJ. Lumbar facet joint osteoarthritis: a review. Semin Arthritis Rheum 2007;37(2):69–80

Kalichman L, Suri P, Guermazi A, Li L, Hunter DJ. Facet orientation and tropism: associations with facet joint osteoarthritis and degeneratives. Spine 2009;34(16):E579–E585

Lindgren E. Röntgenologie einschliesslich Kontrastmethoden. In: Olivecrona H, Tönnis W, eds. Handbuch der Neurochirurgie. Berlin: Springer; 1954

Simril WA, Thurston D. The normal interpediculate space in the spines of infants and children. Radiology 1955;64(3):340–347

Ward CV, Latimer B, Alander DH, et al. Radiographic assessment of lumbar facet distance spacing and spondylolysis. Spine 2007;32(2):E85–E88

Zehnder SW, Ward CV, Crow AJ, Alander D, Latimer B. Radiographic assessment of lumbar facet distance spacing and pediatric spondylolysis. Spine 2009;34(3):285–290

Nomenclature and Classification of Degenerative Disc Changes

Pathoanatomic Classification of Posterior Disc Displacement

The following classification of posterior disc displacement is based entirely on pathoanatomic criteria, and was traditionally applied to radiologic interpretation in many English-speaking countries (**Fig. 8.27**).

- *Annular bulge:* "Bulging" refers to a diffuse or circumscribed extension of disc material beyond the posterior margin of the vertebral body while the annular fibers remain intact.
- *Disc protrusion:* A disc protrusion is present when nucleus pulposus tissue has entered a tear in the annulus fibrosus, resulting in the posterior displacement of disc material. By definition, at least some peripheral portions of the annulus fibrosus must still be intact.
- *Disc extrusion:* An extrusion is present when disc material has herniated into the spinal canal through a perforation in the annulus fibrosus. An extrusion beneath the intact posterior longitudinal ligament is called a subligamentous extrusion. If the posterior longitudinal ligament and adjacent epidural membrane are perforated, the disc material lies uncontained in the epidural space.
- *Sequestration:* Strictly speaking, sequestration refers to a fragment of disc material that is displaced into the spinal canal and has lost all continuity with the parent disc. The term has various definitions in the literature, however, and in some cases it includes disc material displaced into the epidural space and extrusions that have migrated upward or downward but are still in contact with the parent disc.

!

This classification, based entirely on pathoanatomic criteria, is often difficult to use in the interpretation of magnetic resonance and computed tomography images because anatomic structures relevant for making distinctions (e.g., the nucleus pulposus and annulus fibrosus) cannot always be positively identified. Therefore, this classification should be replaced by the nomenclature presented in the next section, which is based on the recommendations of the North American Spine Society, American Society of Spine Radiology, and the American Society of Neuroradiology.

Type of displacement	Description	
Annular bulge	The annular fibers remain intact but are protruded into the spinal canal	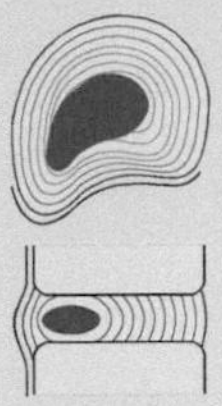
Disc protrusion (prolapse)	The displaced nucleus is still confined by the intact outermost annular fibers	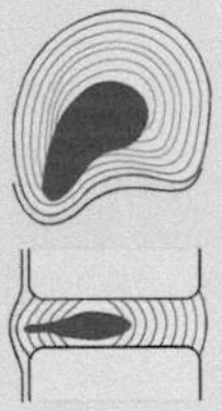
Disc extrusion	The displaced nucleus penetrates all annular fibers but is still confined by the posterior longitudinal ligament	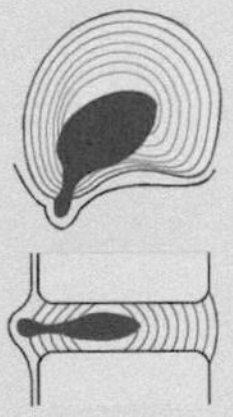
	The displaced nucleus has penetrated the posterior longitudinal ligament and lies within the epidural space	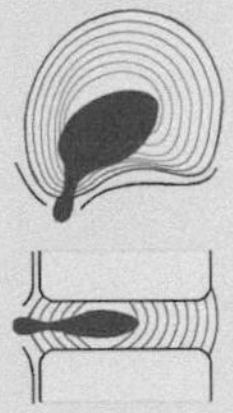
Sequestration	A fragment of the displaced disc has migrated in a cephalad or caudad direction and is separated from the parent disc	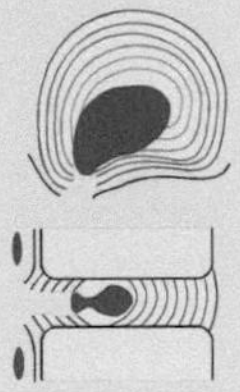

Fig. 8.27 Classification of posterior disc displacement (after Resnick; slightly modified).

Resnick D, Niwayama G. Degenerative diseases of the spine. In: Resnick D. Diagnosis of Bone and Joint Disorders. 3rd ed. Philadelphia: WB Saunders; 1995: 1372–1462

Nomenclature and Classification of Lumbar Disc Pathology

In 2001 a combined task force of the North American Spine Society (NASS), American Society of Spine Radiology (ASSR), and American Society of Neuroradiology (ASNR) issued recommendations on the terminology and classification of disc pathology based on radiologic findings to establish a more precise and uniform nomenclature. The goal was to link the interpretation of sectional imaging findings as closely as possible to the underlying pathoanatomy.

The consensus definitions are presented below (**Fig. 8.28**). A key element for classification purposes is to divide the intervertebral disc into four quadrants, each encompassing 90° or 25% of the disc circumference.

■ Definitions

Bulging

Bulging refers to a slight, *generalized* expansion of disc tissue past the circumference of the vertebral body. "Generalized" in this context means that the bulge

Spine

8

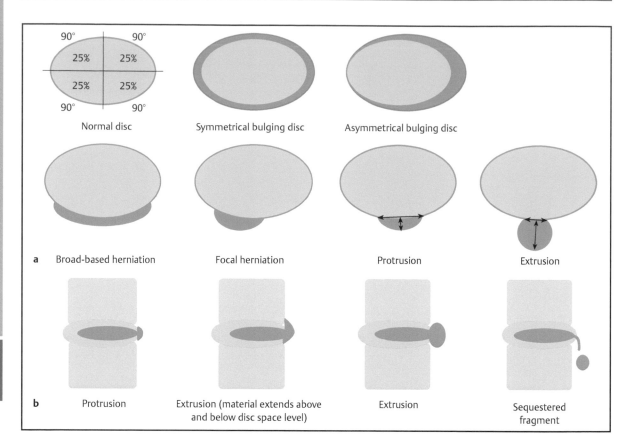

Fig. 8.28a,b Classification of disc pathology based on the recommendations of the North American Spine Society and other organizations.

a Types of posterior herniation on transverse sections.

b Types of posterior herniation on sagittal sections.

involves more than 50% or 180° of the disc circumference. Normally the bulge measures < 3 mm. A bulge may be described as symmetrical or asymmetrical, depending on its extent. An asymmetrical bulging disc, for example, is often found in scoliosis as a result of localized compression.

Herniation

Herniation is defined as a *localized* displacement of disc material. Unlike a generalized bulge, this localized displacement involves less than 50% or 180° of the disc circumference. The herniated disc material may consist of nucleus pulposus, annular tissue, cartilage, or fragmented apophyseal bone. Herniations may be classified as focal or broad-based:

- *Focal herniation:* A focal herniation involves less than 25% or 90° of the disc circumference.
- *Broad-based herniation:* A broad-based herniation involves 25–50% or 90–180° of the disc circumference.

A herniated disc may take the form of a protrusion or extrusion, based on the shape of the displaced disc material:

- *Protrusion:* A protrusion is present when the greatest diameter of the disc material displaced beyond the disc space is less than the diameter of its base. This must hold true for all imaging planes. Following the classification of herniations described above, a protrusion may be classified as broad-based (25–50% of the disc circumference) or focal (< 25% of the disc circumference).
- *Extrusion:* An extrusion is present when, in at least one plane, the greatest diameter of the herniated disc material is greater than the diameter of its base. A herniation should also be classified as an extrusion if the displaced disc material extends beyond the level of the disc space. This criterion applies only to images in the sagittal plane, not to transverse images.
- *Sequestration:* This is a subtype of extrusion in which the displaced disc material has lost all continuity with the parent disc.

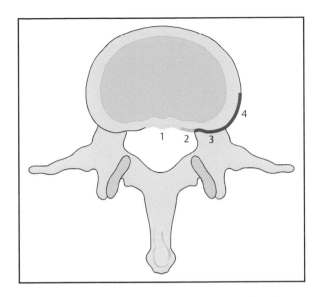

Fig. 8.29 Anatomic zones on transverse images based on the recommendations of the North American Spine Society and other organizations. Schematic representation.
1 = Central zone
2 = Subarticular zone
3 = Foraminal zone
4 = Extraforaminal zone

- *Migration:* This refers to the upward or downward displacement of disc material away from the extrusion site, regardless of whether the material is sequestered or not. Because the displaced material extends above or below the level of the disc space, this is by definition a subtype of extrusion.

Containment

"Containment" describes the integrity of the outer portions of the annulus fibrosus. With a contained herniation, the displaced nucleus pulposus tissue is held within an intact outer annulus. Containment is often difficult to evaluate by imaging, because the extent of an annular tear cannot always be defined due to difficulties in distinguishing among the nucleus pulposus, annulus fibrosus, and posterior longitudinal ligament. Herniated disc material can be characterized as "contained" or "uncontained."

Location

The use of anatomic landmarks is recommended so that the location of a disc herniation can be described as accurately and reproducibly as possible. Four anatomic zones are identified on transverse images (**Fig. 8.29**):
- *Central zone:* bounded laterally by the medial edge of the articular facets.

- *Subarticular zone:* from the lateral boundary of the central zone to the medial border of the pedicles. This zone corresponds to the lateral recess zone.
- *Foraminal zone:* located between the medial and lateral borders of the pedicles.
- *Extraforaminal zone:* the most lateral zone extending forward from the lateral border of the pedicle.

Based on this subdivision into zones, the location of a disc herniation can be described as follows (moving from central to right lateral as an example): central, right central, right subarticular, right foraminal, or right extraforaminal. Analogous terms would be used on the left side.

In the craniocaudal direction, location can be described in terms of levels as shown in **Fig. 8.30**. The following levels are distinguished based on the upper and lower borders of the pedicles and the vertebral endplates:
- Disc level
- Suprapedicular level
- Pedicular level
- Infrapedicular level

These terms are useful for describing the level of a disc herniation on sagittal images.

> **!**
> The NASS, ASSR and ASNR classification is based largely on morphologic criteria. This makes sense because the anatomic structures used in older classifications (nucleus pulposus, annulus fibrosus, etc.) cannot always be clearly distinguished on sectional images, and so findings often could not be positively identified or could only be crudely assessed. The different use and definition of the term "protrusion" may seem confusing at first sight. "Protrusion" in the newest classification is a focal disc herniation that does not meet the criteria for an extrusion. The new definition of the pathoanatomic term protrusion is that of a "contained" disc, or a bulging disc or broad-based herniation when morphologic criteria are applied. We recommend that the new classification be used in radiologic reporting, as it provides a less ambiguous nomenclature that has already become widely accepted.

Fardon DF, Milette PC; Combined Task Forces of the North American Spine Society, American Society of Spine Radiology, and American Society of Neuroradiology. Nomenclature and classification of lumbar disc pathology. Recommendations of the Combined Task Forces of the North American Spine Society, American Society of Spine Radiology, and American Society of Neuroradiology. Spine 2001;26(5):E93–E113

Wiltse LL, Berger PE, McCulloch JA. A system for reporting the size and location of lesions in the spine. Spine 1997;22(13):1534–1537

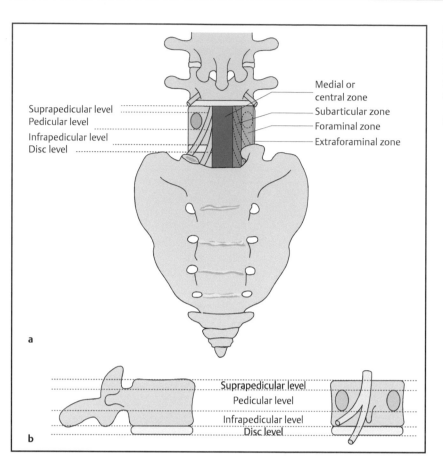

Suprapedicular level
Pedicular level

Infrapedicular level
Disc level

Medial or central zone
Subarticular zone
Foraminal zone
Extraforaminal zone

a

Suprapedicular level
Pedicular level
Infrapedicular level
Disc level

b

Fig. 8.30a,b Anatomic zones and levels based on the recommendations of the North American Spine Society and other organizations.
a Schematic representation of the zones and levels.
b Anatomic levels on craniocaudal images (sagittal and coronal).

Spine

8

9 Craniocervical Junction and Cervical Spine

Atlantodental Interval

■ Anterior and Posterior Atlantodental Intervals

The anterior and posterior atlantodental intervals are measured on a lateral radiograph of the cervical spine in patients with suspected anterior atlantoaxial subluxation. The indications for this study include the evaluation of cervical spine trauma and inflammatory joint diseases (especially rheumatoid arthritis).

● *Measuring the anterior atlantodental interval* (**Fig. 9.1**): A line is drawn along the anterior arch of the atlas connecting the most posterior points of its superior and inferior borders. Then a second, parallel line is drawn along the anterior aspect of the dens. The distance between the two lines is the anterior atlantodental interval (AADI), which can be measured in the neutral position and also in flexion and extension. Values > 3 mm are considered suspicious. Widening of the AADI to > 5 mm strongly suggests rupture or inflammatory damage to the transverse atlantal ligament. In children under 8 years of age, an AADI of 4 mm is

considered the upper limit of normal, especially during flexion, because the ligaments are slightly more lax in children.

● *Measuring the posterior atlantodental interval* (**Fig. 9.2**): A line is drawn along the posterior arch of the atlas connecting the most anterior points of its superior and inferior borders. The distance between that line and a parallel line along the posterior aspect of the dens is the posterior atlantodental interval (PADI). In patients with atlantoaxial instability due to rheumatoid arthritis, values < 10 mm are critical in terms of spinal canal encroachment and possible spinal cord compression.

■ Lateral Atlantodental Interval

Two techniques are available for evaluating atlantodental dislocation in the coronal plane. Both are based on a transoral odontoid view.

● *Evaluation of the lateral atlantodental interval* (**Fig. 9.3**): Draw a line tangent to the most medial point on the left and right lateral masses of C1. Measure its distance from the dens on each side, and compare the

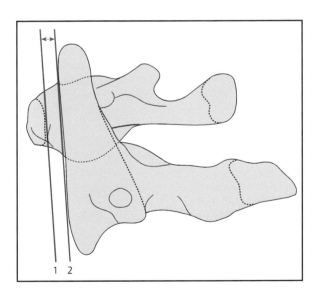

Fig. 9.1 Anterior atlantodental interval. The AADI is measured as the distance between a line along the anterior arch of the atlas (1) and a parallel line along the anterior border of the dens (2).

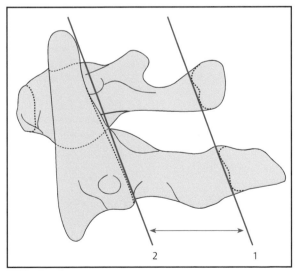

Fig. 9.2 Posterior atlantodental interval. The PADI is measured as the distance between a line along the posterior arch of the atlas (1) and a parallel line along the posterior border of the dens (2).

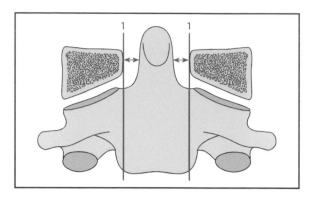

Fig. 9.3 Measurement of the lateral atlantodental interval.
1 = Line tangent to the most medial part of the lateral mass

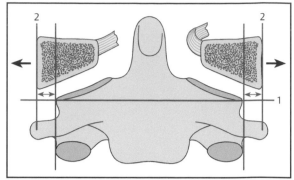

Fig. 9.4 Displacement of the C1 lateral masses.
1 = Horizontal line through the lateral margins of the articular facets of C2
2 = Line tangent to the lateral borders of C1

sides. Definitive cutoff values have not been published in the literature, but it should be noted that only a true anteroposterior (AP) transoral odontoid view will permit a reliable evaluation.

- *Measuring the displacement of the C1 lateral masses* (**Fig. 9.4**): This method is more practical and dependable. Lateral displacement signifies a possible rupture of the transverse ligament due to a Jefferson fracture. The offset of a line tangent to the lateral aspects of C1 is measured along a horizontal line drawn through the lateral margins of the articular facets of C2. Normally the lateral margins of the atlas and axis should line up with each other, even during slight neck rotation. Displacement of the C1 lateral masses by > 7 mm (adding both sides) suggests the presence of a Jefferson fracture accompanied by rupture of the transverse ligament.

!

Measuring the anterior atlantodental interval and evaluating displacement of the C1 lateral masses are particularly important in patients with cervical spine injuries. The posterior atlantodental interval is a key parameter in patients with destructive changes caused by inflammatory joint disease, but its role in selecting patients for surgery has been diminished by the increasing use of magnetic resonance imaging (MRI) for the detection of associated myelopathy.

El-Khoury GY, Wener MH, Menezes AH, Dolan KD, Kathol ME. Cranial settling in rheumatoid arthritis. Radiology 1980;137(3):637–642
Haaland K, Aadland HA, Haavik TK, Vallersnes FM. Atlanto-axial subluxation in rheumatoid arthritis. A study of 104 hospital patients. Scand J Rheumatol 1984;13(4):319–323
Halla JT, Hardin JG, Vitek J, Alarcón GS. Involvement of the cervical spine in rheumatoid arthritis. Arthritis Rheum 1989;32(5):652–659

Locke GR, Gardner JI, Van Epps EF. Atlas–dens interval (ADI) in children: a survey based on 200 normal cervical spines. Am J Roentgenol Radium Ther Nucl Med 1966;97(1):135–140
Steel HH. Anatomical and mechanical considerations of the atlantoaxial articulations. J Bone Joint Surg Am 1968;50:1481–1482

Vertebral Alignment

Lateral Radiograph

Four contour lines can be used to evaluate vertebral alignment on a lateral radiograph of the cervical spine (**Fig. 9.5**). Each of the lines should form a smooth, gentle curve with no steps or discontinuities. Approximately 20% of children have a physiologic anterior offset of C2 relative to C3 through ~ 7 years of age ("pseudosubluxation"), but good spinolaminar alignment should still be preserved.

- *Anterior vertebral line:* formed by the anterior borders of the vertebral bodies. On radiographs it can be traced from the anterior arch of the atlas through C7. Physiologic notches or bevels in the anterior vertebral margins (apophyseal region) may create slight irregularities.
- *Posterior vertebral line:* formed by the posterior borders of the vertebral bodies, marks the anterior boundary of the spinal canal. It can be traced from the base of the atlas through C7. An electronic display with windowing options can often show the posterior margin of the dens as an upward prolongation of the line.
- *Spinolaminar line:* formed by the junction of the C1 through C7 spinous processes and laminae, marks the posterior boundary of the spinal canal. The posterior arch of C1 may be a few millimeters anterior to the spinolaminar line as a normal variant. The line extends upward to the posterior rim of the foramen magnum.

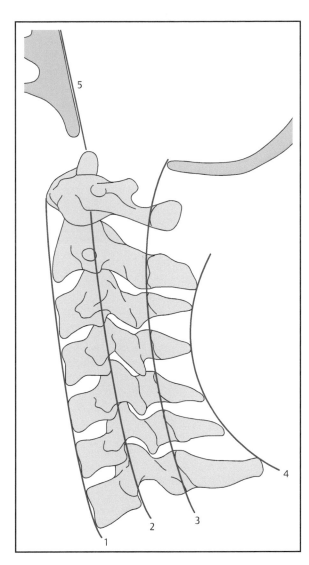

Fig. 9.5 Contour lines on a lateral radiograph of the cervical spine.
1 = Anterior vertebral line
2 = Posterior vertebral line
3 = Spinolaminar line
4 = Posterior spinous line
5 = Wackenheim clivus line

- *Posterior spinous line:* formed by the tips of the C2 through C7 spinous processes. The distance between the C2 and C3 spinous processes is physiologically smaller than in the other segments.

Thiebaut and Wackenheim described the basilar line, also called the Wackenheim clivus line, which represents a downward extension of the posterior surface of the clivus. This line should be tangent to the posterior cortex of the tip of the dens or should cross the dens at the junction of the anterior and middle thirds of the tip. Deviations from this alignment are evidence of atlanto-occipital

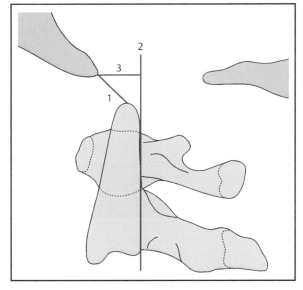

Fig. 9.6 Basion–dens interval and basion–axial interval.
1 = Basion–dens interval
2 = Line along the posterior border of the dens
3 = Basion–axial interval

dislocation. The normal variability of the clivus slope makes this technique very unreliable, however.

A practical alternative for the diagnosis of atlanto-occipital dislocation is to measure the basion–dens interval and basion–axial interval (**Fig. 9.6**). Harris in 1994 evaluated these intervals on lateral radiographs of 37 patients with known atlanto-occipital dislocation and a control group of 400 adults with no occipitovertebral abnormalities. The basion–dens interval is determined by measuring the distance between the basion (caudal tip of the clivus) and the highest point on the dens. The basion–axial interval is measured between the basion and a line along the posterior surface of the dens. For both measurements, an interval > 12 mm is considered evidence of atlanto-occipital dislocation. This is a valid cutoff value for the basion–axial interval even on flexion and extension views. In rare cases the clivus may be physiologically up to 4 mm behind the line along the posterior cortex of the dens. Because the dens is not fully ossified until about age 12 years, it is recommended that the basion–dens interval be measured only in patients aged 14 years or older. By contrast, the basion–axial interval can be measured in younger children.

Wackenheim A. Roentgen Diagnosis of the Cervical Vertebral Region. New York: Springer; 1974

Thiebaut F, Wackenheim A, Vrousos C. La ligne basilaire: etude d'une ligne d'orientation verticale pour la reconnaissance des displacements anterieurs et posterieurs de la dent de l'axis dans des malformations et traumatismes de la charniére cervico-occipitale. Sem Hop Paris 1963;3–4:43–46

Anteroposterior Radiograph

Three additional lines can be used to evaluate vertebral alignment on an AP radiograph of the cervical spine (**Fig. 9.7**):

- *Contour line of the spinous processes:* A line drawn along the C2 through C7 spinous processes on a transoral odontoid view should, when extended upward, pass through the tip of the dens. The line may be slightly irregular in patients with bifid spinous processes.
- *Contour line of the lateral vertebral bodies:* Lines drawn along the lateral margins of the C2 through C7 vertebral bodies should diverge slightly outward in the craniocaudal direction.
- *Contour line of the vertebral arches:* A line drawn along the outer borders of the C2 through C7 vertebral arches should form a gentle curve that is tangent to the lateral masses of C1.

> **!**
> Besides prevertebral soft-tissue measurements (see below), the analysis of vertebral alignment in two planes is the most important step in the radiographic evaluation of cervical spine trauma. It is essential to recognize normal variants such as pseudodislocation of C2/C3 in children or the C1 posterior arch located a few millimeters anterior to the spinolaminar line.

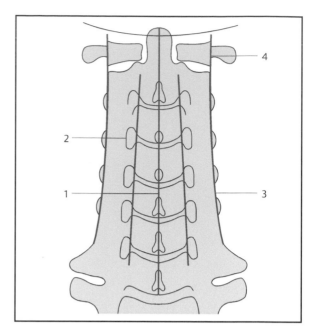

Fig. 9.7 Contour lines of the cervical spine on anteroposterior radiographs.
1 = Contour line of the spinous processes
2 = Contour line of the lateral vertebral bodies
3 = Contour line of the vertebral arches
4 = Contour line of the lateral masses

Daffner RH, Deeb ZL, Rothfus WE. "Fingerprints" of vertebral trauma—a unifying concept based on mechanisms. Skeletal Radiol 1986;15(7):518–525

Harris JH Jr, Carson GC, Wagner LK. Radiologic diagnosis of traumatic occipitovertebral dissociation: 1. Normal occipitovertebral relationships on lateral radiographs of supine subjects. AJR Am J Roentgenol 1994;162(4):881–886

Harris JH Jr, Carson GC, Wagner LK, Kerr N. Radiologic diagnosis of traumatic occipitovertebral dissociation: 2. Comparison of three methods of detecting occipitovertebral relationships on lateral radiographs of supine subjects. AJR Am J Roentgenol 1994;162(4):887–892

Harris JH Jr. The cervicocranium: its radiographic assessment. Radiology 2001;218(2):337–351

Holdsworth F. Fractures, dislocations, and fracture-dislocations of the spine. J Bone Joint Surg Am 1970;52(8):1534–1551

Roche C, Carty H. Spinal trauma in children. Pediatr Radiol 2001;31(10):677–700

Prevertebral Soft-Tissue Measurements

The width or thickness of the prevertebral soft tissues is measured on a lateral radiograph of the cervical spine (**Fig. 9.8**). This measurement is useful for detecting hematoma formation as an indirect sign of cervical spine injury. A widened prevertebral soft-tissue shadow is very specific for fracture diagnosis, although it is not very sensitive. The same measurements can be performed on sagittal computed tomography (CT) images.

- *Nasopharyngeal soft-tissue shadow:* The width of this shadow is measured as the horizontal distance between the nasopharynx and the anterior arch of the atlas.
- *Retropharyngeal soft-tissue shadow:* Measured as the horizontal distance between the antero-inferior border of the axis and the posterior pharyngeal wall.
- *Retrotracheal soft-tissue shadow:* Defined by a horizontal line between the anterior margin of the lower endplate of C6 and the posterior border of the trachea.

Prevertebral soft-tissue measurements

- *Normal width of nasopharyngeal soft-tissue shadow:* < 10 mm
- *Normal width of retropharyngeal soft-tissue shadow:* ≤ 7 mm
- *Normal width of retrotracheal soft-tissue shadow:*
  - Adults: ≤ 22 mm
  - Children: ≤ 14 mm

Displacement of the prevertebral fat stripe in front of the anterior longitudinal ligament can provide an additional indirect sign.

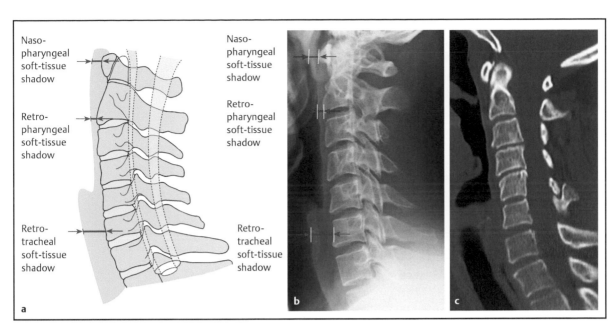

Fig. 9.8a–c Prevertebral soft-tissue measurements.

a Schematic representation. **b** Conventional radiograph. **c** Computed tomography.

> ! False-positive findings may occur in children whose lymphatic tissue forms a prevertebral soft-tissue mass that is mistaken for a hematoma. Equivocal cases can be resolved by MRI.

DeBehnke DJ, Havel CJ. Utility of prevertebral soft tissue measurements in identifying patients with cervical spine fractures. Ann Emerg Med 1994;24(6):1119–1124

Whalen JP, Woodruff CL. The cervical prevertebral fat stripe. A new aid in evaluating the cervical prevertebral soft tissue space. Am J Roentgenol Radium Ther Nucl Med 1970;109(3):445–451

Basilar Impression

Congenital or acquired deformities of the occipital bone (e.g., hypoplasia of the clivus) may lead to basilar impression. In this condition the atlas is located closer to the skull. The dens of C2 enters the foramen magnum and may compress the medulla oblongata during movements of the head. Basilar impression may occur congenitally in conditions such as achondroplasia, trisomy 21, or Klippel–Feil syndrome. Acquired basilar impression is also called vertical subluxation of the dens. Most cases are caused by inflammatory joint diseases (especially rheumatoid arthritis) and less commonly by Paget disease, osteomalacia, or hyperparathyroidism. Congenital basilar impression is frequently associated with platybasia (abnormally shallow posterior fossa).

A lateral radiograph of the skull is needed to evaluate for possible basilar impression. The McRae, Chamberlain and McGregor lines can be drawn on the skull radiograph. The Ranawat method can also detect upward displacement of the dens on a lateral radiograph of the cervical spine.

- *McRae line:* The McRae line (**Fig. 9.9a**) defines the opening of the foramen magnum and connects its anterior and posterior rims. The tip of the dens should be at or below this line. A vertical line drawn from the tip of the dens to the McRae line should intersect the anterior third of the line. If the tip of the dens protrudes above the line, basilar impression is diagnosed.
- *Chamberlain line:* The Chamberlain line (**Fig. 9.9b**) is drawn from the posterior rim of the foramen magnum to the posterior edge of the hard palate. The dens should project no more than 3 mm above this line. Various studies have shown a large range of variation, so different values are stated in the literature for the diagnosis of basilar impression. Most authors agree that a value ≥ 4 mm is suggestive of basilar impression while a value ≥ 6.6 mm is a strong indicator.
- *McGregor line:* The McGregor line (**Fig. 9.9c**) is drawn from the posterosuperior edge of the hard palate to the lowest point on the occipital squama of the skull. Normally the tip of the dens is no more than 4.5 mm above this line. A value > 5 mm is considered evidence of basilar impression.

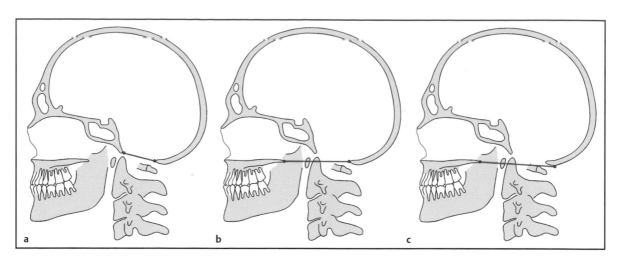

Fig. 9.9a–c Reference lines for evaluating basilar impression on the lateral radiograph.

a McRae line.   **b** Chamberlain line.   **c** McGregor line.

Since the hard palate often cannot be identified on a lateral radiograph of the cervical spine, Ranawat et al developed an alternate method for detecting upward displacement of the dens (**Fig. 9.10**). The coronal axis of C1 is defined by drawing a line connecting the centers of its anterior and posterior arches. A second line is then drawn from the center of the C2 pedicle to the first line along the dens axis, and the length of the second line is measured.

Normal lengths of the Ranawat line	
• *Normal value in men:*	17 mm (± 2 mm)
• *Normal value in women:*	15 mm (± 2 mm)

A decreased distance suggests upward displacement of the C2 vertebra and is suspicious for basilar impression.

! The Chamberlain line is the recommended reference line for practical use. The measurement is relatively easy to perform and has been most thoroughly evaluated in clinical studies. In principle, the above reference lines can also be evaluated on midsagittal reformatted CT images.

Chamberlain WE. Basilar impression (platybasia): a bizarre developmental anomaly of the occipital bone and upper cervical spine with striking and misleading neurologic manifestations. Yale J Biol Med 1939;11(5):487–496

El-Khoury GY, Wener MH, Menezes AH, Dolan KD, Kathol ME. Cranial settling in rheumatoid arthritis. Radiology 1980;137(3):637–642

McGregor M. The significance of certain measurements of the skull in the diagnosis of basilar impression. Br J Radiol 1948;21(244):171–181

McRae DL. Bony abnormalities in the region of the foramen magnum: correlation of the anatomic and neurologic findings. Acta Radiol 1953;40(2-3):335–354

Ranawat CS, O'Leary P, Pellicci P, Tsairis P, Marchisello P, Dorr L. Cervical spine fusion in rheumatoid arthritis. J Bone Joint Surg Am 1979;61(7):1003–1010

Schmitt HP, Tamáska L. Significance of occipito-cervical malformations for forensic pathology. [Article in German] Z Rechtsmed 1973;72(2):140–150

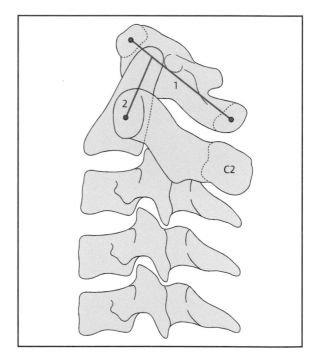

Fig. 9.10 Ranawat method for detecting upward displacement of the dens.
1 = Line connecting anterior and posterior C1 arches
2 = Line along dens axis from center of C2 pedicle

Radiographic Criteria of Cervical Instability According to Panjabi

The diagnosis of instability is an important issue in the evaluation of cervical spine injuries. Authors have published various radiologic measurements for diagnosis of instability on conventional radiographs or sagittal reformatted CT images. The best-known works were published by Panjabi and White, who performed numerous biomechanical studies on cadaveric spines as well as retrospective clinical reviews. These authors defined three criteria for evaluating the lower cervical spine (C3–C7) on the lateral radiograph. Each of these criteria is suggestive of cervical instability (**Fig. 9.11**):

- *Relative sagittal-plane displacement of adjacent vertebrae:* Posterior vertebral body margins are displaced more than 3.5 mm relative to each other
- *Segmental kyphosis:* More than 11° of relative sagittal-plane angulation between the lower and upper endplates of adjacent vertebrae
- *Facet joint subluxation:* Facet joints overlap by less than 50%

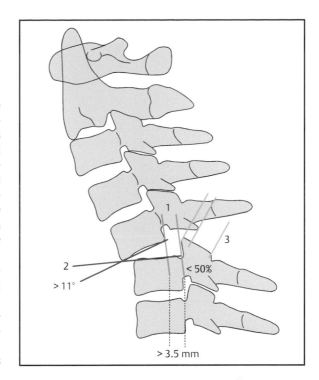

Fig. 9.11 Panjabi instability criteria.
1 = Relative displacement of adjacent vertebrae in the sagittal plane
2 = Relative angulation in the sagittal plane between two adjacent vertebrae
3 = Subluxation of facet joints

Daffner RH, Deeb ZL, Rothfus WE. "Fingerprints" of vertebral trauma—a unifying concept based on mechanisms. Skeletal Radiol 1986;15(7):518–525

Holdsworth F. Fractures, dislocations, and fracture-dislocations of the spine. J Bone Joint Surg Am 1970;52(8):1534–1551

Panjabi MM, White AA III, Keller D, Southwick WO, Friedlaender G. Stability of the cervical spine under tension. J Biomech 1978;11(4):189–197

Panjabi MM, White AA III. Basic biomechanics of the spine. Neurosurgery 1980;7(1):76–93

White AA, Southwick WO, Panjabi MM. Clinical instability in the lower cervical spine. Spine 1976;1(1):15–27

White AA, Panjabi MM. The problem of cervical instability in the human spine: a systematic approach. In: White AA, Panjabi MM, eds. Clinical Biomechanics of the Spine. Philadelphia: Lippincott; 1990

Craniocervical Junction and Cervical Spine

9

10 Musculoskeletal Tumors

Histopathologic Classification

The World Health Organization (WHO) published a revised version of the histopathologic classification of bone and soft-tissue tumors in 2002.

Bone Tumors

Bone tumors are classified either by their tissue of origin (e.g., cartilage and osteogenic tumors) or by their characteristic cell type (e.g., giant cell tumor) (**Table 10.1**). Exceptions are tumors of the Ewing group and "miscellaneous tumors" whose origin is uncertain. The classification also includes miscellaneous *tumorlike* (nonneoplastic) lesions, omitting some typical entities in this category such as nonossifying fibroma. Synovial osteochondromatosis is listed as a joint lesion that, although it may cause secondary bone involvement, primarily represents a soft-tissue process.

Soft-Tissue Tumors

The WHO classification of soft-tissue tumors (**Table 10.2**) lists more than 120 different entities in its original version, including many rare lesions and subtypes. The tumors are classified on the basis of histologic differentiation and are divided into *benign*, *intermediate*, and *malignant* subgroups. Intermediate lesions are benign tumors with locally aggressive behavior such as desmoid-type fibromatosis or low-grade malignancies such as well-differentiated liposarcoma. The classification also includes *soft-tissue tumors of unknown origin. Neurogenic soft-tissue tumors* have been disregarded in the WHO classification of soft-tissue tumors because they are classified as tumors of neural origin. Entities in this category that are relevant to soft-tissue imaging were adopted from Enzinger and Weiss and added to **Table 10.2**.

Fletcher CDM, Unni KK, Mertens F, eds. Pathology and genetics of tumours of soft tissue and bone. In: World Health Organization Classification of Tumours. Lyon: IARC Press; 2002
Weiss SW, Goldblum JR, eds. Enzinger and Weiss's Soft Tissue Tumors. 4th ed. St. Louis: Mosby; 2001

Staging

Staging of Malignant Bone Tumors

In Europe the clinical staging of a malignant bone tumor is usually based on the classification of the American Joint Committee on Cancer (AJCC) adopted by the Union internationale contre le cancer (UICC) (**Table 10.3**). This is a TNM system that has been expanded by adding the grade of histologic tumor differentiation (G), which is a key determinant of prognosis. Only the tumor diameter (T1/T2) and the presence of skip lesions (T3) are relevant for describing local tumor extent. Skip lesions, which are bony metastases occurring in the same bone as the primary tumor, are best detected or excluded by magnetic resonance imaging (T1-weighted spin-echo sequence). Regional lymph node metastases (N1) are very rare with bone tumors. Distant metastasis occurs predominantly to the lung (M1a) and rarely to other organs (M1b).

Staging of Soft-Tissue Sarcomas

As far as local tumor extent is concerned, the staging system for soft-tissue sarcomas (**Table 10.4**) differs only in its designation of tumor size (T1/T2) and lesion location relative to the muscle fascia (a/b). Superficial tumors are subcutaneous lesions that are entirely superficial to the muscle fascia and show no fascial invasion. Deep tumors may be entirely beneath the fascia, above the fascia and invading it, or both above and beneath the fascia. Retroperitoneal, mediastinal, and pelvic soft-tissue sarcomas are classified as deep tumors.

> **!** Lymph node metastases (N1) are rare with soft-tissue sarcomas. Distant metastasis (M1) occurs predominantly to the lung.

AJCC. Cancer Staging Manual. 7th ed. New York, NY: Springer, 2010
Peabody TD, Gibbs CP Jr, Simon MA. Evaluation and staging of musculoskeletal neoplasms. J Bone Joint Surg Am 1998; 80(8):1204–1218

Table 10.1 World Health Organization classification of bone tumors (Fletcher et al 2002)

Classification	Classification
Cartilage tumors	**Hematopoietic tumors**
• Osteochondroma	• Plasma cell myeloma
• Chondroma	• Malignant lymphoma, NOS
• Enchondroma	**Giant cell tumor**
• Periosteal chondroma	• Giant cell tumor
• Multiple chondromatosis	• Malignancy in giant cell tumor
• Chondroblastoma	**Notochordal tumors**
• Chondromyxoid fibroma	• Chordoma
• Chondrosarcoma	**Vascular tumors**
• Central, primary and secondary	• Hemangioma
• Peripheral	• Angiosarcoma
• Dedifferentiated	**Smooth muscle tumors**
• Mesenchymal	• Leiomyoma
• Clear cell	• Leiomyosarcoma
Osteogenic tumors	**Lipogenic tumors**
• Osteoid osteoma	• Lipoma
• Osteoblastoma	• Liposarcoma
• Osteosarcoma	**Neural tumors**
• Conventional	• Neurilemmoma
• Chondroblastic	**Miscellaneous tumors**
• Fibroblastic	• Adamantinoma
• Osteoblastic	• Metastatic malignancy
• Telangiectatic	**Miscellaneous/Tumorlike lesions**
• Small cell	• Aneurysmal bone cyst
• Low-grade central	• Simple bone cyst
• Secondary	• Fibrous dysplasia
• Parosteal	• Osteofibrous dysplasia
• Periosteal	• Langerhans cell histiocytosis
• High-grade surface	• Erdheim–Chester disease
Fibrogenic tumors	• Chest wall hamartoma
• Desmoplastic fibroma	**Joint lesions**
• Fibrosarcoma	• Synovial chondromatosis
Fibrohistiocytic tumors	
• Benign fibrous histiocytoma	
• Malignant fibrous histiocytoma	
Ewing sarcoma and PNET	
• Ewing sarcoma	

NOS = Not otherwise specified
PNET = Primitive neuro-ectodermal tumor

Musculoskeletal Tumors

10

Table 10.2 World Health Organization classification of soft-tissue tumors (Fletcher et al 2002)

Classification	Classification
Adipocytic tumors *Benign* • Lipoma and variants *Intermediate* • Well-differentiated liposarcoma *Malignant* • Liposarcoma (subtypes)	**Smooth muscle tumors** • Angioleiomyoma and variants • Leiomyosarcoma (excluding skin) • Pericytic (perivascular) tumors • Glomus tumor and variants • Malignant glomus tumor • Myopericytoma
Fibroblastic and myofibroblastic tumors *Benign* • Nodular fasciitis • Proliferative fasciitis • Proliferative myositis • Myositis ossificans • Ischemic fasciitis • Elastofibroma • Fibrous hamartoma • Fibromatosis (subtypes) • Fibroma, fibroblastoma (subtypes) *Intermediate (locally aggressive)* • Superficial fibromatosis • Desmoid-type fibromatosis • Lipofibromatosis *Intermediate (rarely metastasizing)* • Solitary fibrous tumor and hemangiopericytoma • Inflammatory myofibroblastic tumor • Low-grade myofibroblastic sarcoma • Myxoinflammatory fibroblastic sarcoma • Infantile fibrosarcoma *Malignant* • Fibrosarcoma (subtypes)	**Pericytic (perivascular) tumors** • Glomus tumor and variants • Malignant glomus tumor • Myopericytoma
	Skeletal muscle tumors *Benign* • Rhabdomyoma and variants *Malignant* • Rhabdomyosarcoma (subtypes)
	Vascular tumors *Benign* • Hemangioma and variants • Angiomatosis • Lymphangioma *Intermediate (rarely metastasizing)* • Hemangioendothelioma and variants • Kaposi sarcoma *Malignant* • Epithelioid hemangioendothelioma • Angiosarcoma of soft tissue
Fibrohistiocytic tumors *Benign* • Giant cell tumor of tendon sheath (GCTTS) • Diffuse giant cell tumor (PVNS) • Deep benign fibrous histiocytoma *Intermediate (rarely metastasizing)* • Plexiform fibrohistiocytic tumor • Giant cell tumor of soft tissues *Malignant* • Malignant fibrous histiocytoma (MFH; subtypes)	**Chondro-osseous tumors** • Soft-tissue chondroma • Mesenchymal chondrosarcoma • Extraskeletal osteosarcoma
	Tumors of uncertain differentiation *Benign* • Myxoma and variants • Pleomorphic hyalinizing angiectatic tumor • Ectopic hamartomatous thymoma *Intermediate (rarely metastasizing)* • Angiomatoid fibrous histiocytoma • Ossifying fibromyxoid tumor • Mixed tumor/myoepithelioma/parachordoma *Malignant* • Synovial sarcoma • Epithelioid sarcoma • Alveolar soft part sarcoma • Clear cell sarcoma of soft tissue • Extraskeletal myxoid chondrosarcoma • Extraskeletal Ewing tumor/PNET • Desmoplastic small round cell tumor • Extrarenal rhabdoid tumor • Malignant mesenchymoma • Intimal sarcoma
Neurogenic tumors* *Benign* • Neuroma and variants • Neurofibroma and variants • Benign schwannoma (neurinoma) and variants • Perineuroma and variants *Malignant* • Malignant peripheral nerve sheath tumors (MPNST) and variants	

* From Enzinger and Weiss classification of neurogenic tumors, simplified.

Table 10.3 American Joint Committee on Cancer/Union internationale contre le cancer 2010 staging system for bone tumors

Stage	T (primary tumor)	N (regional lymph nodes)	M (distant metastasis)	G (grade)
IA	T1	N0	M0	G1–2 low grade, GX
IB	T2	N0	M0	G1–2 low grade, GX
	T3	N0	M0	G1–2 low grade, GX
IIA	T1	N0	M0	G3–4 high grade
IIB	T2	N0	M0	G3–4 high grade
III	T3	N0	M0	G3–4
IVA	Any T	N0	M1a	Any G
IVB	Any T	N1	Any M	Any G
		Any N	M1b	Any G

Primary tumor:
T1 = Tumor 8 cm or less in greatest dimension
T2 = Tumor more than 8 cm in greatest dimension
T3 = Discontinuous tumor(s) at the primary bone site, skip
lesion(s)
Regional lymph nodes:
N0 = No regional lymph node metastasis
N1 = Regional lymph node metastasis

Distant metastasis:
M0 = No distant metastasis
M1 = Distant metastasis
M1a = Lung
M1b = Other distant sites
Histologic grade:
G1 = Well-differentiated, low grade
G2 = Moderately differentiated, low grade
G3 = Poorly differentiated, high grade
G4 = Undifferentiated, high grade

Table 10.4 American Joint Committee on Cancer/Union internationale contre le cancer 2010 staging system for soft-tissue sarcomas

Stage	T (primary tumor)	N (regional lymph nodes)	M (distant metastasis)	G (grade)
IA	T1a	N0	M0	G1, GX
	T1b	N0	M0	G1, GX
IB	T2a	N0	M0	G1, GX
	T2b	N0	M0	G1, GX
IIA	T1a	N0	M0	G2, G3
	T1b	N0	M0	G2, G3
IIB	T2a	N0	M0	G2
	T2b	N0	M0	G2
III	T2a, T2b	N0	M0	G3
	Any T	N1	M0	Any G
IV	Any T	Any N	M1	Any G

Primary tumor:
T1 = Tumor 5 cm or less in greatest dimension
T1a = Superficial tumor
T1b = Deep tumor
T2 = Tumor more than 5 cm in greatest dimension
T2a = superficial tumor
T2b = Deep tumor

Regional lymph nodes:
N0 = No regional lymph node metastasis
N1 = Regional lymph node metastasis
Distant metastasis:
M0 = No distant metastasis
M1 = Distant metastasis
Histologic grade (National Federation of French Cancer Centers
[FNCLCC] system preferred): G1–G3.

Table 10.5 Staging system for musculoskeletal tumors of the Musculoskeletal Tumor Society (source: Enneking et al 1980)

Stage	G (grade)	T (primary tumor)	M (distant metastasis)
IA	1	1	0
IB	1	2	0
IIA	2	1	0
IIB	2	2	0
III	1 or 2	1 or 2	1

Grade:
G1 = Low grade
G2 = High grade
Primary tumor:
T1 = Intracompartmental (intra-articular/superficial to deep fascia/paraosseous/intrafascial compartment)

T2 = Extracompartmental (soft-tissue extension/intrafascial extension/intraosseous or extrafascial extension/extrafascial compartment)
Distant metastasis:
M0 = No distant metastasis
M1 = Distant metastasis

Enneking Staging System

The staging system of the Musculoskeletal Tumor Society introduced by Enneking (**Table 10.5**) is applicable to bone and soft-tissue tumors and has a more surgical orientation than the systems cited above. Possible regional lymph node involvement is disregarded in this system because of its relative rarity. The T stage (T1/T2) is determined by whether the tumor is *intracompartmental* or *extracompartmental*, rather than by tumor size.

Enneking WF, Spanier SS, Goodman MA. A system for the surgical staging of musculoskeletal sarcoma. Clin Orthop Relat Res 1980;153(153):106–120
Weiss SW, Goldblum JR, eds. Enzinger and Weiss's Soft Tissue Tumors. 4th ed. St. Louis: Mosby; 2001

■ Intracompartmental Tumors

Intracompartmental tumors are confined to a single anatomic compartment, whereas extracompartmental tumors (or their reactive zone = peritumoral "edema") have spread past the boundaries of the original compartment. The anatomic compartments relevant for this classification (**Figs. 10.1 and 10.2**) are as follows:
- Skin and subcutaneous tissue
- Muscle compartments
- Paraosseous space
- Bone
- Joints

■ Extracompartmental Tumors

Some anatomic spaces have ill-defined or undefined boundaries and are collectively referred to as extracompartmental spaces. Tumors that arise within these areas are classified as *primary extracompartmental* tumors. The extracompartmental spaces include the following:
- Head and neck
- Paraspinal tissues
- Periclavicular tissue
- Axilla
- Antecubital fossa
- Wrist
- Dorsum of the hand
- Groin: inguinal and femoral regions
- Popliteal fossa
- Ankle
- Dorsum of the foot

Secondary extracompartmental tumors are primary intracompartmental lesions that have spread to other anatomic compartments as a result of fractures (bone tumors), hemorrhage, technically poor biopsies, or unplanned resections.

Anderson MW, Temple HT, Dussault RG, Kaplan PA. Compartmental anatomy: relevance to staging and biopsy of musculoskeletal tumors. AJR Am J Roentgenol 1999;173(6):1663–1671

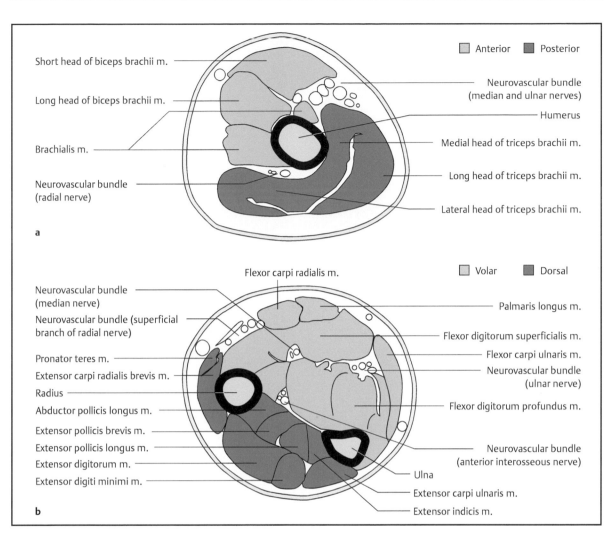

Fig. 10.1a,b Anatomic compartments of the upper limb.

a Upper arm.   **b** Forearm.

Musculoskeletal Tumors

10

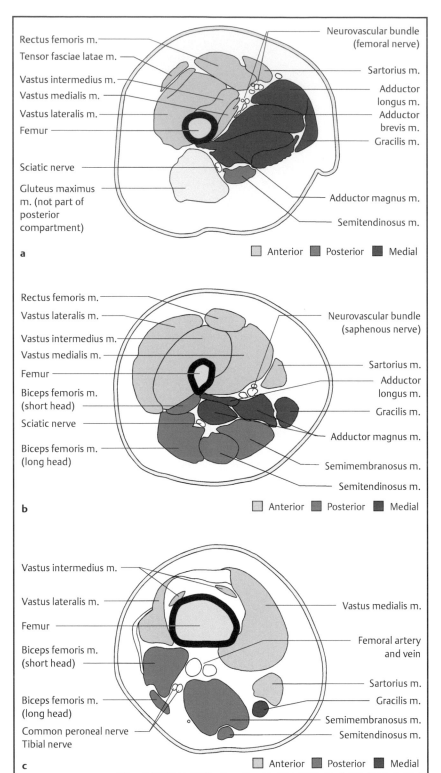

Fig. 10.2a–c Anatomic compartments of the lower limb.
a Proximal thigh.
b Mid-thigh.
c Distal thigh.

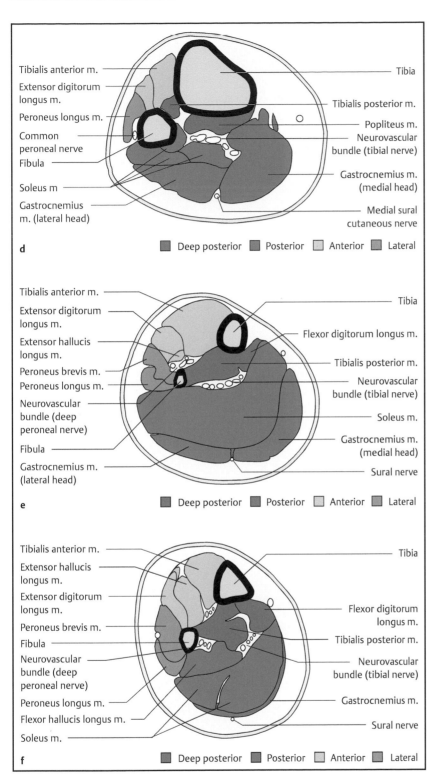

Fig. 10.2d–f *Continued*
d Proximal lower leg.
e Mid-lower leg.
f Distal lower leg.

In figure d:
Tibialis anterior m.
Extensor digitorum longus m.
Peroneus longus m.
Common peroneal nerve
Fibula
Soleus m
Gastrocnemius m. (lateral head)
Tibia
Tibialis posterior m.
Popliteus m.
Neurovascular bundle (tibial nerve)
Gastrocnemius m. (medial head)
Medial sural cutaneous nerve

d — ■ Deep posterior ■ Posterior ☐ Anterior ■ Lateral

In figure e:
Tibialis anterior m.
Extensor digitorum longus m.
Extensor hallucis longus m.
Peroneus brevis m.
Peroneus longus m.
Neurovascular bundle (deep peroneal nerve)
Fibula
Gastrocnemius m. (lateral head)
Tibia
Flexor digitorum longus m.
Tibialis posterior m.
Neurovascular bundle (tibial nerve)
Soleus m.
Gastrocnemius m. (medial head)
Sural nerve

e — ■ Deep posterior ■ Posterior ☐ Anterior ■ Lateral

In figure f:
Tibialis anterior m.
Extensor hallucis longus m.
Extensor digitorum longus m.
Peroneus brevis m.
Fibula
Neurovascular bundle (deep peroneal nerve)
Peroneus longus m.
Flexor hallucis longus m.
Soleus m.
Tibia
Flexor digitorum longus m.
Tibialis posterior m.
Neurovascular bundle (tibial nerve)
Gastrocnemius m.
Sural nerve

f — ■ Deep posterior ■ Posterior ☐ Anterior ■ Lateral

Musculoskeletal Tumors

10

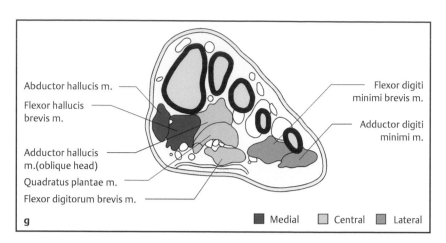

Abductor hallucis m.

Flexor hallucis brevis m.

Adductor hallucis m.(oblique head)

Quadratus plantae m.

Flexor digitorum brevis m.

Flexor digiti minimi brevis m.

Adductor digiti minimi m.

■ Medial   □ Central   ■ Lateral

g

Fig. 10.2g *Continued*
g Foot.

Surgical Margins, Resection Status

Four types of surgical margins are distinguished in the resection of musculoskeletal tumors (**Figs. 10.3 and 10.4**):

- *Intralesional:* The tumor is shelled out of its capsule or pseudocapsule (e.g., curettage of a bone tumor) or at least opened somewhere on its surface during the resection.
- *Marginal:* The tumor is removed en bloc but is covered (in at least one site) by only its capsule or pseudocapsule.
- *Wide:* The tumor is removed en bloc together with a continuous rim of normal tissue that fully encompasses the specimen.
- *Radical:* The tumor is removed en bloc together with the entire compartment or all involved compartments, respectively.

Intralesional and marginal-type resections as a primary surgical treatment are generally reserved for benign bone and soft-tissue tumors but are occasionally a palliative option for malignancies (e.g., removal of metastases, tumor debulking). The goal of the surgical treatment of bone and soft-tissue sarcomas is to achieve a complete tumor removal while preserving limb function. Whenever possible, therefore, malignant tumors are removed by a wide excision with adequate margins and not by a radical excision, which is often tantamount to amputation.

!
In the case of subcutaneous tumors, a wide excision is one that includes the muscle fascia and < 5 cm of normal skin and subcutaneous tissue around the tumor. The radical excision of a subcutaneous tumor would remove > 5 cm of skin and subcutaneous tissue along with the tumor.

As in other types of surgery, the resection status of musculoskeletal tumors is classified as R0, R1, or R2 (**Table 10.6**).

Enneking WF. Musculoskeletal Tumor Surgery. Edinburgh: Churchill-Livingstone; 1983
AJCC. Cancer Staging Manual. 7th ed. New York, NY: Springer, 2010

Table 10.6 Resection status

Resection	Description
R0	Complete tumor resection with all margins negative. Microscopic examination shows no tumor cells in the specimen margins.
R1	Incomplete tumor resection with microscopic involvement of a margin (gross total marginal resection).
R2	Incomplete tumor resection with gross residual tumor that was not resected

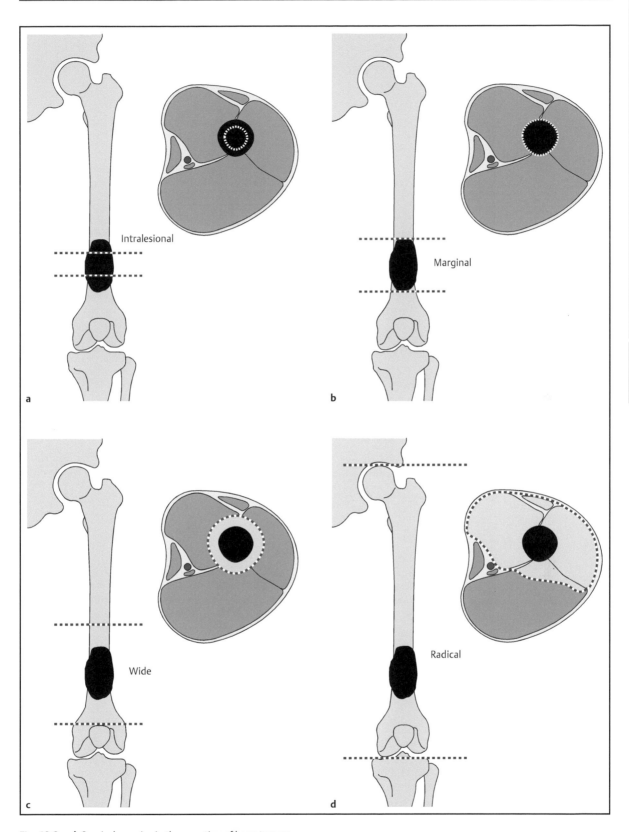

Fig. 10.3a–d Surgical margins in the resection of bone tumors.

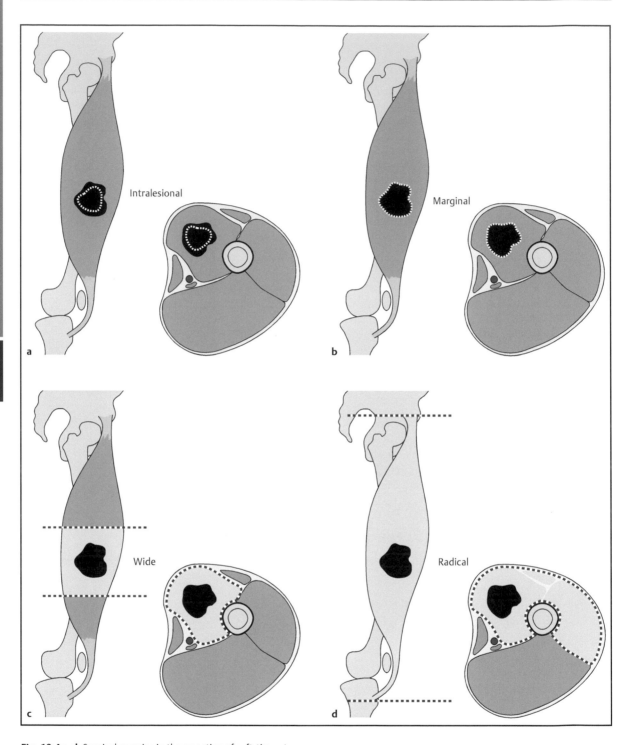

Fig. 10.4a–d Surgical margins in the resection of soft-tissue tumors.

Radiographic Evaluation of Bone Tumors

Pattern of Bone Destruction

The pattern of bone destruction depicted on conventional radiographs is useful for assessing the growth rate (aggressiveness) of an osteolytic bone tumor. Three main patterns of destruction are distinguished:

- *Geographic destruction:* This pattern is characterized by a single osteolytic area that is clearly demarcated from healthy bone. The transition zone with healthy bone tissue is of variable width and may have sharp or ill-defined margins.
- *Moth-eaten destruction:* A moth-eaten pattern of bone destruction may be found in both trabecular and cortical bone. It consists of multiple osteolytic sites of varying size that tend to develop separately rather than from a central lesion and may coalesce.
- *Permeative destruction:* This pattern occurs exclusively in cortical bone. It consists of multiple small, oval or linear osteolytic lesions caused by bone destruction from within the cortex (i.e., via the haversian canals).

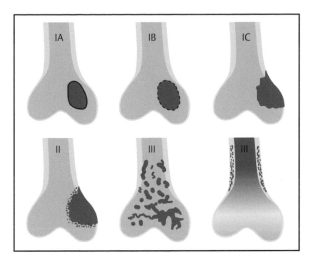

Fig. 10.5 Lodwick classification (after Lodwick and Freyschmidt).

Lodwick Classification

Lodwick developed a system for grading the growth rate of osteolytic bone tumors based on these three patterns of bone destruction. Besides the pattern of destruction, the Lodwick classification (**Table 10.7** and **Fig. 10.5**) also takes into account the radiographic appearance of the

Table 10.7 Lodwick classification of bone destruction (after Lodwick et al, 1980 and Freyschmidt et al, 2010)

Grade	Pattern of bone destruction	Edge characteristics	Penetration of cortex	Sclerotic rim	Expanded shell
IA	Mandatory geographic	One of three patterns: • regular or • lobulated or • multicentric	None or partial	Mandatory	Optional, only 1 cm or less
IB	Mandatory geographic	One of four patterns: • regular or • lobulated or • multicentric or • ragged/poorly defined	None or partial	Optional	If sclerotic rim is present, expanded shell > 1 cm
IC	Mandatory geographic	One of four patterns: • regular or • lobulated or • multicentric or • ragged/poorly defined but not moth-eaten	Mandatory total	Optional	Optional
II	Mandatory geographic combined with moth-eaten and/or permeative		Total by definition	Optional, but unlikely	Optional, but unlikely
III	Moth-eaten and/or permeative		Total by definition	Optional, but unlikely	Optional, but unlikely

transition zone and the integrity of the cortical bone bordering the tumor. The aggressiveness of a bone lesion in this classification increases from grade I through grade III.

> ! It is important to note that the biological activity does not necessarily correlate with the dignity of a bone tumor. Lesions assigned to Lodwick grade IC have an equal likelihood of being benign or malignant. Lesions graded IA or IB are, however, mostly benign, while the vast majority of grade II and III lesions are malignant tumors. The Lodwick classification was developed for conventional radiographs and must not be applied to CT or even MRI, as this could lead to significant misinterpretation.

Lodwick GS, Wilson AJ, Farrell C, Virtama P, Smeltzer FM, Dittrich F. Estimating rate of growth in bone lesions: observer performance and error. Radiology 1980;134(3):585–590
Freyschmidt J, Ostertag H, Jundt G. Knochentumoren. 3rd ed. Heidelberg: Springer; 2010

Classification of Periosteal Reactions

Periosteal reactions are a common radiographic sign of bone tumors but also occur after trauma and in response to inflammatory processes, perfusion deficits, local hypoxia, metabolic disorders, and in the setting of primary periosteal diseases. The mineralization pattern of the reaction reflects the aggressiveness and chronicity of the underlying process and so provides a measure for the biological activity of bone tumors.

Ragsdale developed a widely used classification of periosteal reactions (**Fig. 10.6**) that defines three main types:

- Continuous periosteal reactions (with or without destruction of the underlying cortex)
- Interrupted periosteal reactions
- Complex periosteal reactions

Periosteal shells represent a continuous periosteal reaction caused by periosteal new bone formation (neocortex) in response to endosteal resorption of the original cortex. This type of periosteal reaction occurs almost exclusively in association with bone tumors. Continuous periosteal reactions with an intact cortex may be a radiographic manifestation of many different systemic and focal bone diseases. Although the solid type of periosteal reaction and a single lamella suggest that the underlying bone lesion is benign, a lamellated (onion-skin) or spiculated (hair-on-end) reaction is also seen with

malignancies. Note that the term "intact cortex" denotes the apparent integrity of the cortex on a conventional radiograph and generally is not confirmed by histologic examination. It would be more correct, therefore, to speak of an "apparently intact cortex."

> ! Interrupted and complex periosteal reactions signify a very aggressive bone process in most cases.

Ragsdale BD, Madewell JE, Sweet DE. Radiologic and pathologic analysis of solitary bone lesions. Part II: periosteal reactions. Radiol Clin North Am 1981;19(4):749–783

Patterns of Matrix Mineralization

Osteogenic and chondrogenic tumors produce an intracellular substance called "matrix" that may be visible on radiographs when it undergoes mineralization (calcification or ossification). The patterns of matrix mineralization are helpful in evaluating the composition of the matrix and identifying the tumor entity.

Sweet et al classified the radiographic appearance of mineralized matrix patterns that form in association with bone-producing and cartilage-producing bone tumors (**Fig. 10.7**):

- *Mineralized tumor osteoid* may produce a solid (sharp-edged), cloud-like (ill-defined margins) or ivory-like pattern of increased density.
- *Mineralized tumor cartilage* may have a stippled, flocculent, or ring-and-arc appearance on radiographs. The latter pattern results from peripheral ossification of the cartilage lobules in more highly differentiated cartilage tumors or elements of those tumors.

> ! In unambiguous cases, the detection of the above-described mineralization patterns can be helpful in narrowing the differential diagnosis (e.g., osteoblastic osteosarcoma). Often, however, it is quite difficult to positively identify matrix calcifications and ossifications, to definitively classify them as chondrogenic or osteogenic, and to distinguish them from reactive or regressive calcific deposits. Furthermore, there is no correlation between the presence of matrix mineralizations and the dignity of a bone tumor.

Sweet DE, Madewell JE, Ragsdale BD. Radiologic and pathologic analysis of solitary bone lesions. Part III: matrix patterns. Radiol Clin North Am 1981;19(4):785–814

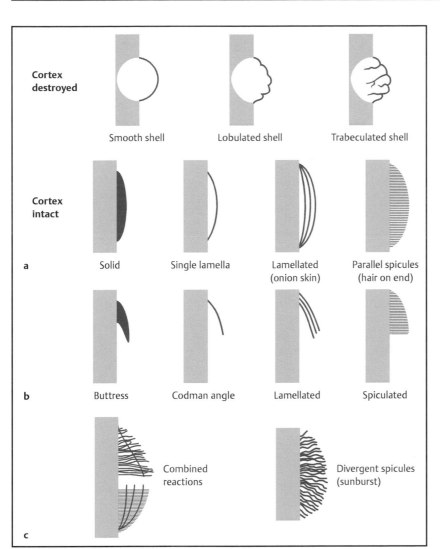

Fig. 10.6a–c Radiographic classification of periosteal reactions (after Ragsdale).
a Continuous periosteal reactions.
b Interrupted periosteal reactions.
c Complex periosteal reactions.

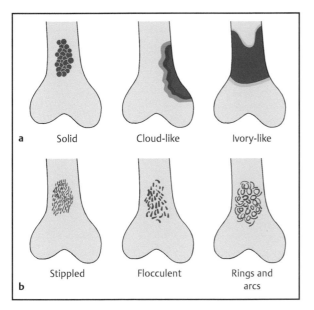

Fig. 10.7a,b Radiographic patterns of matrix mineralization (after Sweet and Freyschmidt).
a Bone-forming tumors.
b Cartilage-forming tumors.

11 Osteoporosis

Bone Densitometry

The basis for the radiologic diagnosis of osteoporosis is the measurement of bone mineral density (BMD). The standard clinical tests for this purpose are dual X-ray absorptiometry (DXA) and quantitative computed tomography (CT).

Dual X-Ray Absorptiometry

Dual X-ray absorptiometry has become established as the standard procedure for measuring BMD because of its high reproducibility, standardized methodology, and lower radiation exposure compared with quantitative CT.

In 1994 the World Health Organization (WHO) issued a definition for osteoporosis based entirely on bone densitometry by DXA. According to this definition, osteoporosis is present when the BMD is more than 2.5 standard deviations below the mean value for a healthy young reference population. The BMD expressed in relative standard deviations from the mean is called the T-score. Strictly speaking, the WHO definition applies only to density measurements performed in the lumbar spine (anteroposterior and posteroanterior projections) and proximal femur.

Bone mass is determined in relation to surface area and is expressed in g/cm^2.

WHO definition of osteoporosis	
• *Normal:*	T-score > − 1
• *Osteopenia:*	− 2.5 < T-score < − 1
• *Osteoporosis:*	T-score < − 2.5

Besides the T-score, which states the deviation of BMD from a healthy young reference population, DXA also provides a Z-score, which states the deviation from a reference population of the same age and gender.

> ❗ The T-score is the most important parameter for predicting fracture risk and should direct treatment in consideration of other factors. The Z-score is of minor importance since it does not provide a direct measure of individual fracture risk.

Quantitative Computed Tomography

Bone densitometry by quantitative CT (QCT) is performed in the lumbar spine. The L1 through L3 vertebral bodies are scanned in transverse midvertebral sections (section thickness: 8–10 mm). A relatively large section thickness is used because averaging over a larger volume improves the reproducibility of the test. If the scout view shows the presence of a vertebral body fracture, an adjacent vertebra should be used for densitometry.

After the examination, a region of interest (ROI) is selected in the bone and the corresponding attenuation value is measured in Hounsfield units (HU). Conversion to an absolute density value is aided by using a reference phantom that is scanned with the patient. The result is expressed in mg/mL, i.e., bone mass relative to volume. The following cutoff values are used in the diagnosis of osteoporosis and osteopenia:

BMD values
• *Osteoporosis:* < 80 mg/mL
• *Osteopenia:* 80 mg/mL < BMD < 120 mg/mL

> ❗ The T-scores and Z-scores established for DXA are not directly applicable to QCT. QCT specifically measures the density of trabecular bone, which is the most sensitive indicator of physiologic bone loss, so that the average yearly bone loss determined by QCT is greater than that determined by DXA. Because QCT is more sensitive, a BMD of 80 mg/mL would correspond to a T-score of approximately − 3. The absolute density values should therefore be used in making a diagnosis.

Felsenberg D, Gowin W. Bone densitometry by dual energy methods. [Article in German] Radiologe 1999;39(3): 186–193

WHO. Technical report: assessment of fracture risk and its application to screening for postmenopausal osteoporosis. A report of a WHO study group. Geneva: World Health Organization; 1994

Classification of Osteoporotic Vertebral Body Fractures

Various classifications have been devised for evaluating the severity of osteoporosis based on the extent of osteoporotic vertebral body fractures. The following classifications are most commonly used within the framework of studies and clinical routine.

Spinal Fracture Index of Genant

The spinal fracture index (SFI) of Genant is a semiquantitative method used to evaluate the T4 through L4 vertebral bodies on conventional lateral radiographs of the thoracic and lumbar spine. First a morphologic type of deformity (wedge fracture, biconcave fracture, crush fracture) is determined for each of the fractured vertebrae. For grading, all the vertebral bodies are evaluated for the height difference between the anterior, middle and posterior thirds. Then one of four severity grades is assigned based entirely on this height difference, regardless of morphologic type (**Fig. 11.1**).

Changes that are intermediate between two grades are stated in 0.5 increments. The SFI is then obtained by adding together all grades of deformity assigned to the vertebral bodies and dividing the sum by the number of vertebral bodies evaluated.

> **!**
> The International Osteoporosis Foundation currently recommends the SFI as the standard method for evaluating osteoporotic vertebral body fractures. It has high reproducibility and has been used successfully in many pharmacologic and epidemiologic studies.

Genant HK, Wu CY, van Kuijk C, Nevitt MC. Vertebral fracture assessment using a semiquantitative technique. J Bone Miner Res 1993;8(9):1137–1148

Spine Deformity Index

The spine deformity index (SDI) is also determined on conventional lateral radiographs of the thoracic and lumbar spine. The heights of the T4 vertebra are measured in the anterior, central and posterior thirds of the vertebral body to establish a reference. Values are then measured for the other vertebral bodies included in the evaluation (T5 through L5) and are divided by the reference heights measured for T4. The values obtained for each vertebral body are added together to yield the vertebral deformity index. The sum of the indices for all vertebral bodies yields the SDI.

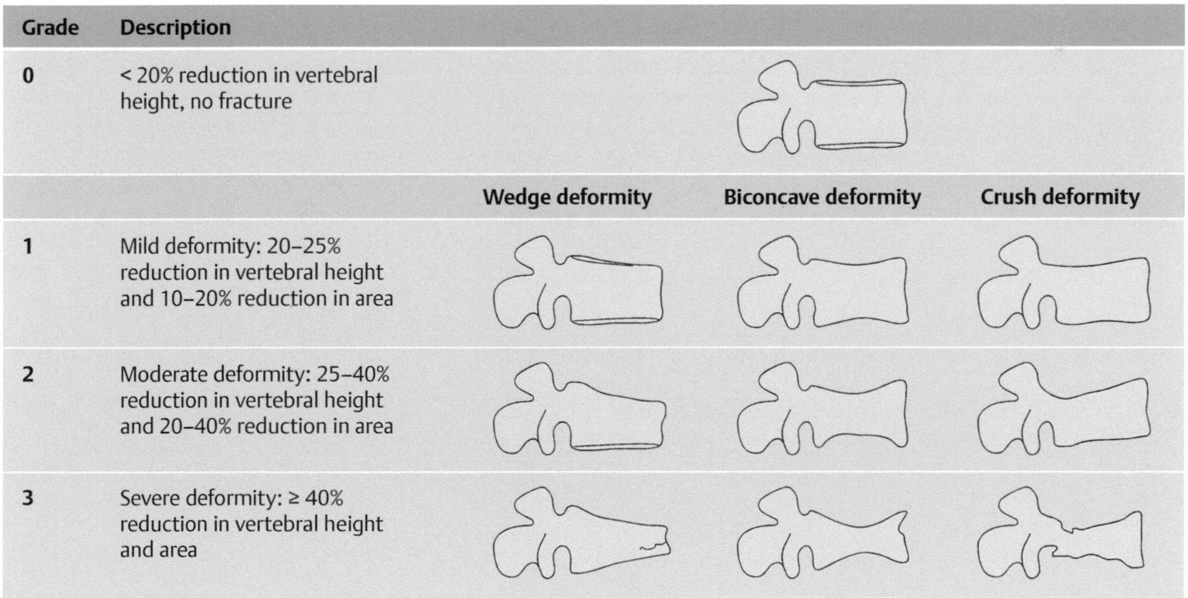

Osteoporosis

11

Grade	Description	Wedge deformity	Biconcave deformity	Crush deformity
0	< 20% reduction in vertebral height, no fracture			
1	Mild deformity: 20–25% reduction in vertebral height and 10–20% reduction in area			
2	Moderate deformity: 25–40% reduction in vertebral height and 20–40% reduction in area			
3	Severe deformity: ≥ 40% reduction in vertebral height and area			

Fig. 11.1 Spinal fracture index of Genant.

! The T4 vertebral body is used as a reference because it is rarely affected in patients with spinal osteoporosis. The advantage of the SDI is that the heights of the examined vertebral bodies relative to T4, or the vertebral deformity index, is independent of body height. This method is demanding, however, as it requires a normal population to diagnose an osteoporotic fracture. If the vertebral deformity index is below the normal range, it indicates the presence of an osteoporotic fracture.

Leidig-Bruckner G, Genant HK, Minne HW, et al. Comparison of a semiquantitative and a quantitative method for assessing vertebral fractures in osteoporosis. Osteoporos Int 1994;4(3):154–161

Minne HW, Leidig G, Wüster C, et al. A newly developed spine deformity index (SDI) to quantitate vertebral crush fractures in patients with osteoporosis. Bone Miner 1988;3(4):335–349

12 Osteoarthritis

Kellgren–Lawrence Score

Although many new and modified scores have been published for the quantification or semiquantification of radiologic findings in osteoarthritis, the grading system introduced by Kellgren and Lawrence in 1957 and 1963 is still widely used today. It is easy to use (even in routine clinical work) and yields reproducible results. The Kellgren–Lawrence score was recognized at a 1961 World Health Organization conference as the standard for grading osteoarthritis in large epidemiologic studies.

The Kellgren–Lawrence classification is based on the interpretation of conventional radiographs. In the original 1957 publication, the score was determined from radiographs of the hands, knee joints, cervical and lumbar spine, and hip joints.

A corresponding radiographic atlas published in 1963 established a system for classifying osteoarthritic changes into five distinct stages based on the following radiographic signs (**Fig. 12.1**):

- Osteophytes
- Joint-space narrowing
- Subchondral sclerosis
- Deformity of the bone ends
- Cyst formations (hip joint, first carpometacarpal joint, proximal interphalangeal joint, distal interphalangeal joint)

Kellgren JH, Lawrence JS. Radiological assessment of osteoarthrosis. Ann Rheum Dis 1957;16(4):494–502

Kellgren JH, Jeffrey MR, Ball J. The epidemiology of chronic rheumatism. Atlas of Standard Radiographs of Arthritis. Oxford, UK: Blackwell Scientific Publications; 1963: 1–13

Schiphof D, Boers M, Bierma-Zeinstra SMA. Differences in descriptions of Kellgren and Lawrence grades of knee osteoarthritis. Ann Rheum Dis 2008;67(7):1034–1036

Osteoarthritis Research Society Atlas of Altman

The newer osteoarthritis scores are based on the interpretation of specific, reproducible criteria. In the scale published by the Osteoarthritis Research Society (OARS), the size of osteophytes and the degree of joint-space narrowing are graded separately (grades 0–3) on conventional radiographs. In addition, other radiographic criteria of osteoarthritis such as subchondral sclerosis, subchondral cysts, and angular deformity are evaluated as present or absent (yes/no). The OARS atlas published by Altman et al provides a reference image for each grade of change in the criteria evaluated. It presents radiographs of the hands, knee, and hip joints. Studies using the atlas have shown very good to excellent intraobserver and interobserver reliabilities in the interpretation of specific criteria.

However, for the overall assessment of a joint the OARS atlas recommends assigning a Kellgren–Lawrence grade instead of determining an overall score for a joint with OARS criteria.

!

At present, only the Kellgren–Lawrence score can be recommended for the routine quantitative assessment of osteoarthritic changes on conventional radiographs. The use of this score permits a relatively fast and reliable overall evaluation of the radiographic changes in a joint.

The OARS atlas is recommended in situations where changes must be graded with somewhat higher precision, as in epidemiologic or pharmacologic studies.

A general problem in the radiologic evaluation of osteoarthritis is that clinical symptoms often do not correlate with radiologic findings. For this reason, imaging findings should always be supplemented by an accurate clinical evaluation (e.g., using the WOMAC [Western Ontario and McMaster Universities Osteoarthritis Index] score).

Altman RD, Gold GE. Atlas of individual radiographic features in osteoarthritis, revised. Osteoarthr Cartil 2007; 15: A1–A56

Grade of osteoarthritis	Radiographic features	Illustrative knee radiograph
0 None	Normal findings	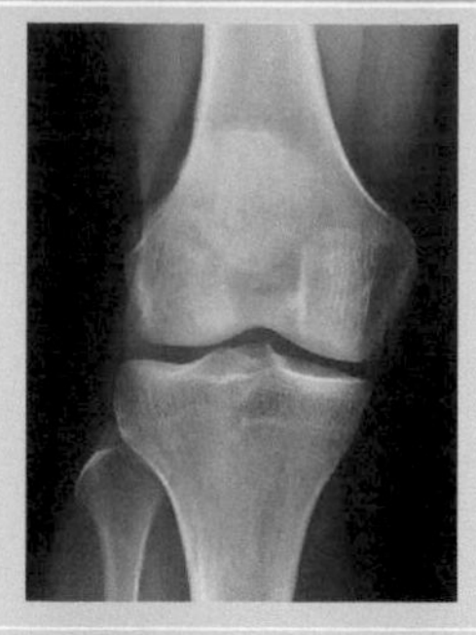
1 Doubtful	Doubtful joint space narrowing and possible osteophytic lipping	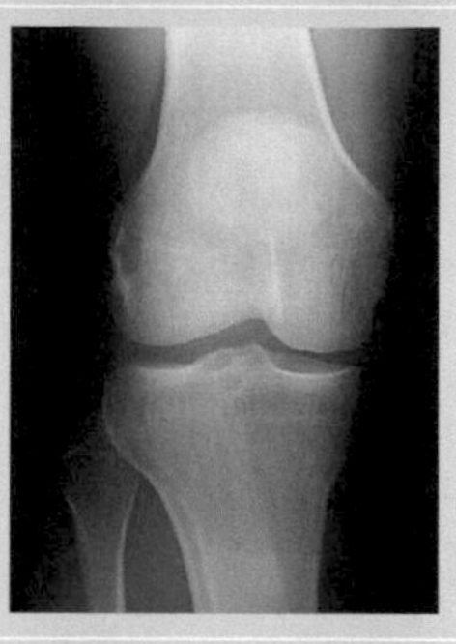
2 Minimal	Definite osteophytes and possible joint space narrowing	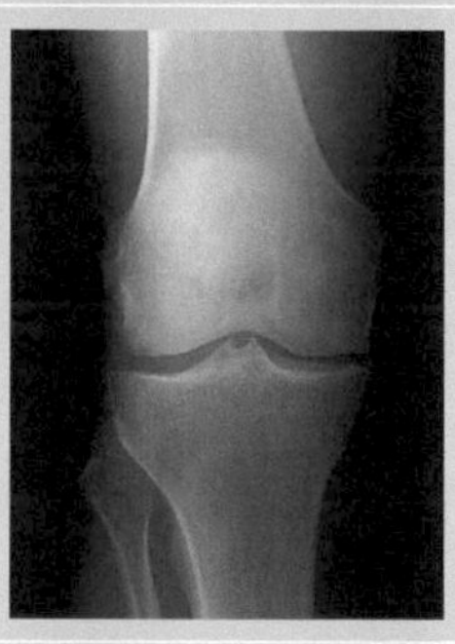
3 Moderate	Moderate multiple osteophytes, definite joint space narrowing, some sclerosis and possible deformity of bone ends	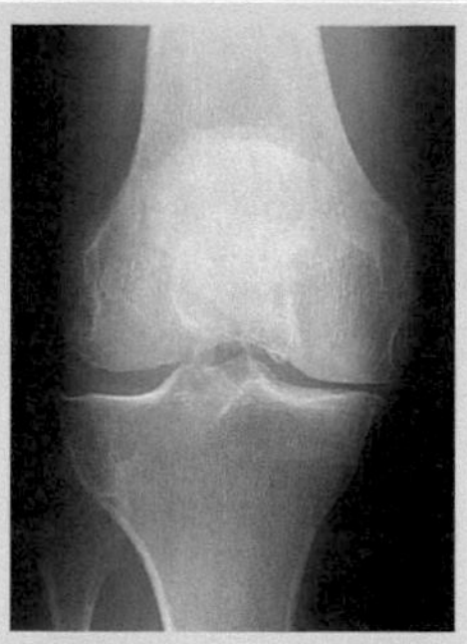
4 Severe	Large osteophytes, marked joint space narrowing, severe sclerosis and definite deformity of bone ends	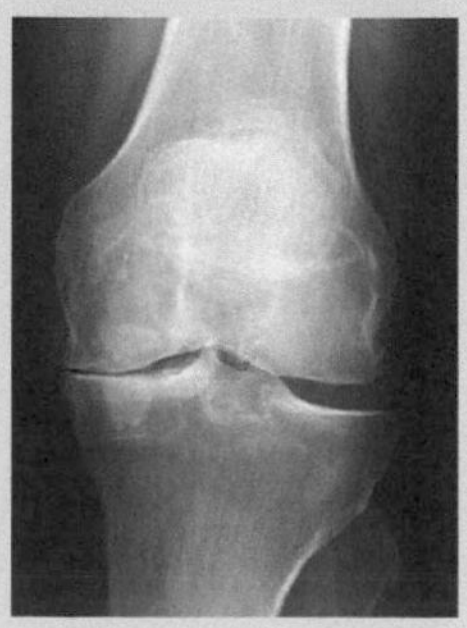

Fig. 12.1 Kellgren–Lawrence score for grading osteoarthritis of the knee on conventional radiographs.

13 Articular Cartilage

Grading of Cartilage Lesions

The radiologic grading of articular cartilage lesions by magnetic resonance imaging (MRI), MR arthrography, or computed tomographic (CT) arthrography in the clinical setting is based on surgical and arthroscopic classification systems. Cartilage lesions can be classified according to their morphologic appearance, depth, size, and location. Various authors have proposed clinical classification systems that take into account one or more of these features.

Outerbridge Classification

The classic Outerbridge classification defines four grades of chondromalacia (**Table 13.1**).

> **!** The Outerbridge classification implies a staged progression of cartilage damage and is therefore limited to the description of degenerative cartilage lesions. Because Outerbridge developed this classification for the progression of chondromalacia patellae, its original version can be strictly applied only to the patellar cartilage. Ultimately, however, all arthroscopic classifications are based on this grading system to some degree.

Outerbridge RE. The etiology of chondromalacia patellae. J Bone Joint Surg Br 1961;43-B:752–757

Table 13.1 Outerbridge classification of articular cartilage lesions

Grade	Description
1	Softening and swelling (closed chondromalacia)
2	Fragmentation and fissuring < ½ inch (< 1.3 cm) in diameter
3	Fragmentation and fissuring > ½ inch (> 1.3 cm) in diameter
4	Erosion of cartilage down to bone

Shahriaree Classification

The grading system proposed by Shahriaree builds directly on the Outerbridge classification. It comprises four grades of chondromalacia, and distinguishes between a more localized basal degeneration and superficial degeneration that usually involves extensive surfaces of the articular cartilage (**Table 13.2**). In the original article, the author assumed that this categorization might facilitate differentiation between traumatic and degenerative lesions. However, over the years, this classification, like the Outerbridge system, turned out to be applicable only to degenerative cartilage lesions.

Shahriaree H. Chondromalacia. Contemp Orthop 1985;11: 27–39

Table 13.2 Shahriaree system for the arthroscopic classification of cartilage lesions

Grade	Basal degeneration	Superficial degeneration
1	Softening	Fibrillation
2	Blister formation	Fissure formation
3	Ulceration and "crabmeat" formation	Fragmentation
4	Crater formation and eburnation	Crater formation and eburnation

Noyes and Stabler Classification

The Noyes and Stabler classification (**Table 13.3**) was developed for the knee joint and basically defines only three different lesion grades. Grade 1 indicates softened cartilage with an intact surface. Grades 2 and 3 describe superficial defects of varying depth, irrespective of defect morphology. The size and location of the cartilage lesions are also classified. Additionally, the examiner states the degree of knee flexion where the lesion is in weight-bearing contact (e.g., 20–45° of flexion).

Noyes FR, Stabler CL. A system for grading articular cartilage lesions at arthroscopy. Am J Sports Med 1989;17(4):505–513

Table 13.3 Noyes and Stabler system for the arthroscopic classification of cartilage lesions

Grade	Extent of involvement	Surface description	Diameter (all grades)	Location (all grades)
1A	Definite softening with some resilience remaining	Cartilage surface intact	< 10 mm ≤ 15 mm ≤ 20 mm ≤ 25 mm > 25 mm	Patella: Proximal, middle, distal third Medial facet, ridge, lateral facet Trochlea:
1B	Extensive softening with loss of resilience (deformation)			• Medial femoral condyle: 　• Anterior third 　• Middle third
2A	< Half thickness	Cartilage surface damaged; cracks, fissures, fibrillation, or fragmentation		• Posterior third
2B	≥ Half thickness			• Lateral femoral condyle: 　• Anterior third 　• Middle third
3A	Bone surface intact	Bone exposed		• Posterior third
3B	Bone surface cavitation			• Medial tibial condyle: 　• Anterior third 　• Middle third 　• Posterior third • Lateral tibial condyle: 　• Anterior third 　• Middle third 　• Posterior third

Bauer and Jackson Classification

Bauer and Jackson developed a descriptive arthroscopic classification for chondral lesions of the femoral condyles of the knee joint. **Table 13.4** lists the morphologic lesion types that are distinguished in this system.

> !
> • While types I–V in the Bauer and Jackson classification describe the morphology of traumatic (acute) chondral lesions, type VI covers all degrees of degenerative cartilage changes, from softening to surface defects.

Bauer M, Jackson RW. Chondral lesions of the femoral condyles: a system of arthroscopic classification. Arthroscopy 1988;4(2): 97–102

Table 13.4 Bauer and Jackson classification of chondral lesions

Type	Description
I	Linear crack
II	Stellate fracture
III	Flap
IV	Crater
V	Fibrillation
VI	Degrading

International Cartilage Repair Society Classification of Cartilage Lesions

The classification proposed by the International Cartilage Repair Society (ICRS) in 1997 is applicable to degenerative and traumatic cartilage lesions of the knee joint. The system is part of the ICRS Cartilage Injury Evaluation Package (ICRS 2000) and was also integrated into the documentation form of the International Knee Documentation Committee (IKDC 2000). The ICRS classification documents the grade, size, and location of chondral and osteochondral lesions. The five-part grading system (**Table 13.5**) is based on known classifications.

The precise anatomic location of cartilage defects is documented on the femoral condyles, tibial plateau, and patella in relation to the sagittal and coronal planes (**Fig. 13.1**). Defect size is stated in millimeters.

The ICRS classification differs from older classification systems in that only very superficial lesions are classified as grade 1. Deeper fissures are classified as ICRS grade 2 or 3, and blisters are generally classified as ICRS grade 3. Cartilage defects that have been previously treated, are also categorized according to the ICRS classification system. Hence, the ICRS classification focuses more on the therapeutic relevance and surgical treatability of a given lesion than on grading the stage of its progression.

Articular Cartilage

13

Table 13.5 International Cartilage Repair Society (ICRS) grading scheme for (osteo)chondral lesions

ICRS grade	Status	Defect morphology
0	Normal	None
1	Nearly normal	Superficial lesions. Soft indentation (A) and/or superficial fissures and cracks (B)
2	Abnormal	Lesions extending down to <50% of cartilage depth
3	Severely abnormal	Cartilage defects • extending down > 50% of cartilage depth (A) • extending down to calcified layer (B) • extending down to but not through the subchondral bone (C) • blisters (D)
4	Severely abnormal	Osteochondral defects • extending through subchondral bone (A) • extending down to trabecular bone (B) Defects previously treated by drilling are considered osteochondral lesions and are classified as ICRS 4C

Articular Cartilage

13

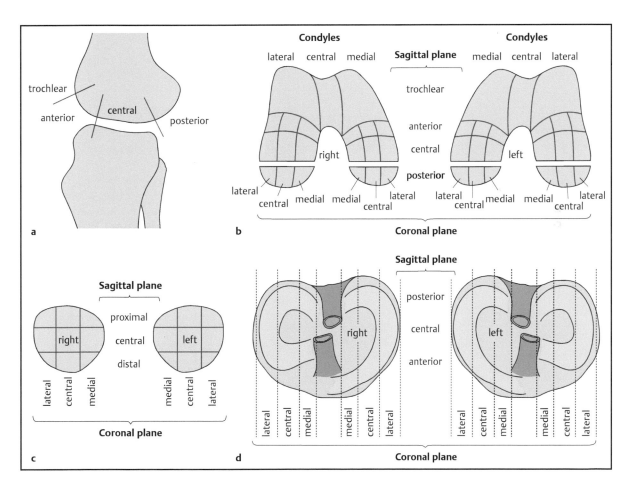

Fig. 13.1a–d Diagram for documenting the location of (osteo)chondral lesions of the knee joint (source: ICRS 2000).

a Femoral condyles, sagittal.
b Femoral condyles, coronal/sagittal.
c Patella.
d Tibial plateau.

International Cartilage Repair Society (ICRS). ICRS Cartilage Injury Evaluation Package 2000. Website: http://www.cartilage.org/_files/ contentmanagement/ICRS_evaluation.pdf; status: 18 December 2010

Classification of Acute Chondral and Osteochondral Injuries

At present there is no standard terminology for describing traumatic lesions of the articular cartilage and chondroosseous junction. Bohndorf (1999) and Wörtler (2008) proposed MRI-based classifications for these injuries. The latter classification distinguishes between purely chondral and osteochondral patterns of injury (**Fig. 13.2**).

Bohndorf K. Imaging of acute injuries of the articular surfaces (chondral, osteochondral and subchondral fractures). Skeletal Radiol 1999;28(10):545–560

Wörtler K. MRI of the knee joint. [Article in German] Orthopade 2008;37(2):157–172

Classification of Chronic Osteochondral Lesions

Chronic articular surface lesions that have a traumatic etiology and involve both the cartilage and subchondral bone and the chronic osteochondritis dissecans are currently referred to collectively as "osteochondral lesions." This is because the precise etiology of a focal osteochondral defect is often uncertain in any given case and has little impact on treatment planning.

Berndt and Harty Classification

Almost all systems for classifying and staging osteochondral lesions are based on the Berndt and Harty classification (**Fig. 13.3**). The authors originally developed this system to describe posttraumatic osteochondral lesions of the talus. The terms "transchondral fracture" and "osteochondritis dissecans" were already used synonymously in the original 1959 publication. The classification defines four stages.

> **!** The Berndt and Harty stages can be applied directly to conventional radiographs. Stage I denotes an absence of radiographic abnormalities.

Berndt AL, Harty M. Transchondral fractures (osteochondritis dissecans) of the talus. J Bone Joint Surg Am 1959; 41:988–1020

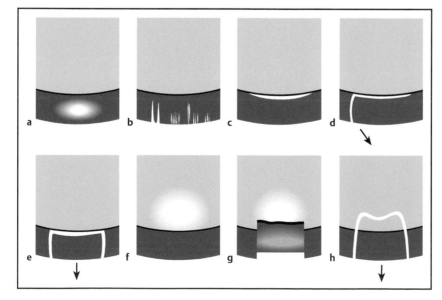

Fig. 13.2a–h Magnetic resonance imaging classification of traumatic cartilage and bone lesions. Chondral injuries (a–e) and osteochondral injuries (f–h; after Wörtler). The diagrams represent findings displayed by fat-suppressed magnetic resonance images with T2 contrast.
a Cartilage contusion.
b Traumatic fissuring or fibrillation.
c Delamination.
d Chondral flap.
e Chondral flake fracture.
f Osteochondral contusion (cartilage injury often undetectable initially).
g Osteochondral impaction.
h Osteochondral flake fracture.

Articular Cartilage

13

Stage	Description	
1	Intact cartilage with small area of subchondral "compression"	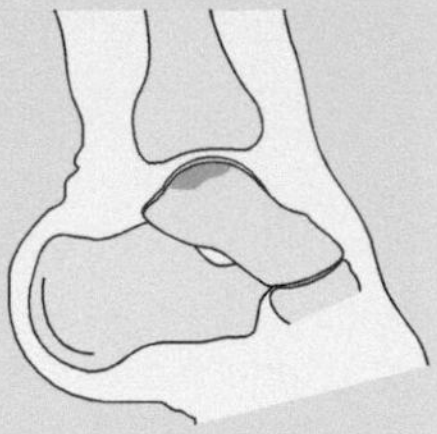
2	Partially detached osteochondral fragment	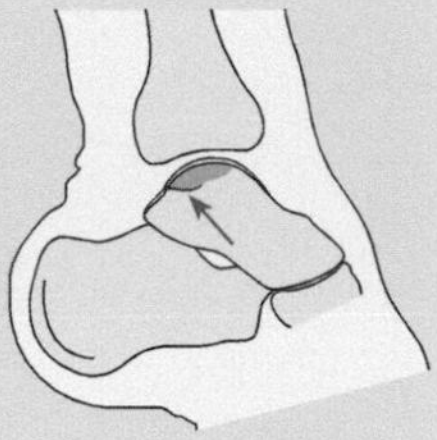
3	Completely detached osteochondral fragment, not displaced	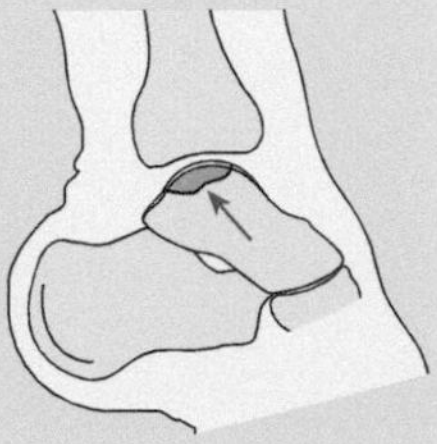
4	Osteochondral fragment displaced within the joint (intra-articular loose body)	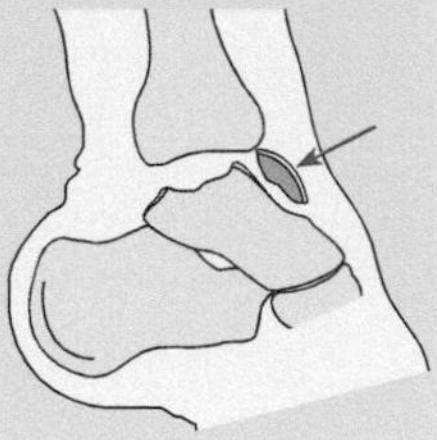

Fig. 13.3 Berndt and Harty classification of osteochondral lesions.

International Cartilage Repair Society Classification of Osteochondritis Dissecans

The ICRS uses a four-stage arthroscopic classification for osteochondritis dissecans of the knee (**Table 13.6**). This classification is often applied to other joint regions and is part of the ICRS Cartilage Injury Evaluation package (ICRS 2000). The ICRS classification has the same basic structure as the Berndt and Harty classification.

International Cartilage Repair Society (ICRS). ICRS Cartilage Injury Evaluation Package 2000. Website: http://www.cartilage.org/_files/ contentmanagement/ICRS_evaluation.pdf; status: 18 December 2010

Table 13.6 International Cartilage Repair Society classification of osteochondritis dissecans (OCD); (source: ICRS 2000)

Stage	Arthroscopic findings
OCD I	Stable, no discontinuity; softened area covered by intact cartilage
OCD II	Partial discontinuity, stable on probing
OCD III	Complete discontinuity, "dead in situ," not displaced
OCD IV	Displaced fragment, loose within the bed or empty defect • Subgroup A: defect < 10 mm in depth • Subgroup B: defect > 10 mm in depth

Magnetic Resonance Imaging Staging System of Nelson and Dipaola

The staging system proposed by Nelson for describing osteochondritis dissecans of the knee and ankle joints combined MRI findings with arthroscopic findings and radiographic findings (based on the Berndt and Harty stages). Dipaola later modified the system somewhat for the characterization of osteochondral lesions. The findings are assigned to four stages (**Table 13.7**).

> **!** According to text of the original publication, the articular cartilage in stage 2 is not necessarily breached, provided that a demarcated subchondral fragment can definitely be detected.

All other MRI-based classification systems follow this classification to a greater or lesser degree. Treatment decisions depend mainly on the stability and viability of the bone fragment, the integrity of the overlying cartilage, and on the integrity of the opposing articular surface.

> **!** Both MR and CT arthrography have advantages over conventional MRI for evaluating the integrity of the articular cartilage and the stability of the fragment (e.g., intra-articular contrast medium can demonstrate partial or complete detachment) and therefore help in distinguishing between stages 2 and 3.

Dipaola JD, Nelson DW, Colville MR. Characterizing osteochondral lesions by magnetic resonance imaging. Arthroscopy 1991;7(1):101–104

Nelson DW, Dipaola J, Colville M, Schmidgall J. Osteochondritis dissecans of the talus and knee: prospective comparison of MR and arthroscopic classifications. J Comput Assist Tomogr 1990;14(5):804–808

Articular Cartilage

13

Table 13.7 Nelson and Dipaola classification of osteochondral lesions

Stage	Arthroscopy	Magnetic resonance imaging	Radiographs (Berndt and Harty)
1	Irregularity and softening of articular cartilage, no definable fragment	Thickening of articular cartilage and low-signal (subchondral) changes	Compression lesion, no visible fragment
2	Articular cartilage may be breached, definable fragment, not displaceable	Articular cartilage may be breached, low-signal rim behind fragment indicating fibrous attachment	Partially detached osteo-chondral fragment
3	Articular cartilage breached, definable fragment, displaceable, but attached by some overlying articular cartilage	Articular cartilage breached, high-signal changes behind fragment indicating synovial fluid between the fragment and underlying subchondral bone	Nondisplaced fragment without attachment
4	Loose body	Loose body	Displaced fragment

14 Hemophilia

In patients with severe or moderately severe hemophilia (decreased activity of coagulation factor VIII [hemophilia A] or IX [hemophilia B]), recurrent episodes of intra-articular bleeding during childhood and adolescence can produce mild to irreversible joint changes. The joints most commonly affected by hemophilic arthropathy are the knees, elbows, and ankles. The early initiation of pro-phylactic treatment with factor VII–IX concentrates has been recommended since the 1980s for the prevention of hemophilic arthropathy. Clinically, the severity of the disease is typically determined by the degree of ankle joint involvement.

Two main types of scoring system are used in the radiologic evaluation of hemophilic arthropathy: progressive scores (e.g., the Arnold–Hilgartner score), in which the finding with the highest grade determines the final score, and additive scores (e.g., the Pettersson score), in which each finding is scored separately and the values are added together to yield a final score.

Pettersson Score

Pettersson et al published a score in 1980 that has become the most widely established system for evaluating hemophilic arthropathy on conventional radiographs. The Pettersson score has also been recommended for follow-ups by the World Federation of Hemophilia since 1981 and is applicable to all large joints.

The Pettersson score (**Table 14.1**) covers eight parameters that are scored on radiographs of the affected joint taken in two planes. The extent of irreversible joint changes is assessed by scoring each of the parameters on a 0–2-point scale. Essentially reversible findings such as soft-tissue swelling or synovial thickening are disregarded. The maximum possible score for a given joint is 13 points. The score describes the natural progression of hemophilic arthropathy and has proven more accurate than other classifications (e.g., the Arnold–Hilgartner score) in discriminating among the various stages of the disease.

Table 14.1 Pettersson score (source: Pettersson et al 1980)

Radiographic parameter	Finding	Score
Osteoporosis	Absent	0
	Present	1
Enlarged epiphysis	Absent	0
	Present	1
Irregular subchondral surface	Absent	0
	Slight	1
	Pronounced	2
Narrowing of joint space	Absent	0
	< 50%	1
	> 50%	2
Subchondral cyst formation	Absent	0
	One cyst	1
	More than one cyst	2
Erosions at joint margins	Absent	0
	Present	1
Gross incongruence of articulating bone ends (angulation/displacement)	Absent	0
	Slight	1
	Pronounced	2
Joint deformity	Absent	0
	Slight	1
	Pronounced	2

Possible joint score = 0–13 points.

> **!** Because synovial and cartilaginous changes precede irreversible bone changes, the Pettersson score tends to underestimate the severity of arthropathy in the early stages of the disease (total score: 0–4).

Pettersson H, Ahlberg A, Nilsson IM. A radiologic classification of hemophilic arthropathy. Clin Orthop Relat Res 1980;149:153–159

Magnetic Resonance Imaging Scores

Since the 1990s, magnetic resonance imaging (MRI) has been used increasingly to detect synovial proliferation, incipient cartilage damage, and hemosiderin deposition in patients with hemophilic arthropathy. Although numerous scores have been proposed for this imaging modality, most are still undergoing clinical validation and no single score has yet been established as a standard method.

Denver Score

The Denver score (**Table 14.2**) is a simple scoring system for everyday clinical practice and has already been used successfully in large clinical therapeutic trials. It is a progressive system in which the final score equals the highest grade that is assigned to any finding. It includes the assessment of effusion, hemarthrosis, synovial hypertrophy, hemosiderin deposits, subchondral cysts, and erosive changes. Articular cartilage loss is considered the end stage and receives the highest score.

Since the Denver score was introduced, the authors of that score as well as other authors have described several modifications and expansions, although none are used as frequently as the original score. Additive scales like that developed by Mathew et al (2000) are also used at selected centers but yield a cumulative score based on the sum of individual changes.

Table 14.2 Denver score

Findings	Stage	Scale
None	Normal joint	0
Effusion/hemarthrosis	Small	1
	Moderate	2
	Large	3
Synovial hypertrophy/ hemosiderin	Small	4
	Moderate	5
	Large	6
Cysts/erosions	One cyst or partial surface erosion	7
	More than one cyst or full surface erosion	8
Cartilage loss	< 50% cartilage loss	9
	≥ 50% cartilage loss	10

Final score = highest grade assigned to any finding.

Funk MB, Schmidt H, Becker S, et al. Modified magnetic resonance imaging score compared with orthopaedic and radiological scores for the evaluation of haemophilic arthropathy. Haemophilia 2002;8(2):98–103.

Lundin B, Pettersson H, Ljung R. A new magnetic resonance imaging scoring method for assessment of haemophilic arthropathy. Haemophilia 2004;10(4):383–389.

Manco-Johnson MJ, Abshire TC, Shapiro AD, et al. Prophylaxis versus episodic treatment to prevent joint disease in boys with severe hemophilia. N Engl J Med 2007;357(6):535–544.

Mathew P, Talbut DC, Frogameni A, et al. Isotopic synovectomy with P-32 in paediatric patients with haemophilia. Haemophilia 2000;6(5):547–555.

Hemophilia Score of the Expert MRI Working Group

Since no single, standard score has yet been established for MRI, the use of many different systems has made it difficult to compare the results of different clinical studies. For this reason, the Expert MRI Working Group of the International Prophylaxis Study Group proposed a consensus classification that permits both an additive and a progressive assessment (**Table 14.3**).

> One limitation of almost all MRI scores is that they are influenced by acute, reversible changes such as joint effusion and hemarthrosis. These changes may mask the true extent of chronic destructive processes in the joint. For this reason, the MRI scoring of hemophilic arthropathy should be performed no earlier than 6 weeks after the last bleeding event.

Lundin B, Babyn P, Doria AS, et al. International Prophylaxis Study Group. Compatible scales for progressive and additive MRI assessments of haemophilic arthropathy. Haemophilia 2005;11(2):109–115

Nuss R, Kilcoyne RF, Geraghty S, et al. MRI findings in haemophilic joints treated with radiosynoviorthesis with development of an MRI scale of joint damage. Haemophilia 2000;6(3):162–169

Using the Scores

At present, the Pettersson score is the only internationally accepted scoring system recommended for the radiographic evaluation of hemophilic arthropathy—both for studies and for routine clinical assessments.

But given the trend toward the early evaluation of hemophilic arthropathy by MRI and the lack of an established standard, the consensus classification of the Expert MRI Working Group of the International Prophylaxis Study Group can provide an effective scoring system for clinical studies. Because this system has both an additive and a progressive scale, it also enables comparisons with

Table 14.3 Hemophilia score of the Expert MRI Working Group of the International Prophylaxis Study Group

Hemophilia		Progressive scale	Additive scale
Effusion, hemarthrosis	• Small	1	
	• Moderate	2	
	• Large	3	
Synovial hypertrophy	• Small	4	1
	• Moderate	5	2
	• Large	6	3
Hemosiderin deposits	• Small	4	1
	• Moderate	5	
	• Large	6	
Changes of subchondral bone or joint margins	• Any surface erosion	7	1
	• Any surface erosion in at least two bones		1
	• Half or more of the articular surface eroded in at least one bone	8	1
	• Half or more of the articular surface eroded in at least two bones		1
	• At least one subchondral cyst	7	1
	• More than one subchondral cyst	8	1
	• Subchondral cysts in at least two bones		1
	• Multiple subchondral cysts in each of at least two bones		1
Cartilage loss	• Any loss of joint cartilage height	9	1
	• Any loss of joint cartilage height in at least two bones		1
	• Any loss of joint cartilage height involving more than one-third of the joint surface in at least one bone		1
	• Any loss of joint cartilage height involving more than one-third of the joint surface in at least two bones	10	1
	• Full-thickness loss of joint cartilage in at least some area in at least one bone		1
	• Full-thickness loss of joint cartilage in at least some area in at least two bones		1
	• Full-thickness loss of joint cartilage involves at least one-third of the joint surface in at least one bone		1
	• Full-thickness loss of joint cartilage involves at least one-third of the joint surface in at least two bones		1
Score		Highest value (maximum of 10)	Sum of individual scores (maximum of 20)

older works. During the next few years, studies might tell us whether the additive or progressive scale is better for making a long-term assessment and prognosis. One continuing problem with most MRI scores is that they are influenced by reversible changes such as hemarthrosis, which can mask the true extent of hemophilic arthropathy.

15 Rheumatoid Arthritis

Radiographic Scoring

The modification of radiographic progression is the main criterion for evaluating the efficacy of disease-modifying drugs in rheumatoid arthritis. Since the mid-20th century, various scoring methods have been developed for quantifying the changes depicted by radiographs. The main goal of radiographic scoring in rheumatoid arthritis is the quantification of joint destruction, a largely irreversible process that is the primary measure of disease progression. So far, attempts to measure joint destruction with computer techniques have met with little success. Semiquantitative scoring methods are based largely on erosive changes, and some methods score the percentage of articular surface destruction or the reduction of joint-space width as an indicator of cartilage destructioh.

> **!**
>
> The reliability of radiographic scores depends critically on the quality (readability) of the image. A technically sound radiograph should meet the following criteria:
>
> - Use of a high-resolution screen-film combination
> - Optimum positioning (true dorsoplantar or dorsopalmar projection):
>   - Hands placed flat on the cassette
>   - Patient sitting with the forefeet placed on a cassette lying on the floor
> - 18 × 24-cm format for each hand or for both forefeet
> - Beam centered on the third metacarpophalangeal joints or between the metatarsophalangeal joints of the big toes
> - Alternative method: both hands are placed on a 24 × 30-cm cassette and exposed separately
> - Collimate to include the whole hand and the distal ends of the radius and ulna
> - Constant exposure parameters
> - Semioblique views are not strictly necessary

The best approach to radiographic scoring is to include all radiographs of one patient in the evaluation, doing so either in chronological or random order. The latter method is preferred as it reduces misinterpretations based on the assumption of constant progression.

Several different methods of radiographic scoring are presented in the literature:

- Global scoring of the patient as a whole
- Global scoring of each joint
- Separate scoring of erosions and joint-space narrowing

Whereas the first method (e.g., the Kellgren score) is no longer used because it provides only a global assessment, the Larsen scoring system (global score for each joint) or the Sharp system (separate scoring of erosions and joint-space narrowing) are most used in everyday practice and especially within the framework of studies. The Ratingen score is commonly used in everyday practice (outside studies) owing to its relative simplicity. It grades only destructive changes, yielding a separate score for each joint but it does not score joint-space narrowing.

Larsen Score

The original 1977 version of the Larsen scoring system focused mainly on erosive destruction. The severity of changes is graded on a 0–5 scale as shown in **Fig. 15.1**.

The definitions in the Larsen score relate mainly to radiographic changes of the hands and feet. The following joints are evaluated in the standard protocol:

- Second through fifth proximal interphalangeal joints
- First interphalangeal joint (thumb)
- First through fifth metacarpophalangeal joints
- Wrist
- First through fifth metatarsophalangeal joints

A total of 32 joints are scored, and the individual joint scores are added together to give a total score between 0 and 160. Originally the different grades of severity were illustrated by standard reference films, but Larsen later replaced the reference films with schematic drawings (see **Fig. 15.1**).

The method was modified several times by Larsen himself and by other authors, but no change was made in the list of joints that are scored. In 1995 Larsen introduced a modification for long-term studies that addressed the difficulty of scoring soft-tissue swelling and articular osteoporosis because of the variable quality of radiographs. This prompted Larsen to redefine grade 1 (one or more erosions < 1 mm in diameter or joint-space narrowing) and grade 2 (one or more small erosions > 1 mm in diameter) (see **Fig. 15.1**). The following joints are scored in this modification (**Fig. 15.2**):

- Second through fifth proximal interphalangeal joints
- Second through fifth metacarpophalangeal joints
- Radial and ulnar compartments of the wrist

Larsen score, 1977 version				Modification for long-term studies (Larsen 1995)	
Score	Definition	Findings	Diagram	Findings	Diagram
0	Normal conditions	Normal conditions. Abnormalities not related to arthritis, such as marginal bone deposition, may be present	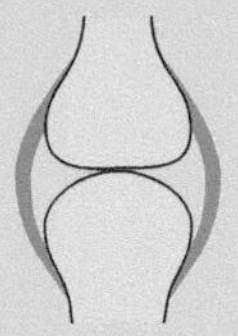	Same as 1977 version	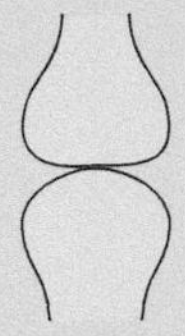
1	Slight abnormality	One or more of the following lesions is present: periarticular soft-tissue swelling, periarticular osteoporosis, and slight joint-space narrowing	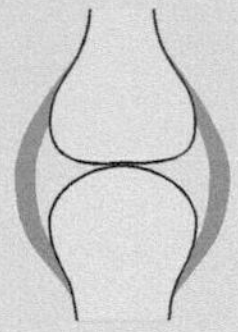	≥ 1 erosion less than 1 mm in diameter or joint space narrowing	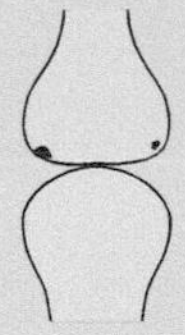
2	Definite abnormality	≥ 1 small erosion; joint-space narrowing is not obligatory	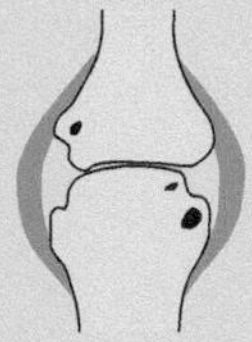	≥ 1 erosion, diameter more than 1 mm	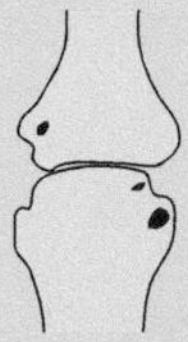
3	Marked abnormality	Marked erosions. Erosion and joint-space narrowing must be present	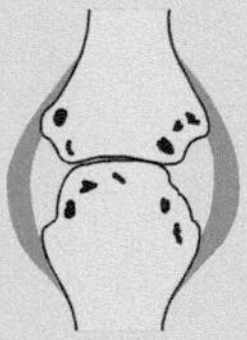	Marked erosions	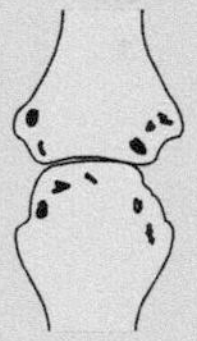
4	Severe abnormality	Severe erosions. There is usually no joint space left. Original bony outlines are partly preserved	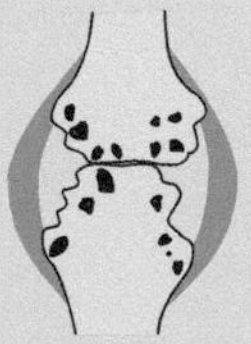	Severe erosions. There is usually no joint space left. Original bony outlines are partly preserved	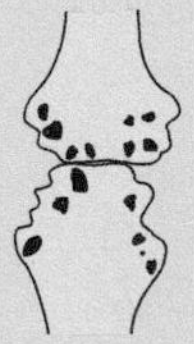
5	Mutilating abnormality	Original articular surfaces have disappeared. Gross bone deformation may be present	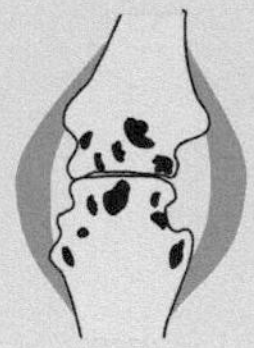	Mutilating changes: The original bony outlines have been destroyed	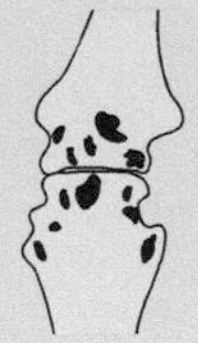

Fig. 15.1 Larsen score.

- Radial and ulnar compartments of the carpometacarpal joint
- Second through fifth metatarsophalangeal joints

Again, a total of 32 joints are counted to yield a total score between 0 and 160.

Larsen A, Dale K, Eek M. Radiographic evaluation of rheumatoid arthritis and related conditions by standard reference films. Acta Radiol Diagn (Stockh) 1977;18(4):481–491

Larsen A, Thoen J. Hand radiography of 200 patients with rheumatoid arthritis repeated after an interval of one year. Scand J Rheumatol 1987;16(6):395–401

Rheumatoid Arthritis

15

Rheumatoid Arthritis

15

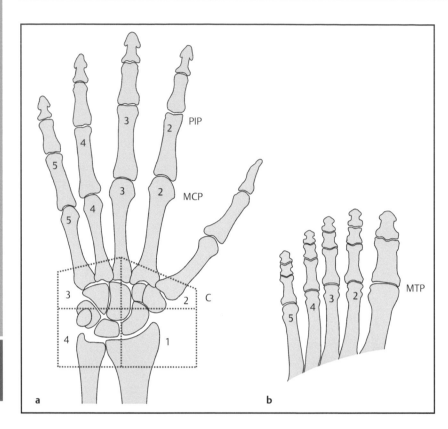

Fig. 15.2a,b Joints and joint regions scored in the 1995 modification of the Larsen score (source: Rau et al 2008).

a Hand.
  C   = Carpus
  MCP = Metacarpophalangeal joint
  PIP = Proximal interphalangeal joint
b Foot.
  MTP = Metatarsophalangeal joint

Larsen A. How to apply Larsen score in evaluating radiographs of rheumatoid arthritis in long-term studies. J Rheumatol 1995;22(10):1974–1975

Rau R, Herborn G, Wassenberg S. Atlas radiologischer Scoringmethoden bei der rheumatoiden Arthritis. Stuttgart: Thieme; 2008

Rau R, Herborn G, Wassenberg S. Atlas radiologischer Scoringmethoden bei der rheumatoiden Arthritis. Stuttgart: Thieme; 2008

Sharp JT, Young DY, Bluhm GB, et al. How many joints in the hands and wrists should be included in a score of radiologic abnormalities used to assess rheumatoid arthritis? Arthritis Rheum 1985;28(12):1326–1335

Sharp Scoring System

Another method useful in clinical studies is the 1985 modification of the Sharp scoring system (**Table 15.1**). This score, which grades possible erosions in a total of 17 joints and joint-space narrowing in 18 joints, proved to be simpler and more accurate compared with a previously published method that scored a total of 27 joint regions. Erosions (0–5 points) are counted independently of their size. With erosions that are poorly defined (e.g., confluent lesions), the percentage of the affected joint surface is also scored (< 50% versus > 50% of the joint surface). Joint-space narrowing is scored at 0–4 points according to severity (see **Table 15.1**). Subluxations or dislocations are not scored. The joints that are scored are shown in **Fig. 15.3**. The maximum erosion score for 34 joints is 170 (34 × 5; see **Fig. 15.3b**). The maximum joint-space narrowing score for 36 joints is 144 (36 × 4; see **Fig. 15.3a**). Hence, the maximum total score is 314.

Ratingen Score

The Ratingen score provides an easy-to-use method for routine clinical purposes (**Table 15.2**). Unlike the Larsen method, it scores only destructive changes in bone. Reversible indicators of disease activity such as soft-tissue swelling and osteoporosis are disregarded. Joint-space narrowing is not scored either. As in the Sharp method, the wrist is divided into several regions.

The Ratingen method scores the surfaces of both bone ends within the joint space enclosed by the synovial membrane. The hand score is assessed in the following joints:
- Second through fifth proximal interphalangeal joints
- First interphalangeal joint (thumb)
- First through fifth metacarpophalangeal joints
- Four regions in the wrist (scaphoid, lunate, distal radius, distal ulna)

Table 15.1 Sharp score, 1985 modification

Score	Erosive changes	Joint-space narrowing
0	No erosions	No narrowing
1	One discrete erosion	Focal narrowing
2	Two discrete erosions	Diffuse narrowing of less than 50% of the original joint space
3	Three discrete erosions	Definite narrowing with loss of more than 50% of the normal joint space
4	Four discrete erosions	Absence of a joint space, presumptive evidence of ankylosis
5	Extensive destruction—more than 50% bone loss of either articular bone	

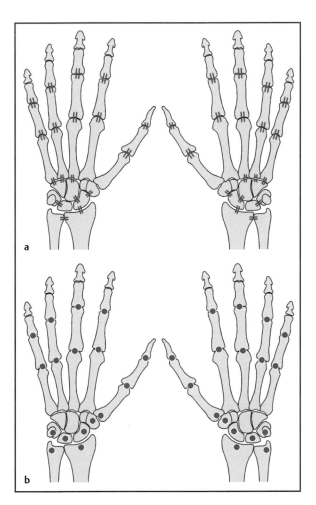

a
b

Fig. 15.3a,b Joints scored in the 1985 modification of the Sharp score. Schematic drawing (source: Rau et al 2008).
a Joints scored for joint-space narrowing.
b Joints or joint regions scored for erosions.

At the feet the following joints are scored: the second through fourth metatarsophalangeal joints and the first interphalangeal joint (of the great toe), resulting in a total of 38 joints to yield a total score between 0 and 190.

Table 15.2 Ratingen score

Score	Extent of destruction
0	Normal joint
1	One or more erosions; < 20% destruction of the joint surface
2	Joint-surface destruction of 21–40%
3	Joint-surface destruction 41–60%
4	Joint-surface destruction 61–80%
5	Joint-surface destruction > 80%

> **!** One advantage of the Ratingen score over the Sharp score is that the grading system (with each grade representing 20% of the articular surface) ensures a good correlation between the extent of joint destruction and the score value throughout the entire course of the disease.

Kellgren JH. Radiological signs of rheumatoid arthritis; a study of observer differences in the reading of hand films. Ann Rheum Dis 1956;15(1):55–60

Rau R, Wassenberg S, Herborn G, Stucki G, Gebler A. A new method of scoring radiographic change in rheumatoid arthritis. J Rheumatol 1998;25(11):2094–2107

Magnetic Resonance Imaging Scores

With the increasing utilization of magnetic resonance imaging (MRI) for the earlier detection of synovial proliferations, incipient cartilage damage, and also periarticular soft-tissue changes, it is inevitable that powerful scores will be established for this modality as well. The most important method developed to date is the OMERACT RA MRI scoring system (**Table 15.3**). The object of this system is to better describe the inflammatory and destructive

Table 15.3 OMERACT RA MRI scoring system. Basic magnetic resonance imaging sequences: T1-weighted sequences in two planes before and after intravenous contrast administration and a T2-weighted fat-saturated or STIR sequence in one plane (after Østergaard M et al 2003)

Pathology	Definition of important RA pathologies	Remarks on scoring system	Score
Synovitis	An area in the synovial compartment that shows above-normal postgadolinium enhancement of a thickness greater than the width of the normal synovium	Is assessed in three wrist regions (the distal radioulnar joint, the radiocarpal joint, the intercarpal and carpometacarpal joints) and in each MCP joint. The first carpometacarpal joint and first MCP joint are not scored	0 (normal) 1 (mild) 2 (moderate) 3 (marked)
Bone erosion	A sharply marginated bone lesion, with correct juxta-articular localization and typical signal characteristics, which is visible in two planes with a cortical break seen in at least one plane	Each bone (wrists: carpal bones, distal radius, distal ulna, metacarpal bases; MCP joints: metacarpal heads, phalangeal bases) is scored separately. The scale is 0–10, based on the proportion of eroded bone compared with the "assessed bone volume," judged on all available images—0: no erosion; 1: 1–10% of bone eroded; 2: 11–20%, etc. For long bones, the "assessed bone volume" is from the articular surface (or its best estimated portion if absent) to a depth of 1 cm, and in carpal bones it is the whole bone	0–10
Bone marrow edema	A lesion within the trabecular bone, with ill-defined margins and signal characteristics consistent with increased water content	Each bone is scored separately (as for erosions). The scale is 0–3, based on the proportion of bone with edema as follows—0: no edema; 1: 1–33% of bone edematous; 2: 34–66% of bone edematous; 3: 67–100%	0–3

MCP = Metacarpophalangeal
OMERACT RA MRI = Outcome measures in rheumatology. Clinical trials. Rheumatoid arthritis magnetic resonance imaging score
RA = Rheumatoid arthritis

changes in rheumatoid arthritis. The scoring system and requisite MRI sequences are summarized in **Table 15.3**. As the table indicates, the system assigns a possible total score of 0–21 for synovitis, 0–230 for bone erosions, and 0–69 for bone marrow edema.

Østergaard M, Peterfy C, Conaghan P, et al. OMERACT Rheumatoid Arthritis Magnetic Resonance Imaging Studies. Core set of MRI acquisitions, joint pathology definitions, and the OMERACT RA-MRI scoring system. J Rheumatol 2003;30(6):1385–1386

Østergaard M, Edmonds J, McQueen F, et al. An introduction to the EULAR-OMERACT rheumatoid arthritis MRI reference image atlas. Ann Rheum Dis 2005;64(Suppl 1):i3–i7

Rau R, Herborn G, Wassenberg S. Atlas radiologischer Scoringmethoden bei der rheumatoiden Arthritis. Stuttgart: Thieme; 2008

Using the Scores

Radiographic scoring methods should be used in all therapeutic studies that span a period of 1 year or longer.

The Ratingen score can also be used in everyday practice owing to its simple methodology. It is best to document radiographic findings on a standard form, which can display the findings and their progression better than a detailed verbal description. The use of scores has yielded important new discoveries on the progression of rheumatoid arthritis and the efficacy of various disease-modifying antirheumatic drugs.

One disadvantage of radiographic scoring methods is that the one-dimensional X-ray image can detect only defects at a marginal location. Moreover, radiographic features reflect current disease activity with a time lag of ~ 6–12 months. Hence it takes 6 months to document the inhibition of destructive changes.

The literature (e.g., Rau et al 2008) may be consulted for images that illustrate the various grades of findings in different scoring systems.

For the present, MRI scoring is performed only at specialized centers because the scores have yet to be fully validated.

Rau R, Herborn G, Wassenberg S. Atlas radiologischer Scoringmethoden bei der rheumatoiden Arthritis. Stuttgart: Thieme; 2008

Rheumatoid Arthritis

15

16 Muscle Injuries

Müller-Wohlfahrt Classification

The terminology used in the literature for classifying muscle injuries is highly diverse, and many proposed classifications are unsuitable for evaluating injuries with respect to their management and prognosis.

In 2010, Müller-Wohlfahrt introduced a new classification that precisely defines the different types of muscle injury while also taking into account factors that are relevant to treatment, such as the size of the tear. The classification also includes "functional minor injuries," which cause no structural damage and usually produce no imaging abnormalities but account for a large percentage of muscle injuries in general. Most stage II–IV injuries in this classification can be reliably differentiated on magnetic resonance imaging (MRI).

The best imaging modalities for diagnosing muscle injuries are MRI and ultrasound. Ultrasound imaging requires an experienced examiner, and the findings are depicted less clearly and objectively than by MRI. For this reason, MRI has become the imaging modality of choice for the differentiation of muscle injuries. A quality examination requires the correct pulse sequences and the highest possible spatial resolution. This chapter describes the typical patterns of MRI findings that are associated with different types of muscle injury. For details on sonographic findings, we refer the reader to the specialized literature.

Table 16.1 summarizes the Müller-Wohlfahrt classification with special emphasis on MRI findings.

> **!**
> To understand the classification, it is necessary to know the structure of muscle tissue and the imaging appearance of its various elements. The muscle fibers (multinucleated muscle cells) are grouped by connective tissue (epimysium and perimysium) into primary and secondary bundles. Only the secondary bundles can be directly visualized by MRI. They are important functional units that measure a few millimeters in diameter and consist of multiple primary bundles sheathed by perimysium. They can be palpated by an experienced examiner and appear as "muscle fibers" on MR images.

Painful Muscle Hardening (Type I Lesion)

Two types of muscle hardening are distinguished: type Ia (fatigue-induced) and type Ib (neurogenic). Both are classified as minor injuries because muscle hardening is a functional lesion that occurs in the absence of underlying structural damage. While a type Ia injury is caused by fatigue or overuse, a type Ib injury is based on a neurogenic increase in muscle tone. The result of the injury is a hardening or firmness that extends the full length of the affected muscle. Complaints range from an aching or tight sensation to significant pain. MRI, which is rarely performed for these injuries, typically shows no abnormalities. However, in some cases of type I lesions rapidly reversible intramuscular edema may develop, and subfascial edema may also be present with a type Ib lesion.

Muscle Strain (Type II Lesion)

Muscle strain is caused by a dysregulation of muscle tone that usually occurs suddenly, often at the start of exercise. The injury is most commonly located in the area of the muscle belly. Typically a localized swelling is found on physical examination. Since the integrity of the tissue is intact, all fibers visible on MRI (secondary bundles) appear to be intact, and images typically show edematous changes around the intact fiber structures, which have a feathery appearance.

Muscle-Fiber and Muscle-Bundle Tears (Type III Lesions)

■ Muscle Fiber Tear (Type IIIa Lesion)

A muscle fiber tear involves the rupture of one or more secondary bundles. The usual site of occurrence is at the musculotendinous junction. MRI reveals a circumscribed discontinuity in the fibers caused by a wavy pattern of the torn secondary bundles, which are consistently demarcated by intramuscular hematoma or edema.

Tears smaller than 5 mm are classified as a muscle fiber tear. The size of the tear is measured perpendicular to the course of the muscle fibers. Differentiation from a

Table 16.1 Müller-Wohlfahrt classification of muscle injuries (source: Müller-Wohlfahrt et al 2010)

Type of lesion	Ia Painful muscle hardening (fatigue-induced)	Ib Painful muscle hardening (neurogenic)	II Muscle strain	IIIa Muscle fiber tear	IIIb Muscle bundle tear	IV Complete muscle tear or tendon avulsion
Classification	Minor injury; functional	Minor injury; functional	Minor injury; functional	Major injury; structural, mechanical	Major injury; structural, mechanical	Major injury; structural, mechanical
Location	Up to full muscle length	Muscle bundle or larger group involving the full muscle length	Usually involves 15-cm length of the muscle belly	Most common site: musculotendinous junction	Most common site: musculotendinous junction	Musculotendinous junction or, more commonly, tendon avulsion
MRI	Usually negative; may show rapidly reversible edema	Usually negative; may show rapidly reversible edema and subfascial fluid	Edematous changes between secondary bundles in localized muscle area; all visible fibers are intact; no confluent hematoma	Discontinuity in a few secondary bundles; transverse diameter of tear < 5 mm; intramuscular hematoma is typical	Discontinuity in a larger group of secondary bundles; transverse diameter of tear > 5 mm; intramuscular hematoma is typical, often accompanied by an intermuscular or interfascial hematoma	Discontinuity through all secondary bundles; wavy-line pattern plus large intramuscular and intermuscular hematoma
Treatment and its duration	Conservative; usually 1–3 days	Conservative; usually 2–5 days	Conservative; usually 3–5 days	Conservative; usually 10–14 days	Conservative; usually 6 weeks	Tendon avulsion repaired surgically; otherwise conservative; usually 12–16 weeks

muscle bundle tear (see below) is important because of differences in prognosis and treatment: whereas a muscle fiber tear will generally heal completely, a muscle bundle tear will often leave a residual defect with an associated circumscribed scar.

■ Muscle Bundle Tear (Type IIIb Lesion)

A muscle bundle tear involves the rupture of a large group of secondary bundles. By definition, the transverse diameter of the tear is greater than 5 mm. There is often concomitant injury to the stabilizing connective-tissue structures including the muscle fascia—more so than in a muscle fiber tear. As a result, it is common for intramuscular hemorrhage to coexist with larger, intermuscular hematomas. As with a muscle fiber tear, the site of predilection for a muscle bundle tear is the musculotendinous junction. MRI can clearly demonstrate the discontinuity

of the muscle fibers, the size of the defect, and the adjacent hematoma.

Table 16.2 summarizes the Boutin classification, in which muscle bundle tears are further subcategorized according to tear size in relation to cross-section of the muscle.

Complete Muscle Tear or Tendon Avulsion (Type IV Lesion)

In a type IV lesion, the continuity of the muscle is completely disrupted. A full-thickness muscle tear is very rare. It requires a severe traumatizing force and usually occurs at the level of the musculotendinous junction. The discontinuity of the muscle is clearly visible on MRI, and the ruptured fibers typically appear as wavy lines. A complete tendon avulsion is more common. It is important

Table 16.2 Boutin classification of muscle bundle tears

Grade	Description
1	Involves less than one-third of total muscle cross-section
2	Involves between one-third and two-thirds of total muscle cross-section
3	Involves more than two-thirds of total muscle cross-section

Table 16.3 Smigielski classification of muscle injuries

Grade	Description
1	Tear with structural defect involving < 5% of cross-sectional muscle area
2	Tear with structural defect involving > 5% of cross-sectional muscle area
3	Complete muscle tear

in these cases to visualize the retracted portion of the muscle at imaging.

Böck J, Mundinger P, Luttke G. Magnetresonanztomographie. In: Müller-Wohlfahrt H-W, Ueblacker P, Hänsel L. Muskelverletzungen im Sport. Stuttgart: Thieme; 2010: 196–217

Boutin RD, Fritz RC, Steinbach LS. Imaging of sports-related muscle injuries. Magn Reson Imaging Clin N Am 2003;11:341–371

Müller-Wohlfahrt H-W, Ueblacker P, Binder A, et al. Anamnese, klinische Untersuchung und Klassifikation. In: Müller-Wohlfahrt H-W, Ueblacker P, Hänsel L. Muskelverletzungen im Sport. Stuttgart: Thieme; 2010: 136–159

Other Classifications

Many textbooks to date have given a very general classification of muscle injuries in which grade I lesions (muscle strains) are characterized by fiber damage detectable only on a microscopic level. Grade II lesions involve a partial muscle tear (partial disruption), and grade III lesions consist of a complete muscle tear (complete disruption). One disadvantage of this simple classification is that many injuries fall within the grade II category without any further differentiation. The Smigielski classification (**Table 16.3**), commonly used in orthopedics, is similar. It is based on the percentage of cross-sectional muscle area involved by the structural defect. It will be noted that tears of the same size (with approximately the same amount of damage to primary and secondary bundles) can be graded differently by taking into account the cross-sectional area of different muscles.

Disadvantages of the Smigielski classification are lack of precision in estimating the ratio of tear size to muscle area and the absence of subcategories under the heading of grade II lesions.

Smigielski R. Muskulatur und Sehnen. In: Engelhardt M, Krüger-Franke M, Pieper HG, Siebert CH, eds. Praxiswissen Halte- und Bewegungsorgane. Sportverletzungen—Sportschäden. Stuttgart: Thieme; 2005: 82

Muscle Injuries

16

17 Skeletal Age

Basic Principles

Skeletal age is considered the most important and most representative criterion of biological maturity. Skeletal age determination is carried out for the purpose of evaluating growth in pediatric patients and for the diagnosis of many endocrine disorders and pediatric syndromes. It also allows for growth prediction, so skeletal age determination is important for orthopedic procedures in which it is essential to know the remaining potential for longitudinal growth. In rare cases, skeletal age determination is also required in judicial proceedings to determine, for example, whether a suspect should be charged as a juvenile or an adult. Because radiographs alone do not meet the legal requirement of establishing age with a "probability bordering on certainty," these cases additionally require a physical and dental examination (including a panoramic radiograph).

When conventional radiographs are used, present skeletal age and predicted adult height can be calculated on the basis of statistical tables. After 2 months of age, these values can be determined on a radiograph of the left hand because the hand bones, with their numerous secondary ossification centers, are considered representative of the skeletal system as a whole. For decades, skeletal maturity was determined by making a visual assessment of the skeletal development of the hand and wrist. With the development and use of digital imaging techniques, there have been increasing attempts to determine the morphologic hallmarks of ossification using computer-assisted techniques to permit a more effective and objective determination. Practical implementation is difficult, however, because of interindividual differences in the rates of bone growth and the variable shape and size of many ossification centers.

Bone Development

The assessment of skeletal maturity is a process that evaluates the size and shape of bones and their degree of mineralization to predict the time remaining to full maturity. This process requires a fundamental knowledge of bone growth. Basically, the development of the skeleton proceeds in three consecutive stages:

- *Before birth:* Ossification of the skeleton begins during the second month of intrauterine development. At birth, the diaphyses of all the tubular bones are present along with the epiphyseal ossification centers of the distal femur, proximal tibia, talus, calcaneus, and cuboid.
- *After birth:* Postnatal longitudinal growth of the tubular bones parallels the ossification of the epiphyses and apophyses. Maturation of the epiphyses and ossification of the epiphyseal plates follows a timetable that is subject to intraindividual and interindividual variations. The first ossification centers in the wrist become radiographically visible during the third month of life. The epiphyses of the radius and short tubular bones do not appear until the second year of life.
- *Puberty:* Skeletal development concludes with epiphyseal closure during puberty. Sesamoid bones do not appear until after 12 years of age and are variable in their temporal development and number.

Indicators of Skeletal Development in the Hand

The skeletal development of the hand can be divided into six stages. Specific ossification centers in different age groups are the best predictors of skeletal maturity (**Fig. 17.1** and **Table 17.1**). The various methods of determining skeletal age are based on this developmental pattern. **Fig. 17.2** shows the order of appearance of the individual ossification centers, and **Table 17.2** lists the ages at which ossification centers appear in the carpals and metacarpals.

Birkner R. Das typische Röntgenbild des Skeletts: Standardbefunde und Varietäten vom Erwachsenen und Kind. 4th ed. Munich: Elsevier; 2009

Schmitt R, Lanz U. Bildgebende Diagnostik der Hand. Stuttgart: Thieme; 2008

Stuart HC, Stevenson SS. Physical Growth and Development. Textbook of Pediatrics, 7th ed. Philadelphia: Waldo E. Nelson; 1959: 12–61

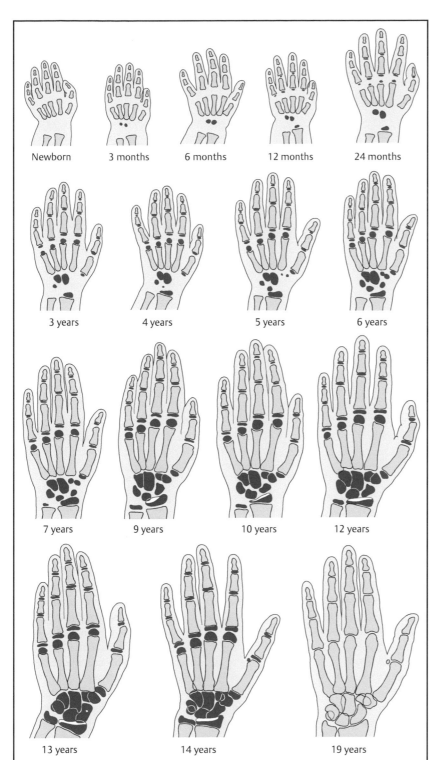

Fig. 17.1 Skeletal development of the hand. Schematic representation (source: Schmitt and Lanz 2008).

Newborn 3 months 6 months 12 months 24 months

3 years 4 years 5 years 6 years

7 years 9 years 10 years 12 years

13 years 14 years 19 years

Table 17.1 Six stages in the ossification of the hand and wrist bones

Group	Age		Ossification centers that best predict skeletal maturity	Developmental stages (relevant to skeletal age determination)
	Girls	Boys		
Infants	Up to 10 months	Up to 14 months	Carpal bones and radial epiphysis	Ossification centers appear first in the capitate and hamate, finally in the distal radial epiphysis
Toddlers	10 months to 2 years	14 months to 3 years	Number of epiphyses visible in the tubular bones of the hand	Ossification follows this scheme: • Proximal phalanges • Metacarpals • Middle phalanges • Distal phalanges (exceptions: distal phalanx of thumb earlier and middle phalanx of fifth ray later than the rest; finally all epiphyses are formed)
Prepuberty	2–7 years	3–9 years	Size of the phalangeal epiphyses	Width of epiphyses approaches width of diaphyses; distal epiphyses are most relevant
Early and mid-puberty	7–13 years	9–14 years	Size of the phalangeal epiphyses	Width of distal and middle epiphyses greater than width of metaphyses
Late puberty	13–15 years	14–16 years	Degree of epiphyseal fusion	Fusion follows this scheme: • Distal phalanges • Metacarpals • Proximal phalanges • Middle phalanges
Postpuberty	15–17 years	17–19 years	Degree of epiphyseal fusion of the radius and ulna	Epiphyseal fusion in the ulna occurs before the radius

Determination of Skeletal Age

Before Three Months

Given the lack of ossification centers, skeletal maturity before age 3 months is often assessed on a conventional lateral radiograph of the lower leg and ankle. An alternative technique is to scan the ossification centers with ultrasound. The radiograph is used in conjunction with clinically validated nomograms to determine skeletal age. Depending on the method, either age (up to 2 years of age; Hernández method) or body weight (up to 1 year of age; Erasmie method) is used as the starting value:

● *Erasmie method:* The sum of the maximum lengths and heights (in mm) of the ossification centers of the talus and calcaneus are calculated as the first step (**Fig. 17.3a**). Next, the ossification centers of the cuboid, third cuneiform, and distal epiphyses of the tibia and fibula and possible accessory ossification centers are graded on a four-point scale. Different scores are assigned based on the maturity of the ossification centers as shown in **Table 17.3**, and the point values are added to yield a total score. The graph in **Fig. 17.3b** is used to determine skeletal maturity. First a vertical line is drawn through the present body weight on the x-axis. Then an upper horizontal line is drawn through the y-axis at the sum of the lengths of the talus and calcaneus. In the lower part of the graph, a horizontal line is drawn through the total maturity score determined for the ossification centers. Each point of intersection with the vertical line indicates the deviation of skeletal maturity from the normal population. This method was evaluated in a total of 115 children.

● *Hernández method:* This is an alternative method for determining skeletal maturity up to 2 years of age by scoring the development of the ossification centers of the calcaneus, cuboid, third cuneiform, distal tibia and fibular epiphysis (**Figs. 17.4 and 17.5**). The percentile of skeletal maturity for a certain age and gender can then be read from a nomogram based on the determined total sum. This method was validated in Bilbao (Spain) in a series of 1,164 radiographs.

Erasmie U, Ringertz H. A method for assessment of skeletal maturity in children below one year of age. Pediatr Radiol 1980;9(4):225–228

Hernández M, Sánchez E, Sobradillo B, Rincón JM, Narvaiza JL. A new method for assessment of skeletal maturity in the first 2 years of life. Pediatr Radiol 1988;18(6):484–489

Table 17.2 Order of appearance of the individual ossification centers of the carpals and metacarpals, listed separately by gender (after Stuart and Stevenson; source: Birkner 2009)

Carpals, metacarpals	Boys		Girls	
	Mean value	Standard deviation	Mean value	Standard deviation
Capitate	2 months	2 months	2 months	2 months
Hamate	3 months	2 months	2 months	2 months
Radial epiphysis	1 year, 1 month	5 months	10 months	4 months
Proximal phalanx II	1 year, 4 months	4 months	11 months	3 months
Proximal phalanx III	1 year, 4 months	4 months	10 months	3 months
Proximal phalanx IV	1 year, 5 months	5 months	11 months	3 months
Distal phalanx I	1 year, 7 months	7 months	1 year	4 months
Metacarpal II	1 year, 6 months	5 months	1 year	3 months
Metacarpal III	1 year, 8 months	5 months	1 year, 1 month	3 months
Proximal phalanx V	1 year, 9 months	5 months	1 year, 2 months	4 months
Metacarpal IV	1 year, 11 months	6 months	1 year, 3 months	4 months
Middle phalanx IV	2 years	6 months	1 year, 3 months	5 months
Middle phalanx III	2 years	6 months	1 year, 3 months	5 months
Middle phalanx II	2 years, 2 months	6 months	1 year, 4 months	5 months
Metacarpal V	2 years, 2 months	7 months	1 year, 4 months	5 months
Distal phalanx IV	2 years, 4 months	6 months	1 year, 6 months	1 year, 3 months
Distal phalanx III	2 years, 4 months	6 months	1 year, 6 months	4 months
Triquetrum	2 years, 6 months	1 year, 4 months	1 year, 9 months	1 year, 2 months
Epiphysis of thumb	2 years, 8 months	9 months	1 year, 6 months	5 months
Proximal phalanx I	2 years, 8 months	7 months	1 year, 8 months	5 months
Distal phalanx II	3 years, 1 month	8 months	1 year, 11 months	6 months
Distal phalanx V	3 years, 1 month	9 months	1 year, 11 months	6 months
Middle phalanx V	3 years, 3 months	10 months	1 year, 10 months	7 months
Lunate	3 years, 6 months	1 year, 7 months	2 years, 2 months	1 year, 1 month
Trapezium	5 years, 7 months	1 year, 7 months	3 years, 11 months	1 year, 2 months
Trapezoid	5 years, 9 months	1 year, 3 months	4 years, 1 month	1 year
Scaphoid	5 years, 6 months	1 year, 3 months	4 years, 3 months	1 year
Ulnar epiphysis	6 years, 10 months	1 year, 2 months	5 years, 9 months	1 year, 1 month
Pisiform	–	–	–	–
Sesamoid I	12 years, 8 months	1 year, 6 months	10 years, 1 month	1 year, 1 month

Three Months and Older

A radiograph of the left hand has become the established tool for determining skeletal age in children aged 3 months and older. This method is easy to perform and requires very little radiation exposure. The technical parameters are as follows:

- Free exposure at 30–45 kV and 3–6 mA
- Film-focus distance of 76 cm (prescribed for the Tanner–Whitehouse method)
- Beam centered on the head of the third metacarpal
- Thumb abducted ~ 30°
- Film speed 400
- Small focus
- No grid

The first radiographic atlas based on the principle of ossification centers was created by Todd in 1937. The atlases of Greulich and Pyle and of Thiemann and Nitz are most widely used at present, along with the Tanner and Whitehouse scoring system.

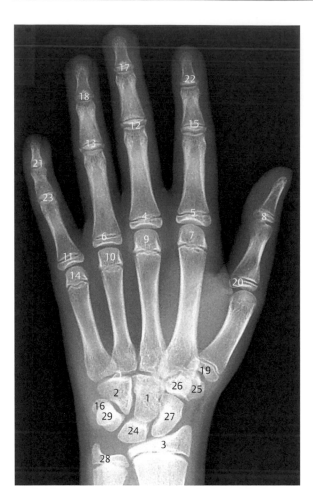

Fig. 17.2 Order in which ossification begins in the hand and wrist bones.

■ Greulich and Pyle Atlas

Published in 1959, the Greulich and Pyle atlas presents standard radiographic plates of the left hand and wrist obtained from 3 months to 16 years of age. The atlas lists 29 standard radiographs for female infants, children and adolescents and 31 standard radiographs for male infants, children and adolescents. The exact ages of the individual ossification centers are indicated for each radiograph and may deviate slightly from one another. Schmid and Moll created a modified, genderless scheme (see **Fig. 17.1**) for faster reference. The second half of the atlas contains drawings and descriptions that illustrate key maturity indicators for specific bones and epiphyses in the hand. The drawings can improve the accuracy of age determination, especially in cases where different developmental stages are seen in one image. To establish their normal population, Greulich and Pyle used radiographs obtained from white, upper-middle-class boys and girls enrolled in the Brush Foundation Growth Study from 1931 to 1942.

The atlas is used by first comparing the radiograph to be assessed with the standards for age and gender. If differences are noted, the image is compared with the

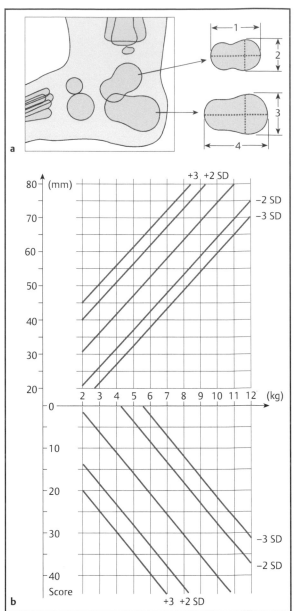

Fig. 17.3a,b Erasmier method of skeletal age determination.
a Measurement of the maximum lengths of the calcaneus and talus (after Erasmier).
b Nomogram. Skeletal maturity is found by drawing a vertical line through present body weight (SD = standard deviation; source: Erasmier and Ringertz 1980). See text for explanation.

next older and younger standards until the best match is found. If significant differences in maturity are found in different ossification centers, the user should perform separate age determinations for the long tubular bones (radius and ulna) and short tubular bones (carpals and metacarpals). In this "bone-by-bone" method, each epiphyseal center can be individually assessed aided by the drawings and descriptions in the second half of the atlas. The mean value of the individual bone ages equals

Table 17.3 Erasmier method. The ossification centers of the cutaneous, third cuneiform, distal tibia and fibula are scored on a four-part scale (all data in mm)

Stage	Definition	Cuboid	Third cuneiform	Distal epiphysis of tibia	Distal epiphysis of fibula	Other ossification centers
A	No signs of an ossification center	0	0	0	0	0
B	Calcium deposition just visible; ill-defined margins	8	5	6	1	1
C	Ossification center clearly visible; soft, continuous margins; greatest diameter is less than half the width of the tibial metaphysis	10	9	13	3	3
D	Greatest diameter of ossification center is more than half the width of the tibial metaphysis	11	–	20	–	–

Stage	Description		Score in boys	Score in girls
B	The ossification center assumes a markedly elongated shape	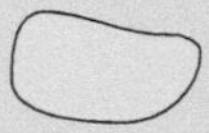	26	24
C	A distinct facet appears on the ventral articular surface; the plantar surface starts to appear as a denser line	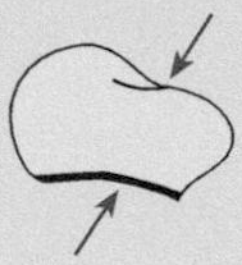	109	63
D	The posterior articular surface is more clearly differentiated and forms an indentation with a double line; sometimes a bulge begins to form on the posterior part of the dorsal articular surface; the linear density on the planar surface becomes thicker	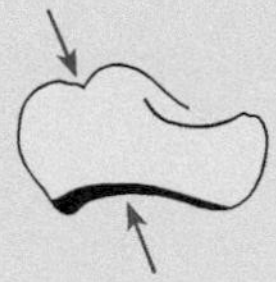	159	90

Fig. 17.4 Hernández method of skeletal age determination. Illustrated for the ossification centers of the calcaneus.

the skeletal age. This method is very time-consuming, however, and is seldom used.

> **!**
> The speed and simplicity of assigning skeletal age has made the Greulich–Pyle atlas the most widely used reference standard in the world. It should be added, however, that the construction of the Greulich–Pyle atlas is based on the assumption that skeletal maturity is uniform in healthy children, that all bones have an identical skeletal age, and that the appearance and development of all ossification centers follow a fixed pattern. But this disregards the genetic differences and the wide range of variation that exist in the ossification patterns of different bones in the same hand. Another problem with the Greulich–Pyle atlas is that some experience in skeletal age determination is needed to minimize intraobserver and interobserver differences.

Greulich W. Radiographic Atlas of Skeletal Development of the Hand and Wrist. 2nd ed. Stanford CA: Stanford University Press; 1959

Loder RT, Estle DT, Morrison K, et al. Applicability of the Greulich and Pyle skeletal age standards to black and white children of today. Am J Dis Child 1993;147(12):1329–1333

Lynnerup N, Belard E, Buch-Olsen K, Sejrsen B, Damgaard-Pedersen K. Intra- and interobserver error of the Greulich–Pyle method as used on a Danish forensic sample. Forensic Sci Int 2008;179(2-3):242.e1-6

Mora S, Boechat MI, Pietka E, Huang HK, Gilsanz V. Skeletal age determinations in children of European and African descent: applicability of the Greulich and Pyle standards. Pediatr Res 2001;50(5):624–628

van Rijn RR, Lequin MH, Robben SGF, Hop WC, van Kuijk C. Is the Greulich and Pyle atlas still valid for Dutch Caucasian children today? Pediatr Radiol 2001;31(10):748–752

Skeletal Age

17

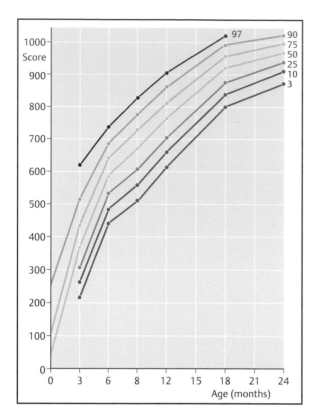

Fig. 17.5 Hernández method of skeletal age determination. Nomogram for assessing skeletal maturity in girls (source: Hernández et al 1988).

■ **Thiemann–Nitz Atlas**

Published in 1986, the Thiemann–Nitz atlas is less widely used than the Greulich–Pyle atlas. It presents hand radiographs obtained in a population of normal children in former East Germany, so establishing standards for conditions in Central Europe. It is used in basically the same way as the Greulich–Pyle atlas.

Thiemann HH, Nitz I. Röntgenatlas der normalen Hand im Kindesalter. 3rd ed. Stuttgart: Thieme; 2006

■ **Tanner–Whitehouse Method**

Tanner and Whitehouse introduced their method of skeletal age determination, based on the summation of maturity scores, in 1962. The original TW1 version of their atlas was published in 1975. They published a partly modified version in 1983, called the TW2 system, which incorporated three different scoring systems (RUS, CARPALS, and TW20; see below). Based on more recent studies showing an increase in the rate of skeletal maturation due to changes in modern society, Tanner and Whitehouse published the last revised version of their atlas (TW3) in 2001. The normal values were derived mainly from longitudinal studies in British children

during the 1960s and 1970s. The Tanner–Whitehouse method can be used in children as young as 1–2 years of age, depending on gender and the particular table that is used (TW2 versus TW3).

In the method developed by Tanner and Whitehouse, the individual ossification centers are analyzed not for their size but for their shape and their tendency to change as maturation proceeds. Three scoring systems are available in the widely used TW2 method:

- *RUS:* radius, ulna, and short bones (first, third and fifth digital rays)
- *CARPALS:* all the carpal bones; no longer useful after 12 years of age
- *TW20:* RUS plus the carpals

The latest TW3 version contains only the RUS and CARPALS scoring systems. On a radiograph of the left hand, the maturity of each epiphyseal center of interest is evaluated and assigned to a stage. Assessment exclusively with the RUS method is acceptable for clinical routine, preferably following a standard protocol and scoring sequence (see numbers in parentheses in **Fig. 17.6**). The plates include drawings and comparative radiographs for all 13 epiphyseal regions that are scored. Different stages are described for all the bones based on their appearance and size, and one, two, or three criteria are defined for each stage. A numerical score—different for male and female hands—is assigned to each stage of bone maturation. The sum of these scores yields a skeletal maturity score (SMS), which is converted to skeletal age using a table. A particular score will yield a different skeletal age depending on whether the TW2 or TW3 system is used.

The image plates and numerical point scales can be found in the publications of Tanner et al. **Fig. 17.7** shows several drawings for the distal radius and the corresponding descriptive criteria.

Ahmed ML, Warner JT. TW2 and TW3 bone ages: time to change? Arch Dis Child 2007;92(4):371–372

Minas K. Bestimmung der Skelettreife nach Tanner-Whitehouse (TW2 und TW3) und Berechnung der prospektiven Erwachsenengrösse. Papenburg: Selbstverlag; 2004

Tanner JM, Whitehouse RH, Takaishi M. Standards from birth to maturity for height, weight, height velocity, and weight velocity: British children, 1965. I. Arch Dis Child 1966;41(219):454–471

Tanner JM, Whitehouse RH, Takaishi M. Standards from birth to maturity for height, weight, height velocity, and weight velocity: British children, 1965. II. Arch Dis Child 1966;41(220):613–635

Tanner J. Assessment of skeletal maturity and prediction of adult height (TW2 method). 2nd ed. London: Academic Press; 1990

Tanner J. Assessment of skeletal maturity and prediction of adult height (TW3 method). 3rd ed. London: Academic Press; 2001

Vignolo M, Naselli A, Magliano P, Di Battista E, Aicardi M, Aicardi G. Use of the new US90 standards for TW-RUS skeletal maturity scores in youths from the Italian population. Horm Res 1999;51(4):168–172

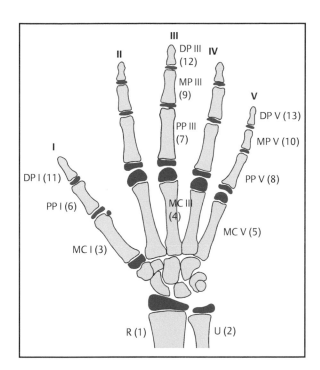

Fig. 17.6 Epiphyseal centers scored in the RUS method (after Minas; schematic representation). Numbers in parentheses indicate the order in which the epiphyseal regions should be scored.

DP = Distal phalanx
MP = Middle phalanx
PP = Proximal phalanx
MC = Metacarpal
U = Ulna
R = Radius

■ Orthodontic Method of Grave and Brown

Grave and Brown introduced a method for orthodontic requirements that can differentiate individual stages relative to the adolescent growth spurt based on a radiograph of the left hand. This method can improve the timing of orthodontic procedures.

Grave KC, Brown T. Skeletal ossification and the adolescent growth spurt. Am J Orthod 1976;69(6):611–619

■ Alternatives

Alternatives to the conventional hand radiograph are currently being evaluated. They include the dual X-ray absorptiometry hand scan and new sonographic techniques involving the wrist (e.g., the BonAge system). The latter method is based on the principle that the velocity of sound conduction is altered by increasing ossification of the epiphyseal plates.

Mentzel HJ, Vogt S, Vilser C, et al. Assessment of skeletal age using a new ultrasound method. [Article in German] Rofo 2005;177(12):1699–1705
Pludowski P, Lebiedowski M, Lorenc RS. Evaluation of practical use of bone age assessments based on DXA-derived hand scans in diagnosis of skeletal status in healthy and diseased children. J Clin Densitom 2005;8(1):48–56

Skeletal Age

17

Fig. 17.7 Examples of staging the ossification center of the distal radius (after Minas).

Stage	Description	
C	• The epiphysis is clearly visible; it is oval in shape and clearly demarcated • The maximum diameter (a) is less than half the width of the metaphysis (b/2)	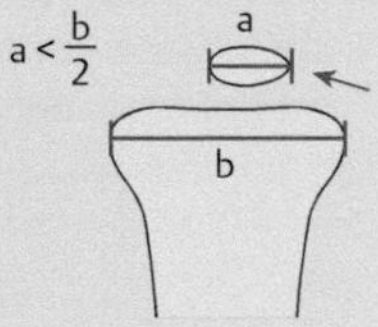 $a < \dfrac{b}{2}$
D	• The maximum diameter (a) of the epiphysis is greater than or equal to half the width of the metaphysis (b/2) • The epiphysis is rounded on the radial side and tapered on the ulnar side • The proximal surface of the epiphysis is flattened; the width of the epiphyseal plate is approximately 1 mm or less	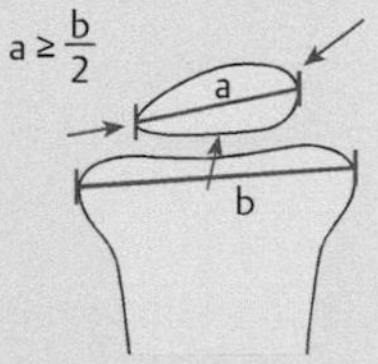 $a \geq \dfrac{b}{2}$
E	• Just proximal to the distal end of the epiphyseal center is a thickened white line representing the palmar border of the epiphysis	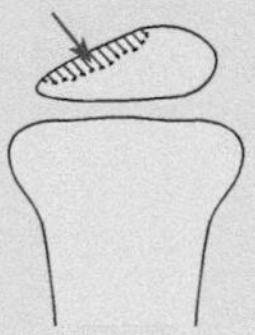

Table 17.4 Limits of normal skeletal development according to Garn (source: Schmitt and Lanz 2008)

Age (years)		Range of normal development (defined by 2 standard deviations)
Boys	**Girls**	**Boys and Girls**
0–1	0–1	± 3–6 months
2–3	3–4	± 1–1.5 years
6–10	7–11	± 2 years
12–13	13–14	± over 2 years

▪ Limits of Normal Skeletal Development

Garn et al published a table of cutoff values that can be used to determine how far a particular skeletal age would fall outside the range of normal skeletal development (**Table 17.4**).

Garn SM, Silverman FN, Rohmann CG. A rational approach to the assessment of skeletal maturation. Ann Radiol (Paris) 1964;7:297–307

Schmitt R, Lanz U. Bildgebende Diagnostik der Hand. Stuttgart: Thieme; 2008

Prediction of Adult Height

Given the strong statistical correlation that exists between skeletal maturation and longitudinal growth, final adult height can be predicted from a patient's present height at any given time. This is of particular clinical interest in patients whose height deviates from the norm. The remaining potential for longitudinal body growth will often direct the further management of patients with scoliosis or leg length discrepancy, for example, and may even be relevant to life-planning issues (e.g., athletic careers).

▪ Bayley–Pinneau Method

Bayley and Pinneau were the first to publish tables for calculating adult height, and their tables were included in the appendix to the final version of the Greulich–Pyle atlas. The tables are based on the assumption that patients at any bone age have already reached a certain percentage of their final adult height. Patients are assigned to one of three categories based on skeletal age: "average" (< 1 year difference between bone age and chronological age), "accelerated" (+1 to +2 years difference), or "delayed" (–1 to –2 years difference). The Greulich–Pyle standard atlas should be used to determine bone age. The Bayley–Pinneau method cannot be used in patients with more than a 2-year discrepancy between chronological age and bone age.

When a child's present height is known, adult height can be predicted by a three-step calculation taking into account the degree of skeletal maturity already achieved (**Table 17.5**). Alternatively, the predicted adult height can be read directly from tables in the original publication. Different tables are used for the different categories; other tables list the standard errors of the method. The accuracy of the prediction increases with the age of the child.

Bayley N, Pinneau SR. Tables for predicting adult height from skeletal age: revised for use with the Greulich–Pyle hand standards. J Pediatr 1952;40(4):423–441

Greulich W. Radiographic atlas of skeletal development of the hand and wrist. 2nd ed. Stanford CA: Stanford University Press; 1959

▪ Tanner–Whitehouse Method

Tanner et al developed an equation that includes the present age of the child, the RUS bone age (see above), present height, and gender. It also takes into account the presence or absence of menarche in girls. The computation system is based on various regression equations in which the individual terms are multiplied by various factors to calculate the predicted adult height for a given chronological age.

> **!** The Tanner–Whitehouse method is considered one of the most accurate height predictors, but it is very time-consuming without a computer because it takes into account numerous tables and requires extensive calculations. Hence it is used only in highly selected cases (with significantly delayed or accelerated growth).

Tanner J. Assessment of skeletal maturity and prediction of adult height (TW2 method). 2nd ed. London: Academic Press; 1990

Tanner J. Assessment of skeletal maturity and prediction of adult height (TW3 method). 3rd ed. London: W.B. Saunders; 2001

▪ Roche–Wainer–Thissen Method

Roche, Wainer, and Thissen developed an equation, similar to that of Tanner and Whitehouse, that takes into account the child's present age, bone age ("bone-by-bone" method of Greulich and Pyle), gender, present height and weight, and mean parental height. This method is time-consuming but is considered the most accurate.

Roche AF, Wainer H, Thissen D. The RWT method for the prediction of adult stature. Pediatrics 1975;56(6):1027–1033

Table 17.5 Bayley and Pinneau method of predicting adult height by determining the percentage of final height reached at a particular bone age

Bone age	Boys			Girls		
	Delayed	Average	Accelerated	Delayed	Average	Accelerated
6.0	68.0			73.3	72.0	
6.3	69.0			74.2	72.9	
6.6	70.0			75.1	73.8	
6.9	70.9			76.3	75.1	
7.0	71.8	69.5	67.0	77.0	75.7	71.2
7.3	72.8	70.2	67.6	77.9	76.5	72.2
7.6	73.8	70.9	68.3	78.8	77.2	73.2
7.9	74.7	71.6	68.9	79.7	78.2	74.2
8.0	75.6	72.3	69.6	80.4	79.0	75.0
8.3	76.5	73.1	70.3	81.3	80.1	76.0
8.6	77.3	73.9	70.9	82.3	81.0	77.1
8.9	77.9	74.6	71.5	83.6	82.1	78.1
9.0	78.6	75.2	72.0	84.1	82.7	79.0
9.3	79.4	76.1	72.8	85.1	83.6	80.0
9.6	80.0	76.9	73.4	85.8	84.4	80.9
9.9	80.7	77.7	74.1	86.6	85.3	81.9
10.0	81.2	78.4	74.7	87.4	86.2	82.8
10.3	81.6	79.1	75.3	88.4	87.4	84.1
10.6	81.9	79.5	75.8	89.6	88.4	85.6
10.9	82.1	80.0	76.3	90.7	89.6	87.8
11.0	82.3	80.4	76.7	91.8	90.6	88.3
11.3	82.7	81.2	77.6	92.2	91.0	88.7
11.6	83.2	81.8	78.6	92.6	91.4	89.1
11.9	83.9	82.7	80.0	92.9	91.8	89.7
12.0	84.5	83.4	80.9	93.2	92.2	90.1
12.3	85.2	84.3	81.8	93.4	93.2	91.3
12.6	86.6	85.3	82.8	94.9	94.1	92.4
12.9	86.9	86.3	83.9	95.2	95.0	93.5
13.0	88.0	87.6	85.0	96.4	95.8	94.5
13.3		89.0	86.1	97.1	96.7	95.5
13.6		90.2	87.5	97.7	97.4	96.3
13.9		91.4	89.0	98.1	97.8	96.8
14.0		92.7	90.5	98.3	98.0	97.2
14.3		93.8	91.8	98.6	98.3	97.7
14.6		94.8	93.6	98.9	98.6	98.0
14.9		95.8	94.3	99.2	98.8	98.3
15.0		96.8	95.8	99.4	99.0	98.6
15.3		97.3	96.7	99.5	99.1	98.8
15.6		97.6	97.1	99.6	99.3	99.0
15.9		98.0	97.6	99.7	99.4	99.2

continued ▷

Table 17.5 (continued)

Bone age	Boys			Girls		
	Delayed	Average	Accelerated	Delayed	Average	Accelerated
16.0		98.2	98.0	99.8	99.6	99.3
16.3		98.5	98.3	99.9	99.6	99.4
16.6		98.7	98.5	99.9	99.7	99.5
16.9		98.9	98.8	99.95	99.8	99.7
17.0		99.1	99.0	100.0	99.9	99.8
17.3		99.3				
17.6		99.4			99.95	99.95
17.9		99.5				
18.0					100.0	

Computer-Assisted Techniques for Determining Skeletal Age

Skeletal age determination using atlases can be very time-consuming, depending on the method used. Since the advent of digital radiography, efforts have been made to provide examiners with digital aids or even semiautomated systems to make the task easier.

As an example, Gilsanz and Ratib created a digital reference atlas, which encompasses 29 reference images drawn from 522 hand radiographs of healthy Caucasian children obtained from 8 months to 18 years of age. Analogous to the Greulich–Pyle atlas, the digital atlas shows a high statistical correlation with chronological age in healthy subjects. The atlas can be installed on a personal computer or personal data assistant, making it easy to compare a hand radiograph with the stored reference images.

Another innovation is the 2004 "Bone-O-Matic" computer program, which can be used for bone age determination and adult height prediction. Bone age is determined by the TW2 method of Tanner. All three scoring systems (RUS, CARPALS and TW20) are available, and the program includes both diagrams and standard reference images. All calculations and tabulations are performed in the background, yielding a consistent result. The methods of Tanner and Whitehouse, Bayley and Pinneau (with tables from the Greulich–Pyle atlas), and Roche–Wainer–Thissen are available for the prediction of adult height.

Additionally, various semiautomated techniques are now being evaluated that use imaging-processing and pattern-recognition processes, plus discoveries on skeletal growth, to analyze specific hand bones, classify their growth and estimate bone age. These methods are based largely on the Greulich–Pyle atlas or the RUS method of Tanner and Whitehouse. Most systems include various components for importing images, selecting image regions relevant to bone growth, identifying specific maturity stages, and calculating the resultant bone age. Some of these systems are already available commercially (e.g., BoneXpert).

Bone-O-Matic. Knochenalterbestimmung. Website: http://www.sukamin.de/ bone-o-matic; status: 18 Dec 2010

BoneXpert. Software for automatic determination of bone age. Website: http://www.bonexpert.com; status: 18 Dec 2010

Gilsanz V. Hand Bone Age: A Digital Atlas of Skeletal Maturity. Berlin: Springer; 2005

Tanner JM, Gibbons RD. Automatic bone age measurement using computerized image analysis. J Pediatr Endocrinol Metab 1994;7(2):141–145

Thodberg HH. Clinical review: An automated method for determination of bone age. J Clin Endocrinol Metab 2009;94(7):2239–2244

Thodberg HH, Kreiborg S, Juul A, Pedersen KD. The BoneXpert method for automated determination of skeletal maturity. IEEE Trans Med Imaging 2009;28(1):52–66

van Rijn RR, Lequin MH, Thodberg HH. Automatic determination of Greulich and Pyle bone age in healthy Dutch children. Pediatr Radiol 2009;39(6):591–597

Practical Aspects of Bone Age Determination

The analysis of left hand radiographs has become the standard method of skeletal age determination in children. The Greulich and Pyle atlas is most widely used because it enables simple and fast assignment of skeletal age. One limitation, however, is that the atlas has not been updated since 1959 and consequently does not reflect the modern trend toward an earlier onset of physical maturation processes. Another difficulty is that the atlas is standardized only for white girls and boys, limiting its usefulness for other ethnic groups. The Greulich–Pyle method has also been found to have a relatively high error rate, especially when used by inexperienced examiners. The Tanner–Whitehouse method yields better results for beginners, although it takes considerably more time. The TW2 version is most widely used in everyday practice. The TW3 version is a 2001 update that takes into account the changes in maturation rates, but so far it has not become widely implemented.

> **!** Because results based on the Greulich–Pyle atlas and Tanner–Whitehouse method cannot be directly compared with each other, only one method should be consistently used in the follow-up of any given patient.

The relatively simple Bayley–Pinneau method is most commonly used for the prediction of adult height and generally yields acceptable results. The more complex Tanner–Whitehouse method is recommended only in patients with markedly delayed or accelerated growth. The Roche–Wainer–Thissen method gives the most accurate height prediction. More recently, several easy-to-use digital systems have been developed that incorporate either an easily available atlas or an automated system for determining skeletal age and predicting adult height. The increasing utilization of digital X-ray systems suggests that these systems will continue to be refined and implemented on a larger scale.

Skeletal Age

17

Index

Note: Illustrations are comprehensively referred to in the text. Therefore, significant items in illustrations have usually been given a page reference only in the absence of their concomitant mention in the text referring to that figure. Page references to tables are in bold and those to figures are in italics. Conventional X-ray radiography (i.e., plain films or radiography) has not been indexed as a main entry on account of the ubiquity of this imaging modality. However, specific radiographic views, e.g., "anteroposterior radiograph," have been indexed.

Index